Client Education

Education

THEORY AND PRACTICE

Mary A. Miller, RN, PhD
Dean Emeritus
School of Nursing, Aurora University
Aurora, Illinois
Associate Dean Emeritus
School of Professional Studies
Metropolitan State College of Denver
Denver, Colorado

Pamella Rae Stoeckel, RN, PhD, CNE
Professor
Loretto Heights School of Nursing
Regis University
Denver, Colorado

JONES & BARTLETT
LEARNING

World Headquarters
Jones & Bartlett Learning
25 Mall Road
Burlington, MA 01803
978-443-5000
info@jblearning.com
www.jblearning.com

Jones & Bartlett Learning books and products are available through most bookstores and online booksellers. To contact Jones & Bartlett Learning directly, call 800-832-0034, fax 978-443-8000, or visit our website, www.jblearning.com.

29883-3

Production Credits
Vice President, Product Management: Marisa R. Urbano
Vice President, Content Strategy and Implementation: Christine Emerton
Outsource Manager, Content Strategy and Design: Carol Brewer Guerrero
Manager, Intellectual Properties and Content Production: Kristen Rogers
Content Production Manager: Belinda Thresher
Content Production Manager, Navigate: Daniel Stone
Senior Digital Project Specialist: Angela Dooley
Senior Product Marketing Manager: Lindsay White

Senior Director of Supply Chain: Ed Schneider
Procurement Manager: Wendy Kilborn
Content Vendor: MPS, Limited
Design: MPS, Limited
Composition and Project Management: S4Carlisle Publishing Services
Media Development Editor: Faith Brosnan
Rights Specialist: Robin Silverman
Cover Image (Title Page, Part Opener, Chapter Opener): © Peter Cade/Stone/Getty Images
Printing and Binding: Sheridan–Kentucky

Library of Congress Cataloging-in-Publication Data
Names: Miller, Mary A. (Mary Alice), author. | Stoeckel, Pamella Rae, author.
Title: Client education : theory and practice / Mary A. Miller, Pamella Rae Stoeckel.
Description: Fourth edition. | Burlington, MA : Jones & Bartlett Learning, [2026] | Includes bibliographical references and index.
Identifiers: LCCN 2024020965 | ISBN 9781284298741 (paperback)
Subjects: MESH: Patient Education as Topic | Models, Educational | Nurse-Patient Relations | Nurses Instruction | BISAC: MEDICAL / Nursing / Nurse & Patient
Classification: LCC RT90 | NLM WA 590 | DDC 615.5071--dc23/eng/20240814
LC record available at https://lccn.loc.gov/2024020965

6048

Printed in the United States of America
28 27 26 25 24   10 9 8 7 6 5 4 3 2 1

For Annie, Mary's beloved sister.

For Dave, Matt, and Josh, Pamella's beautiful loving family.

Brief Contents

Contents

Preface

We are pleased to present the fourth edition of our textbook *Client Education: Theory and Practice* to the nursing community. We have written it for baccalaureate and master's degree nursing students, practicing nurses, nurse educators, and health educators in other health-related fields. We have also written for in-service educators who are responsible for teaching colleagues and health team members.

We are especially delighted to have the text printed in four-color. Now, the book highlights the components of the Miller–Stoeckel Client Education Model (the Model) as they appear throughout the text. We introduce the Model in Chapter 1 and develop the Model's components in each subsequent chapter. Using the four-color format emphasizes how the components in each chapter are woven together to achieve client education outcomes. The Model is comprehensive and thoroughly documented by current literature and applicable research.

Much has happened in our nation since the *Third Edition* of our book was published in 2019. The United States and its healthcare system were overwhelmed by the COVID-19 pandemic, the most serious communicable disease pandemic since the 1918 flu. Health information and guidance was provided by the Centers for Disease Control and Prevention and the White House, but it was not always followed, believed, or trusted by many people. Misinformation (false, inaccurate, or unintentionally misleading information) and disinformation (information created and spread with malicious intent, often with a financial motive) were widespread. Consequently, a hesitancy to receive vaccines or a refusal to receive them resulted. These factors, combined with the political environment, placed a heavy burden on the nation's hospitals, public health departments, and healthcare agencies.

It was amid this environment that we made changes to most chapters in this *Fourth Edition*. You'll find new content, revision of material, and added illustrations and figures to highlight information formerly found solely in text form. Our book has undergone extensive editing and updating consistent with current thinking. The text retains the popular sections on supplemental online resources and evidence-based research examples that educators find especially helpful to students.

Everything in the healthcare environment, from care delivery to the preparation of new nurses was impacted by the pandemic. It became essential to clearly define word usage such as misinformation and disinformation as nurses worked with clients. Nurse educators needed guidance in working with clients confused by the multiple messages confronting them by both the media and social media. Nurse educators also had to consider the issues and cultural characteristics of various racial and ethnic groups. For example, many clients were vaccine hesitant and vaccine avoidant. The importance of clear, accurate information was imperative; therefore, a strong focus of this new edition's text is to offer guidance on working across the human spectrum with different racial and ethnic groups. This is especially true concerning the increased racial discrimination, bias, and violence that arose during the pandemic. Thus, we have provided clear guidance for the nurse educator in these troubling areas.

Nursing is regarded as a stressful occupation. During the pandemic, nurses and healthcare workers were overworked, stressed, and carrying workloads that taxed their physical being. Burnout and exhaustion were prevalent, and sometimes overwhelming. The best care is provided when nurses are functioning at optimal levels of their own wellness. Consequently, we devote a unit of this book to caring for the care giver, an essential part of maintaining one's own health in order to effectively care for others. We discuss examples of self-care for nurses and the importance of building a self-care plan in these pages.

Nursing education itself was impacted during the pandemic. Nursing education programs' enrollments were down and clinical facilities were less available for the education of new nurses. Consequently, simulation became an optional teaching strategy for the education of new nurses and updating working nurses (in-service education). Here, you'll read about simulation, its proper use, and its advantages and disadvantages.

Another important revision in this book concerns the reconceptualization of adherence. Adherence was formerly addressed in the context of nurses educating clients about following the recommendations of healthcare providers. In this edition, we examine the types and causes of nonadherence and introduce a treatment adherence scale to aid the nurse educator. We also introduce the socio-ecological model of adherence, comprised of four distinct foci: individual focused, family social relationship focused, community cultural focused, and system/societal focused. It places adherence in a larger, more realistic context.

We continue our focus on learning, as well as how people think and learn. Since our last edition, two subsequent generations have been identified: Generation Z and Generation Alpha. They have distinct characteristics, and the nurse educator would profit from being aware of these. Constructivism, another theory of learning that is in vogue now, is included, along with how to best apply it in the context of health education.

Our aging population is increasing in numbers and also is living longer. This trend is accompanied by an increased incidence of health and cognitive issues. Suggestions for helping families cope with these changes and specific measures that the nurse educator can offer to assist families are included. Educating the family is essential in working with older adults.

Finally, the most exciting addition to this text is material on artificial intelligence (AI) and its applications in nursing. To help make the best decisions about AI technology use, nurses should engage in all project development phases, from defining the problem to using the tool, to evaluating its impact. Our text provides a basic understanding of AI and its potential use in nursing. We believe AI will continue to develop and ultimately become an established and effective tool for the healthcare sector.

As always, we assume full responsibility for the content of this text and our views on teaching, learning, and client education and welcome your suggestions for improvement.

Mary A. Miller
Pamella Rae Stoeckel

New to the *Fourth Edition*

The fourth edition of *Client Education: Theory and Practice* continues to use the authors' model and conceptual and theoretical support and application. Key chapter revisions include the following:

- Updated to four-color throughout!
- Inclusion of an overview of AI, machine learning, and deep learning in Chapter 1.
- Addition of data on Generation Z and Generation Alpha in Chapter 4.
- Updates to the section on Educating Clients with Disabilities, and an updated discussion of cognitive function and mild cognitive impairment in Chapter 7.
- New material in Chapter 8 discussing the rise of racial discrimination and racially motivated violence toward Asian Americans during the COVID-19 pandemic. Updated data and approaches for educators working with Asian American, Latino, and Native American people.
- New section on nurse educator's self-care and institutional support in Chapter 9.
- Updated information on the use of technology in instructional materials in Chapter 12.
- Enhanced discussion of client adherence in Chapter 14.

The fourth edition of *Client Education: Theory and Practice* is designed for the student. The easy-to-follow layout of the book guides students throughout the text, while also providing them with additional study aids and features to facilitate learning.

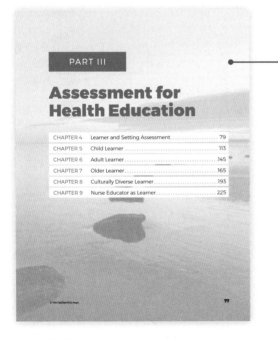

Part Dividers: Each of the five parts are divided up clearly, with an opener page, to make it easier to navigate through the text and find what you are looking for.

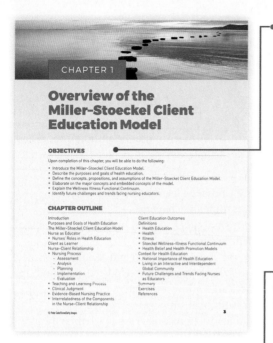

Learning Objectives: Every chapter opens with a list of *Objectives* that allow students to review the important concepts they will encounter in the chapter.

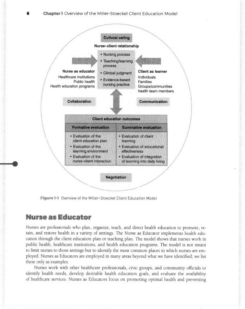

Figures, Tables, and Boxes: *Figures* provide students with visual reinforcement of models and concepts introduced in the text. *Tables* and *Boxes* allow the student to further examine specific aspects of core concepts, review referenced guidelines, and explore the practical application of the authors' model.

nursing students preferred Kolb's diverger and assimilating learning styles. When the clients' thinking and learning styles fit with the learning setting, the task at hand, and the teacher's preferred style, clients thrive. When clients' thinking and learning styles do not fit with these factors, clients may have difficulty grasping the health message (Dunn, 1983; Sternberg, 1997). Clients are best served by having abundant reading materials (books and pamphlets), pictures, videos, interactive instructional materials, demonstrations, and resource persons available. Many choices allow clients to select among the learning options that best suit their own thinking and learning styles because no single option is best for everyone (Moran, Kornhaber, & Gardner, 2006).

Summary

This chapter introduced thinking and learning processes that undergird the nurse–client relationship of the Miller-Stoeckel Client Education Model. It stressed how that knowledge increases the effectiveness of nurses as educators in working with clients. The three domains of learning—cognitive, affective, and psychomotor—provide a framework for developing learning objectives. The cognitive domain involves intellectual activities, the affective domain deals with attitudes and values, and the psychomotor domain involves learning motor skills. Thinking underlies these domains, and a summary of ways of thinking was discussed. In addition to nursing process and clinical judgment, these ways include problem solving, critical thinking, creative thinking, intuition, reflection, fantasy, and reverie. It is important to understand your own thinking and how to promote thinking in clients.

This chapter also examined several styles and models of thinking and learning, including Sternberg's thinking styles, Witkin and Goodenough's Cognitive-Style Dimensions, Kolb's Experiential Learning Model, Gardner's Multiple Intelligences, and the sensory-based learning style. Each view of learning provides insight into the nurse–client relationship and how nurses as educators can best promote learning.

Exercises

Exercise I: Learning Domains

Purpose: Distinguish among cognitive, affective, and psychomotor learning domains.
Directions: Working alone, examine the learning objectives for the course you are taking. Place each objective into one of the learning domains. Then form small groups and compare your answers. Was each learning objective categorized correctly?

Exercise II: Affective Domain

Purpose: Examine the affective domain in teaching and learning.
Directions: Reflect on a client situation in which the client's point of view, attitudes, and beliefs were different from your own. Journal about the following questions:

1. What was the difference between your point of view, attitudes, and beliefs and those of the client?

Chapter Summary: Each chapter concludes with a *Summary*, designed to recap key concepts presented within each chapter.

End of Chapter Exercises: *Exercises* allow students to correlate their professional experience to, and further their knowledge of key concepts presented within the chapter by participating in exercises either singly or in groups.

• How can you use clinical judgment to assess clients and design and implement client education?
• What research that is evidence-based supports your decisions?

Exercise III: Using the Stoeckel Wellness–Illness Continuum

Purpose: Self-analysis of wellness–illness state.
Directions: Chart and analyze your progress on the Stoeckel Wellness–Illness Continuum. Print a copy from the book to plot your score on, or write out your answers.

• Score each factor from 1 to 10: social, physiological, environmental, emotional, and health access.
• Make a summative statement about your overall health.
• Discuss in paragraph form how your personal beliefs, culture, and background affect your views of health, illness, and wellness.

Exercise IV: Ways to Promote Client Education

Purposes:

• Promote creative thinking.
• Raise consciousness regarding client education.

Directions: Form small groups and discuss the following situation. Take notes and prepare a report to be shared with the rest of your peers.

While carrying heavy patient care assignments and responsibilities, some nurses are managing to teach their clients in mutually satisfactory ways. What client teaching have you observed by your clinical instructors, supervisors, primary nurses, or other nursing personnel? What are you doing to promote client teaching? If you are not yet in the clinical area, seek out nurses in your school, hospital, or neighborhood and ask them what they are doing to promote health teaching. Draw on your experiences as a patient, client, relative, or observer. Upon reflection, summarize the nurse's role in client education.

References

Agency for Healthcare Research and Quality. (2002). *Systems to rate the strength of scientific evidence*. Summary, evidence report/technology assessment (No. 47, AHRQ Publication No. 02-E015). Rockville, MD: Author. Retrieved from http://www.thecre.com/pdf/ahrq-system-strength.pdf http://www.ahrq.gov/clinic/epcsums/strengthsum.htm
American Hospital Association. (1992). *A patient's bill of rights*. Retrieved from http://www.ccasino.edu/faculty/dchatman/RT%20106%20AHA%20%20Patient%20Bill%20of%20Rights.pdf
American Nurses Association. (1998). *Standards of clinical nursing practice* (2nd ed.). Washington, DC: Author.
Bastable, S. B., & Alt, M. F. (2014). Overview of education in health care. In S. B. Bastable (Ed.), *Nurse as educator: Principles of teaching and learning for nursing practice* (4th ed., pp. 3–30). Burlington, MA: Jones & Bartlett Learning.
Buchanan, C., Howitt, M. L., Wilson, R., Booth, R. G., Risling, T., & Bamford, M. (2021). Predicted influences of artificial intelligence on nursing education: Scoping review. *JMIR Nursing, 4*(1), e23933. doi:10.2196/23933
Benner, P. (1984). *From novice to expert*. Menlo Park, CA: Addison-Wesley.
Bliss-Holtz, J. (2007). Evidence-based practice: A primer for action. *Issues in Comprehensive Pediatric Nursing, 30*(4), 165–182.
Breckon, D., Harvey, J., & Lancaster, R. (1998). *Community health education: Settings, roles, and skills for the 21st century*. Sudbury, MA: Jones and Bartlett.
Campinha-Bacote, J. (1998). *The process of cultural competence in the delivery of healthcare services* (3rd ed.). Cincinnati, OH: Transcultural C.A.R.E. Associates.
Castellanos, S. (2018) What exactly is artificial intelligence. *The Wall Street Journal*. www.wsj.com/articles/what-exactly-is-artificial-intelligence-1544120887
Chitty, K. K., & Black, B. P. (2007). *Professional nursing: Concepts and challenges* (5th ed.). St. Louis, MO: Elsevier.

References: *References* provide a list of additional resources to help students gain a deeper understanding of the material.

Instructor Resources

- Chapter Quizzes, Midterm Exam, and Final Exam in LMS-compatible formats
- Syllabus

Student Resources

- eBook with Knowledge Check Questions and Quizzes
- Slides in PowerPoint format, including narrated presentations by the authors
- Exercises in writeable PDF format
- Learning Objectives

Acknowledgments

The authors wish to thank the many people who contributed to the creation of this book. We especially thank Marc Bove and Bharathi Sanjeev, and the production staff at Jones & Bartlett Learning, who provided a great deal of advice and encouragement throughout the editing process. We wish to acknowledge the contribution of Dorothy E. Babcock in the initial text of *Client Education: Theory and Practice* published in 1994.

Reviewers

The authors and publisher also wish to thank the reviewers, whose valuable feedback contributed greatly to the preparation of this new edition.

Billie E. Blake, EdD, MSN, BSN, RN, CNE
St. Joseph's College of Maine
Standish, Maine

Janet H. Davis, MSN, MBA, PhD, RN, CNE
Associate Professor College of Nursing
Purdue University Northwest
Hammond, Indiana

Elizabeth Van Dyk, DNP, RN, APN, FNP-C, ANP-BC
Associate Dean, Associate Professor
Felician University
Rutherford, New Jersey

PART I

A Framework for Health Education

Overview of the Miller–Stoeckel Client Education Model

OBJECTIVES

Upon completion of this chapter, you will be able to do the following:

- Introduce the Miller–Stoeckel Client Education Model.
- Describe the purposes and goals of health education.
- Define the concepts, propositions, and assumptions of the Miller–Stoeckel Client Education Model.
- Elaborate on the major concepts and embedded concepts of the model.
- Explain the Wellness Illness Functional Continuum.
- Identify future challenges and trends facing nursing educators.

CHAPTER OUTLINE

Introduction

This chapter introduces the Miller–Stoeckel Client Education Model as the conceptual framework around which this text is written. The use of the model is a unique contribution to understanding the delivery of health education and nursing science. The chapter begins by giving the purposes and goals of health education and then defines the concepts, propositions, and assumptions of the Miller–Stoeckel Client Education Model. Concepts are elaborated on, and the Stoeckel Wellness–Illness Functional Continuum is explained. There is a review of health belief and health promotion models, and then the chapter concludes by reviewing the context for health education and an introduction to artificial intelligence (AI).

Purposes and Goals of Health Education

We view *purpose* and *goal* as having essentially the same meaning (Webster's, 2013) and believe the overall purpose and goal of health education is to promote, retain, and restore health, which is a phrase you will see throughout this text. It involves the prevention, treatment, and management of illness and the preservation of clients' mental and physical well-being. Comprehensive client education includes maintenance and promotion of health, illness prevention, restoration of health, and coping with impaired function. This view of health care can be achieved only by shifting the emphasis away from illness and cure and integrating client education into a comprehensive approach to health maintenance, prevention, and promotion (Davidhizar & Cramer, 2002).

Health education promotes positive, informed changes in lifestyle and involves encouraging behaviors that prevent acute and chronic disease, decrease disability, and enhance wellness. Nurses as educators empower clients to strive for optimal health and well-being. Individuals learn to make informed decisions about personal and family health practices and use health services in the community. From a public health perspective, health education is intended not only to enhance individuals' abilities to make positive lifestyle changes but also to support social and political actions that promote health and quality of life in communities. Hall (2001) notes that effective community education is essential as individuals, communities, and the nation shift focus to wellness and illness prevention. The concept of community empowerment is designed to help individuals and organizations use their abilities and resources in collective efforts to address their health priorities and needs. The ultimate goal of health education is for nurses as educators to help clients make changes in behavior that support healthy living.

The Miller–Stoeckel Client Education Model

The Miller–Stoeckel Client Education Model provides the conceptual framework for understanding the essential, interrelated concepts of health education. The terms *conceptual framework* and *conceptual model* are used interchangeably. Fawcett (2005) defined a conceptual model as:

> A set of relatively abstract and general concepts that address the phenomena of central interest to a discipline, the propositions that broadly describe these concepts, and the propositions that state relatively abstract and general relations between two or more of the concepts. (p. 16)

Conceptual models assist us in identifying concept links that we believe exist and then communicating those concepts to others. Models include concepts, propositions, and assumptions.

Concepts are words or phrases that summarize the essential characteristics or properties of a phenomenon. Propositions are statements about a concept or a statement of the relationship between two or more concepts. Assumptions are "I believe" statements believed to be true. Models have practical value because they guide practice and research. Conceptual models give direction to the search for relevant questions about the phenomena of interest to nursing as a discipline and also suggest solutions to practical problems.

The theoretical basis for the Miller–Stoeckel Client Education Model is drawn from theories of nursing and education: Hildegard Peplau's interpersonal relations theory (1952); Ida Jean Orlando's nursing process discipline theory (1972); Nola Pender's health promotion model (2011); Josepha Campinha-Bacote's model of cultural competence in the delivery of healthcare services model (1998); Christine Tanner's model of clinical judgment in nursing (2006); Bernadette Melnyk and Ellen Fineout-Overholt's process of evidence-based practices (2011); and Malcolm Knowles's adult learning theory—andragogy (1990). These theories provide the theoretical support for the model and are applied throughout the text.

The four major concepts of the Miller–Stoeckel Client Education Model follow:

- **Nurse as Educator**: Nurses are professionals who plan, organize, teach, and direct health education to promote, retain, and restore health in a variety of settings.
- **Client as Learner**: Clients are consumers of health education and include individuals, families, groups and communities, and health team members.
- **Nurse–Client Relationship**: The Nurse–Client Relationship creates the environment for the interaction that focuses on the achievement of health education goals.
- **Client Education Outcomes**: Client Education Outcomes are the results of health education efforts.

The four embedded concepts of the Miller–Stoeckel Client Education Model follow:

- **Cultural Caring**: Behaviors and attitudes exhibited by the nurse that respects and values diversity.
- **Communication**: The exchange of information in spoken, written, and nonverbal forms that is the foundation for clients to understand and act on health information.
- **Negotiation**: The give and take within the relationship that acknowledges the client as a partner with the nurse in achieving mutually acceptable goals.
- **Collaboration**: Sharing, planning, setting goals, solving problems, and working cooperatively together to achieve the goals of health education.

The propositions for the model are as follows:

- The Nurse as Educator and Client as Learner come together in the Nurse–Client Relationship to achieve Client Education Outcomes of promoting, retaining, and restoring health.
- The environment created by the Nurse–Client Relationship is influenced by the embedded concepts of Cultural Caring, Communication, Negotiation, and Collaboration.

The major assumptions of the model are as follows:

- Health status can be improved for most clients through health education.
- Health status is affected by a variety of factors, including lifestyle, heredity, environment, culture, and availability of health care.
- Clients can learn positive health behaviors.
- Clients are responsible for choices under their control that affect their health.
- Nurses are primary providers of health education in a variety of settings (**Figure 1-1**).

The remainder of the chapter will now further elaborate on the concepts of the model.

Figure 1-1 Overview of the Miller–Stoeckel Client Education Model

Nurse as Educator

Nurses are professionals who plan, organize, teach, and direct health education to promote, retain, and restore health in a variety of settings. The Nurse as Educator implements health education through the client education plan or teaching plan. The model shows that nurses work in public health, healthcare institutions, and health education programs. The model is not meant to limit nurses to those settings but to identify the most common places in which nurses are employed. Nurses as Educators are employed in many areas beyond what we have identified; we list these only as examples.

Nurses work with other healthcare professionals, civic groups, and community officials to identify health needs, develop desirable health education goals, and evaluate the availability of healthcare services. Nurses as Educators focus on promoting optimal health and preventing illness, but they also deal with social, cultural, behavioral, legal, and economic issues as they affect health.

Nurses' Role in Health Education

The teaching role of nurses has long been recognized as a function of nursing practice. It has been within the scope of nursing practice since the days of Florence Nightingale. In 1918, the National League of Nursing Education (NLNE), precursor to the present-day National League for Nursing (NLN), defined nursing as the prevention of illness and the promotion of health especially in public health, child welfare, schools, home visiting, industries, hospitals, and social services. Nurses were expected to be responsible for health teaching. Two decades later, in 1937, the NLNE stated that a nurse was essentially a teacher and an agent of health in whatever field nursing practice occurred. In 1998, the American Nurses Association (ANA) stated in the Standards of Clinical Nursing Practice that educating clients is a primary responsibility of nurses. The ANA continues its long-standing support for patient teaching as a primary component of nursing care. Today, all state nurse practice acts in the United States include client teaching within the scope of nursing practice. Further support for the role of Nurse as Educator is found in the Patient's Bill of Rights, which was first adopted by the American Hospital Association (AHA) in 1973. The current bill was approved by the AHA board of trustees in 1992 and states that patients have the right to "relevant, current, and understandable information concerning diagnosis, treatment, and prognosis" (AHA, 1992, Right #2). The Joint Commission, the organization that accredits hospitals, revised its patient education standards to include follow-up treatment and services in 2009 (The Joint Commission, 2009). Many practicing nurses and nurse educators support client education as an essential role for nurses (Bastable & Alt, 2014; Pender, 2011; Redman, 2006).

Just as important as educating clients, nurses also have a professional responsibility to educate colleagues and health team members. The healthcare environment changes rapidly and requires colleagues and team members to stay current in their knowledge and skills. Nursing team members have differing levels of education and training and may require additional education. The Nurse as Educator is often the primary educator and resource for the team (Donner, Levonian, & Slutsky, 2005). Lifelong learning is essential for those in the healthcare professions and requires all providers to stay current with their knowledge and skills.

Nurses coordinate client health education because they are the healthcare providers who have the most continuous contact with clients. Nurses are with clients at teachable moments and do much of the health education. As a nurse, your educational background in anatomy, physiology, nutrition, psychology, sociology, anthropology, and other social and physical sciences enhances your role as an educator. Your education has taught you how the body can and should function and about the interplay among mind, body, and spirit. Your understanding of the importance of using current research helps you assist clients in choosing and maintaining healthy behaviors.

Nurses have earned the public's trust, and by modeling healthy habits, they are more believable when they teach. Clients are entering the healthcare system better informed about health issues. This means they will be demanding more knowledgeable caregivers, and they expect to be provided with current, sound information. Many clients have done considerable reading about their particular health problem and consequently ask informed, sophisticated questions. Your credibility will be established by your answers and ability to access information.

Client as Learner

We chose the word *client* to describe the learner in this text because the client is the consumer of health education and is the focus of our teaching efforts. We define clients as individuals, families, groups and communities, and health team members, which covers the scope of humanity. Clients are everywhere and include everyone in need of health information. The word *client* connotes someone who is free to come and go from your presence; someone who is free to accept or refuse the services, counsel, and teaching that nurses offer. We view clients as responsible, thinking individuals who have the right to make choices about their health.

Contrast the view of the client with the view of the individual as a patient. When examined from this perspective, we think of individuals who must depend on nurses for their care and sometimes for their very survival. The term *patient* conjures up an image of someone who is dependent and in need of physical or psychological assistance related to health. A patient is in your presence—on your nursing unit or in your service area—and needs the health education that nurses can deliver.

Clients bring their individual and collective perceptions of what optimal health is to the Nurse–Client Relationship. Perceptions are influenced by their expectations, emotions, and needs. Perceptions about health are determined individually, culturally, environmentally, and socially. Clients' perceptions may not always be the same as nurses' perceptions. In the client education context, we perceive clients as active participants in health education to the extent of their ability and choice.

Nurse–Client Relationship

Between the Nurse as Educator and Client as Learner is the Nurse–Client Relationship. This is the participants' point of contact where the environment between them is created. The Nurse–Client Relationship is built upon the embedded concepts of Cultural Caring, Communication, Negotiation, and Collaboration. These concepts more fully describe the context in which interactions occur within the model. We call them embedded because they permeate the environment in which health education occurs. The concepts are readily understandable and essential to the process of teaching clients.

The Nurse as Educator uses skills in Cultural Caring to be sensitive to clients' needs in all aspects of the model. Cultural Caring is manifest in all verbal and nonverbal Communication in teaching clients. Through Communication we get an understanding of what clients need to learn and how best to structure the teaching, which in itself is a process of Negotiation. To achieve successful outcomes, it is often necessary to Collaborate with others, including the client's family and other health professionals. The embedded concepts are part of the process of creating an environment that supports successful client outcomes.

The Nurse–Client Relationship is therapeutic, promoting a psychological environment that facilitates positive change and growth. This aspect of the model is drawn from Hildegard Peplau's interpersonal nursing theory (1952) that stressed the importance of the therapeutic interpersonal process. Therapeutic communication between the Nurse as Educator and the Client as Learner is collaborative and focuses on the achievement of health education goals. It focuses on the client achieving optimal personal growth and the highest level of wellness possible given the client's situation. An explicit time frame, a goal-directed approach, and the expectation of confidentiality are important to the relationship. The nurse establishes, directs, and takes responsibility for the interaction where the clients' needs take priority over nurses' needs.

Four goal-directed phases characterize the Nurse–Client Relationship. The preinteraction phase occurs before meeting the client and involves gathering all available client information. This gives the nurse time to anticipate health concerns and plan for the initial interaction. The orientation phase occurs when the Nurse as Educator meets the Client as Learner and they get to know

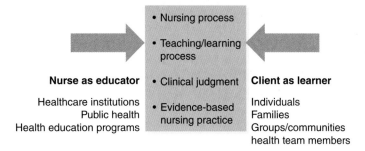

Figure 1-2 Nurse–Client Relationship in the Miller–Stoeckel Client Education Model

one another. The working phase occurs when the Nurse as Educator engages in health teaching and works with the client to solve problems and accomplish goals. Last is the termination phase, which is the process of ending the relationship (Potter & Perry, 2009).

The components that shape the environment of the Nurse–Client Relationship are the Nursing Process, the Teaching and Learning Process, Clinical Judgment, and Evidence-Based Nursing Practice (EBNP). We describe each in order (**Figure 1-2**).

Nursing Process

The Nursing Process is a variation of the scientific reasoning process that allows you to organize your thoughts and systematize nursing practice. Its focus is to address client problems in professional practice in a variety of clinical settings. Steps in the nursing process include assessment, analysis, planning, implementation, and evaluation. Applied to health education, the steps of the nursing process relate directly to the learning needs of clients that are designed to improve clients' health knowledge and promote, retain, and restore health.

The steps of the Nursing Process are iterative because they may overlap or occur simultaneously. Reassessment, reordering of priorities, new goal setting, and revising the client education plan continue as part of the process toward attainment of the health education goals. A discussion of the steps of the nursing process as they apply to health education follows.

Assessment

Assessment is gathering the essential information about the client to identify health education needs. As you assess the physiologic, psychological, sociocultural, developmental, and spiritual influences on each client, it helps to determine each individual's learning style and learning capacity. Assessment includes collecting subjective and objective client data, recording the data, and noting the data that affect learning. Subjective data include clients' perceptions of their condition and health status. How does the client view their situation? How does the client view their health? Is the client's situation conducive or obstructive to learning? Does the client show a readiness to learn? Do you have the requisite knowledge, skills, and attitudes to facilitate each client's learning in the situation at hand?

Analysis

The second step, analysis, is a careful examination and validation of the facts to identify the client's specific health education needs. When possible, you will collaborate with clients to diagnose their learning needs. A clear understanding of these needs becomes the basis for planning, implementing, and evaluating the client education plan. This step includes analyzing both your perceptions and your clients' perceptions of the learning needs to validate them. Assessing and analyzing needs also includes determining the kind of learning clients want. For instance, in which domain do your clients lack information? What do they want to know? Do they lack necessary skills? Is their developmental level a barrier to learning? Do they display attitudes that impair their optimum functioning?

When your client belongs to a specific population, your assessment becomes complex. You may need to conduct a survey as part of the assessment. Another option is to form a focus group composed of individuals who are representative of the large group you are teaching. For smaller groups, interviewing selected members of the group may serve your purpose just as well. In all instances, it is important to avoid making assumptions about what clients need to learn. Ask them and be as thorough in your assessment and analysis as possible.

Another way to approach clients is from the perspective of potential growth. What information do they desire? What new skills do they wish to learn? What opportunities for growth are inherent in their developmental stages? What attitudes are they ready to exhibit? What attitudes do they already possess that could motivate further growth? What strengths of mind, body, and spirit do they manifest that can help them in the inevitable transitions of life?

A nursing diagnosis identifies the human response to the disease process. Standard classifications of nursing diagnosis used to identify dysfunctional patterns include North American Nursing Diagnosis Association (NANDA), Nursing Interventions Classification (NIC), and Nursing Outcomes Classification (NOC) (McFarland & McFarland, 1997). These diagnoses are applicable to health education.

Planning

Planning, the third step of the Nursing Process, is the development of the client education plan. In this step you will outline the learning objectives based on the assessment and analysis of the findings. It involves identifying specific learning objectives and educational outcomes, establishing priorities, and selecting teaching strategies to achieve the outcomes. Planning is deciding what needs to be learned and what strategies and materials will most likely facilitate achievement of the learning objectives. Once these are selected, a written client education plan is devised.

The planning step should involve clients and their families when appropriate. For example, if your client has Alzheimer's disease, then significant others, such as caregivers, a spouse, or family members, must be included in the formation of plans. It is important to get feedback during the planning process about what is to be learned and how this is to be accomplished to discover if you and the client are in accord.

Implementation

Implementing the plan involves acting to accomplish the learning objectives and educational outcomes. You and your clients will carry out the actions that are most likely to facilitate the desired learning. During this step you will need to elicit periodic feedback and stay attuned to behavioral clues that indicate clients' feelings of success or failure. You will use a variety of teaching strategies and instructional materials to facilitate client learning. Ongoing reassessment and continued analysis are part of implementation and involve adapting to feedback as you enact the plan. Note the client's responses to your teaching and modify your approach as needed. Last, it is important to document the health education you provide.

Evaluation

The evaluation phase is the final step of the Nursing Process. This is where you and your clients evaluate teaching effectiveness. Did the clients learn what was expected? Is their behavior more conducive to good health? Has the client's level of wellness improved? Are the problems with which clients needed help diminished, or are they coping with their problems more effectively? Two-way communication with clients helps you to summarize and interpret results.

Although evaluation is presented as the final step of the Nursing Process, evaluation takes place throughout the Teaching and Learning Process. During the assessment phase, for instance, while identifying how clients perceive their problems, you will evaluate how well you communicated. Did you understand what the clients conveyed? To find out, repeat back your interpretation of what they said. Did clients indicate that they were understood correctly? Did clients indicate that your words and actions made sense to them? Such transactions are ongoing throughout each step of the Nursing Process. Evaluation involves determining the overall quality of health education.

Some suggest that the Nursing Process contributes to linear thinking. Chitty and Black state that "the nursing process can be taught, learned, and used in a rigid, mechanistic and linear manner" (2007, p. 194). However, we believe it can be used as a creative approach to health education by attending to feedback throughout the process. The Nursing Process used in health education is ongoing, with constant evaluation and reassessment to meet the ongoing learning needs of clients.

Teaching and Learning Process

The Teaching and Learning Process is the next component of the Nurse–Client Relationship. The process of teaching and learning means to engage with others to acquire new knowledge, behaviors, and skills. Nurses as Educators use "planned learning experiences based on sound theories that provide individuals, groups and communities the opportunity to acquire the information they need to make quality health decisions" (Wurzbach, 2004, p. 6). Learning is a process by which behavior changes as a result of experiences (Ormrod, 2012). In teaching, the Nurse as Educator chooses teaching strategies and selects instructional materials to assist the Client as Learner to make behavioral changes that promote, retain, and restore health.

Learning theories guide teaching practices. They are the foundation of the Teaching and Learning Process. Some learning theories are more applicable than others, depending on the teacher, the client, and the learning context. You will be introduced to behavioral, cognitive, and social theories of learning as they apply to learners at all ages. Learning theories are important and provide the foundation that guides you as educator. Together the Teaching and Learning Process and the Nursing Process provide a holistic approach to address clients' health education needs.

Clinical Judgment

The third component in the Nurse–Client Relationship is the exercise of sound Clinical Judgment during teaching and learning. Clinical Judgment in nursing is the outcome of clinical reasoning, often referred to as clinical decision making. It is a characteristic way of thinking in the nursing discipline. You exercise Clinical Judgment as you assess clients, develop client education plans, select teaching strategies and instructional materials, and evaluate the success of your efforts. Your judgments and decisions impact the outcome of health education.

Some nursing educators believe that critical thinking is "the brain's tool for developing the expert nursing judgment needed to improve patient outcomes" (Scheffer & Rubenfeld, 2006, p. 195). Others believe that forming clinical judgments in the delivery of nursing care is distinct from general critical thinking skills (Tanner, 2005). Regardless, it is essential for nurses to exercise sound Clinical Judgment in the Teaching and Learning Process.

The Teaching and Learning and Nursing Processes provide the structural framework through which Clinical Judgment and clinical reasoning occur. Nurses engage in a variety of thinking patterns because no single pattern characterizes all situations. Tanner (2006) proposed a model with four aspects describing how nurses reason in the clinical area that is applicable to health education situations. The first aspect is noticing, whereby the nurse grasps the situation at hand. The second is interpreting, whereby the nurse develops an understanding of the situation. The third is responding, whereby the nurse decides on an appropriate course of action. The fourth is reflecting, whereby the nurse evaluates the effectiveness of the outcomes. These thinking and reasoning patterns occur within each step of the Teaching and Learning Process and Nursing Process to guide the nurse in the formation of Clinical Judgments related to health education.

Clinical Judgment in nursing develops as nurses gain experience and expertise in a practice area and expand their knowledge, moving from being a novice to being an expert. To become an expert in nursing, a beginning nurse passes through five levels of proficiency: novice, advanced beginner, competent, proficient, and expert (Benner, 1984). The novice has no experience in a situation, relies on rules, and is inflexible. The advanced beginner has more experience and has marginally acceptable performance. The competent nurse has 2 to 3 years of experience in similar situations and brings perspective, abstract, and analytic thinking to problem solving. The proficient nurse sees situations as wholes rather than specific aspects and has learned from past experience what to expect in situations and what to do when things do not go as expected. The expert nurse has a deep understanding and intuitive grasp of situations and no longer needs rules or guidelines. This nurse sees the totality of situations and quickly identifies the nature of the problem and how to solve it. These skill levels apply not only to the delivery of nursing care but also to the delivery of health education.

Evidence-Based Nursing Practice

The last component of the Nurse–Client Relationship is EBNP as it relates to health education. EBNP is the use of current best practices in making decisions about patient care by using a problem-solving approach. This approach incorporates a systematic search for evidence, clinical expertise, and patient preferences and values (Melnyk & Fineout-Overholt, 2004). It is the act of applying current research findings to clinical practice. Applying research to health education is an integral part of the Miller–Stoeckel Client Education Model. It means using the best available and most pertinent research to make health education decisions.

The history of evidence-based research goes back to Dr. Archie Cochrane, an English physician who, in 1972, confronted healthcare professionals about the lack of randomized control studies to support medical practice decisions. Because of his influence, the first electronic database of clinical trials was established in 1988. First called the Oxford Database of Prenatal Trials, it later became The Cochrane Collaboration (Bliss-Holtz, 2007). The Cochrane Collaboration is now an international database that disseminates research worldwide.

The concept of evidence-based practice was embraced by nursing and other healthcare professions in the 1990s. The motivation behind this decision was the realization that many healthcare practices were based on intuition, experience, clinical skills, and guesswork rather than science. EBNP uses a research-based decision-making process to guide the delivery of holistic client-centered nursing care and health education. The specific steps involved in carrying out EBNP include defining the problem and searching for evidence, critically appraising the evidence, applying the findings to practice, taking into account the client–learner's values and preferences, and then evaluating outcomes.

Although EBNP is accepted as a means of promoting best practices, differences of opinion exist among nurses regarding what types of studies constitute the strongest evidence and what weight to give them. The terms *levels of evidence* and *strength of evidence* refer to systems for classifying the evidence in a body of literature through a hierarchy of scientific rigor and quality. Several dozen of these hierarchies exist (Agency for Healthcare Research and Quality, 2002). The reviewers must select the most relevant levels of evidence to meet their needs. The following concise definitions of terms are used in describing the levels of evidence.

- Meta-analysis is a statistical analysis of a collection of quantitative studies.
- Systematic review is a research summary that searches the literature and critically appraises individual quantitative studies to identify valid, applicable evidence.
- Randomized controlled trial is a study in which subjects are randomly assigned to groups; one receives the intervention, and the other is a control group.
- Quasi-experimental design is a modification of an experimental design in which there may not be manipulation of the independent variable, random assignment, or control group.
- Observational study is a study in which researchers have no control; instead, they observe what happens to groups of people.
- Case study (case report, single case report) is an uncontrolled observational study involving an intervention and outcome in a single situation.
- Descriptive study is a statistical study to identify patterns or trends in a situation, but not cause and effect.
- Cohort study is a study that involves the selection of a large population of people who have the same condition, who receive a specific intervention, and who are followed over time and compared with a group that is not affected by the condition.
- Case-controlled study is a study that compares two groups of people: those with the condition, and a similar group without the condition. It is also called a retrospective study.
- Expert opinion is a judgment by people who have experience with a particular subject.
- Qualitative study is a study focused on subjective experiences in naturalistic settings rather than under experimental conditions. There are different types of qualitative studies.

A diagram of the hierarchy of research evidence is included in **Figure 1-3**. It illustrates a research hierarchy in which the lowest tier includes the descriptive studies, case studies, case series, qualitative studies, and expert opinion. The highest tier includes meta-analyses and systematic reviews. Research at this tier has a greater chance of being generalized to a group of clients.

Nurses as Educators should rely on substantiated, critically critiqued research to ensure that the most current health education practices and teaching strategies are provided to clients. Nurses as Educators need a core foundation of health information that reflects quality care and best teaching practices supported by current research. More research is needed on the effectiveness of various teaching strategies and instructional materials for different populations. In addition to using the best available evidence, nurses are called on to exercise their best judgment in clinical and health education situations.

Interrelatedness of the Components in the Nurse–Client Relationship

The components in the Nurse–Client Relationship (Nursing Process, Teaching and Learning Process, Clinical Judgment, and EBNP) are interacting and interdependent. The components complement one another. During assessment and analysis, the client's learning needs are assessed and

Figure 1-3 Levels of Evidence in Research

analyzed to determine the extent of the client's need for health education. In this step, the nurse grasps the client's situation. It may involve looking for applicable literature specific to the client's situation or a group's health education needs.

Planning involves developing individualized care plans drawn from EBNP and setting priorities and learning objectives based on client health education needs. The nurse develops sufficient understanding of the situation and responds by involving the client in designing the client education plan.

Implementation is carrying out the client education plan. The nurse takes action and responds based on EBNP where it exists but also reflects on client responses. Using judgment, the nurse is prepared to alter the client education plan if necessary. The nurse uses judgment in selecting teaching strategies and instructional materials to meet the client's health education needs and preferences.

Evaluation reviews the successes and failures in meeting the learning objectives of the client education plan. Teaching strategies may need to be modified to achieve the objectives. The nurse continually reviews the literature to update the client education plan using current EBNP where available. The client's achievement of the learning objectives is measured and reinforced to help ensure continued success.

The Nurse–Client Relationship is at the heart of the Miller–Stoeckel Client Education Model. To initiate the process, the Nurse as Educator should ask specific questions that guide the process. For example, how am I using the nursing process to initiate and follow through with teaching clients? What are the teaching and learning principles I am using? How am I using clinical judgment in assessing clients and designing and implementing client education? And what research that is evidence-based supports my decisions?

The interrelatedness of the Nursing Process, Teaching and Learning Process, Clinical Judgment, and EBNP components is illustrated in **Table 1-1**.

Table 1-1 Interrelatedness of the Nurse–Client Relationship Components

Nursing Process	Teaching–Learning Process	Clinical Judgment	EBNP Process
Assessment and analysis	Determine learning needs	Noticing	Define problem and search literature
Planning	Develop client education plan	Interpreting	Appraise research findings
Implementation	Use teaching strategies	Responding	Apply to clinical situation
Evaluation	Determine behavior change	Reflecting	Assess the outcomes

Client Education Outcomes

Client Education Outcomes are achieved when health-promoting changes in knowledge, attitudes, and skills occur in clients. The last portion of the Miller–Stoeckel Client Education Model focuses on evaluation. To determine if health education efforts are successful, nurses must evaluate the results. Evaluation of client education outcomes is measuring the degree to which the learning objectives are met.

Evaluation is important to clients and educators because it informs them about their progress and the effectiveness of the Teaching and Learning Process. The Miller–Stoeckel Client Education Model addresses both Formative Evaluation and Summative Evaluation. Both are essential aspects of evaluation that provide a holistic picture of what was achieved (**Table 1-2**).

Formative Evaluation is ongoing during teaching and learning activities. It is important to know if the learning activities are meeting the learning objectives as teaching is progressing. If weaknesses are identified, they can be changed right away. Formative Evaluation addresses three areas: evaluation of the client education plan, evaluation of the learning environment, and evaluation of the nurse–client interaction. The involvement of the Client as Learner and Nurse as Educator is essential to the process.

In Formative Evaluation, evaluation of the client education plan is done by considering concept comprehension and client motivation. The learning environment is evaluated by assessing the effectiveness of the delivery format and the use of technology. The nurse–client interaction is evaluated by determining the level of client engagement and communication. These components of Formative Evaluation seek to answer the question, how are we doing?

Summative Evaluation occurs at the conclusion of the Teaching and Learning Process. It is directed toward measuring the degree to which the learning objectives and overall outcomes are met at the conclusion of the learning activity or program. It addresses three areas: evaluation of client learning, evaluation of educational effectiveness, and evaluation of integration of learning into daily living.

Measurement of learning occurs not only at the conclusion of individual learning activities and programs, but it also involves long-term follow-up of client learning. Results of systematically conducted long-term evaluations are important from an EBNP perspective. Findings from EBNP can serve to guide future health education practices. Summative Evaluation is directed toward outcomes that determine whether clients have learned and if the activities and programs are feasible to continue in the future. Determining feasibility includes examining the effectiveness of learning materials, the costs, the time requirements, the degree of client

Table 1-2 Client Education Outcomes

Formative Evaluation	Summative Evaluation
Evaluation of the client education plan	Evaluation of client learning
Evaluation of the learning environment	Evaluation of educational effectiveness
Evaluation of the nurse–client interaction	Evaluation of learning into daily living

satisfaction, and the long-term benefits of programs. Basically, Summative Evaluation asks the question, how did we do?

Definitions

The following definitions support the Miller–Stoeckel Client Education Model and will broaden your understanding of health education. The most important terms to understand are health education, health, illness, Stoeckel Wellness–Illness Functional Continuum, and Health Belief and Health Promotion Models.

Health Education

Health education enhances the quality of life for people worldwide. It is defined broadly by Green and Kreuter (1991) as any combination of learning experiences designed to encourage voluntary actions that are beneficial to health. Health education is achieved through the use of learning theories combined with teaching strategies to help individuals, families, groups and communities, and health team members to promote, retain, and restore health. It not only involves providing relevant health information, but it also helps clients make appropriate health-related behavioral changes. The term *health education* also refers to the process of educating health team members to become more effective in their roles and responsibilities.

Health

Health, as defined by the World Health Organization in 1948, is "a state of complete physical, mental, and social well-being, not merely the absence of disease or infirmity" (2004). Health is a dynamic state in which individuals adapt to changes in the internal and external environments to maintain a state of well-being in all life dimensions. This is the most popular and comprehensive definition of health worldwide, and it is applicable to individuals, families, groups, and communities. Clients bring their own definitions and perceptions of health to clinical situations. Their perceptions of what is and is not normal health influence their willingness to accept health education teaching.

Illness

Illness is a subjective perception of not being well. It is a mismatch between an individual's needs and their ability to meet those needs. It signals that the present balance to maintain health is not working. During illness, changes may occur in the structure and function of a person's body and mind. Illness has a classifiable set of signs and symptoms resulting from disturbed body functioning. These are associated with characteristic preclinical findings, course, and etiology.

Stoeckel Wellness–Illness Functional Continuum

An individual's level of health is a constantly changing state that moves along a continuum from optimal functioning to a state of total disability. The basic premise of the Stoeckel Wellness–Illness Functional Continuum is that wellness and illness involve a variety of factors: social, physiologic, environmental, emotional, activities of daily living, and health access. The factors in the model can either enhance or distract from the client's health. Disease and illness are a failure of an individual's adaptive mechanisms to adequately counteract changes in functional and structural disturbances. Factors are displayed along a continuum showing incremental increases or decreases in health functioning. Each factor is plotted on the continuum moving from the center (score of 5 is neutral) toward the right (highest score of 10 indicates highest level of wellness) or left (lowest score of 0 indicates lowest level of wellness) and shows changes in the state of health. High-level functioning or wellness involves an increased ability to perform the activities of daily living. Low-level functioning is brought on by illness or disability, resulting in a decreased ability to perform activities of daily living.

This continuum is useful when working with clients to get a holistic picture of their functioning. Clients can place themselves on each factor's continuum to identify their strengths and weaknesses. Each person is unique, with different degrees of wellness and illness. Plotting the continuum for each factor helps the Nurse as Educator determine clients' health perceptions and needs. By using the Stoeckel Wellness–Illness Functional Continuum as an assessment tool when working with clients, you gain a more accurate picture of how the client perceives their state of health. The continuum can also be used to compare a client's previous level of health with the present level, but because of its subjective nature, it cannot be used to compare one client with another. The continuum illustrates the dynamic, ever-changing state of health (**Figure 1-4**).

Figure 1-4 Stoeckel Wellness–Illness Functional Continuum

Health Belief and Health Promotion Models

The Health Belief Model (Rosenstock, 1974) was developed in the 1950s to explain why people did not use preventive health services such as immunizations. The model examines the relationship between a client's beliefs and behaviors, and it helps nurses understand these factors to plan teaching that effectively assists clients in promoting, retaining, and restoring health. An important assumption of this model is that the nurse collaborates with the client to reach mutually agreed-upon goals by understanding the factors that influence health beliefs. The Health Belief Model identifies the following factors that influence health beliefs:

- Personal expectations regarding health and illness
- Perception of the seriousness of the illness
- Likelihood of following prescribed healthcare measures
- Perceived barriers related to such factors as cost, inconvenience, or pain

A criticism of the Health Belief Model is that it is based on the Western cultural health belief system and does not allow for other influences or for the fact that clients do not always act on their belief system. Our approach, shown in **Table 1-3**, uses the basic format of the model, but it includes questions that address the cultural aspects of client teaching. Our approach is a starting point for examining client decision making concerning health education and can be used to develop client education plans. It is important for the nurse to understand client perceptions about health and the likelihood of adhering to health recommendations. This involves examining beliefs through a cultural lens. Communication is targeted at clarifying the nurse's and the client's perceptions and beliefs. Based on this information, nurses use those strategies that are most effective to meet client health education needs.

Table 1-3 Health Belief Model: Perceptions

Client Perceptions	Nursing Application
Need for care	■ Clarifies client concerns and reasons for seeking treatment ■ Explores client experiences with health issues, past and present ■ Asks about family and cultural factors affecting client perceptions
Seriousness and consequences of condition	■ Clarifies client perceptions of harm that the condition can cause ■ Clarifies client perceptions of consequences without treatment ■ Answers questions and clarifies prognosis; describes experiences with similar problems ■ Explores common and different beliefs and values
Value of health intervention	■ Discusses treatment client is seeking ■ Describes treatment: medical treatment, behavior change (lifestyle), medication (side effects), costs, answers questions, and so forth ■ Clarifies client perceptions of treatment
Effectiveness, cost, and barriers of treatment	■ Prepares goals and timeline for client and nurse responsibilities ■ Sets ground rules and boundaries for nurse–client relationship ■ Outlines knowledge and skills for client and nurse ■ Suggests and provides resources for knowledge and skill development ■ Clarifies client understanding of proposed plan

Data from Rankin, S. H., Stallings, K. D., & London, F. (2005). *Patient education in health and illness* (5th ed.). Philadelphia, PA: Lippincott Williams & Wilkins.

Nola Pender's health promotion model (2011) assists nurses in understanding the major determinants of health behaviors as a basis for behavioral counseling to promote healthy lifestyles. Her theory encourages health educators to look at variables that have been shown to impact health behavior. The model uses research findings from nursing, psychology, and public health to understand client health behaviors. This model can be used as a foundation to structure nursing protocols and interventions. This will be further discussed later in the text.

Context for Health Education

Nurses play a vital role in improving health on a local, national, and global scale. Nurses, in partnership with other healthcare professionals, facilitate delivery of health education in different venues to achieve positive client education outcomes. In this section, we address the importance of the wider scope of health education. Nurses should be aware that individual health affects the larger community and eventually affects global health.

National Importance of Health Education

The 1979 surgeon general's report, Healthy People, laid the foundation for a national prevention agenda. Every 10 years since that time, the U.S. Department of Health and Human Services has provided science-based, 10-year national objectives for promoting health and preventing disease. Healthy People 2000 and 2010 established national health objectives that serve as the basis for the development of state and community health initiatives. Currently, Healthy People 2020 (U.S. Department of Health and Human Services, 2012) continues the tradition of improving the health of Americans by establishing benchmarks and monitoring progress over time to encourage collaboration across communities and sectors, empowering individuals toward making informed health decisions, and measuring the impact of prevention activities. Healthy People 2020 contains about 1,200 objectives in 42 topic areas designed to serve as this decade's framework for improving the health of all people in the United States (**Box 1-1**). This information is available at http://www.healthypeople.gov/2020/about/default.aspx on a U.S. government website. Core objectives will remain centered on the prevention of illness and disease as the foundation of health.

Living in an Interactive and Interdependent Global Community

Maintaining health is a global concern. Health issues have global consequences that not only affect the people of developing nations but also the world community. Healthy, productive citizens are essential for global economic growth and security. Stable populations reduce pressures on global

---

Box 1-1 Healthy People 2020 Overarching Goals

- Attain high-quality, longer lives free of preventable disease, disability, injury, and premature death.
- Achieve health equality, eliminate disparities, and improve the health of all groups.
- Create social and physical environments that promote good health for all.
- Promote quality of life, healthy development, and healthy behaviors across all life stages.

economies and the environment. Stable populations also reduce the number and risk of humanitarian crises. Programs to control the spread of infectious diseases reduce the threat of epidemics. With healthcare services placing ever-greater pressures on state and federal health budgets, the economic burden of disease, and the burden to individuals and families, is a cause of great concern for governments and healthcare systems. Health education not only affects the immediate recipients but also future generations that will benefit from improved health habits and efforts to prevent illness. Eventually, improved health behavior will be ingrained when health education is widely available and an accepted part of health care. The prevention of illness and the promotion of health through the delivery of efficient and effective health education lie at the core of society's ability to affect health worldwide.

Future Challenges and Trends Facing Nurses as Educators

Future challenges in health care are difficult to predict, but current demographic and societal trends point to the increased need for Nurses as Educators. Demographic trends indicate an increasing older population and a greater percentage of underrepresented ethnic groups living in the United States that have unique health challenges. Societal trends show changes in social practices, such as cohabitation, acceptance of gay relationships, and more single-parent families. Other trends point to greater access to reliable information using technology, more reliance on alternative medicine, and more questioning of medical advice. Nurses as Educators must be aware of demographic and societal trends. They must adjust to these trends and incorporate the challenges they present into their health education practices.

It is important for nurses to expand their knowledge of health education, their leadership abilities, and their involvement in health policy development. More collaborative networks with other healthcare providers are needed that foster accountability. This collaboration should occur not only on the local level but also within the global community. Basing health education practices on research, demanding adherence to ethical standards, and promoting social justice are escalating challenges and trends. Doing it more, doing it better, and doing it with less are the future challenges.

Doing it more, doing it better, and doing it with less are the future challenges (Breckon, Harvey, & Lancaster, 1998). Novel solutions are urgently needed to improve client care. In healthcare's next chapter, a new type of technology will play a bigger role than ever before. That technology is artificial intelligence or AI. Rooted in the simulation of human intelligence by computer systems and machines, AI has the potential to revolutionize health care and transform nursing.

Artificial intelligence (AI) is defined as technologies that enable a computer system or computer-controlled robot to learn, reason, perceive, infer, communicate, and make decisions similar to or better than a human (Castellanos, 2018). It is predicted that, in the future, artificial intelligence (AI) will transform nursing across all domains of nursing practice, including administration, clinical care, education, policy, and research. In health care, AI is seen as a potential solution for handling anticipated massive increases in complex medical data (McGrow, 2019). Some uses of AI include accelerating innovation, improving decision-making, automating and speeding up processes, and saving overall costs (Buchanan et al., 2021)

The implementation of AI tools will change the way nurses interact with patients and their families and will also change the way educators interact with students. It was proposed at the beginning that AI technologies could substitute for nursing care, but now we know that it can aid nurses in decision making and help them make more self-assured decisions. The fear and distrust that may exist regarding the use of AI technologies is overcome with greater knowledge and an understanding of the existing technology (Fernandes, Santos, Sá, & Neves, 2023). Nurse educators need to have the requisite knowledge to prepare nurses and nursing students to practice safely and efficiently in the age of AI. Nurse educators also need to adopt new and evolving pedagogies that incorporate AI to better support students at all levels of education. The purpose of this review is to give baseline knowledge of AI, beginning with a list of vocabulary to assist with understanding the terminology.

Data: Information such as facts, numbers, speech, text, images, context, and outcomes used to analyze something or make decisions that is in a form that can be processed by a computer.

Input: To enter (data) into a computer or data processing system

Output: The information produced by a computer, includes solutions and outcomes to problems.

Big Data: An accumulation of data that is too large and complex for processing by traditional database management tools

Big Data in Healthcare: Refers to the abundant health data amassed from numerous sources, including electronic health records (EHRs), medical imaging, genomic sequencing, payor records, pharmaceutical research, wearables, and medical devices

Machine Learning (ML): An AI technology that automatically learns and improves from previous sets of experiences without the requirement for explicit programming

Deep Learning (DL): A subset of ML that learns by processing data with the help of artificial neural networks

Natural Language Processing (NLP): A technology that allows computers to comprehend, recognize, interpret, and produce human language and speech

Algorithm: A process or set of rules to be followed by a computer in calculating or problem-solving

ChatGPT: A computer program that simulates human conversation through voice commands or text chats or both

Neural Networks: A type of machine learning process, called deep learning, that uses interconnected nodes or neurons in a layered structure that resembles the human brain

Robotics: A branch of AI that is composed of electrical engineering, mechanical engineering, and computer science for the designing, construction, and application of robots

AI is advanced computer technology that attempts to imitate human thinking and reasoning and encompasses a range of technologies including *machine learning, deep learning,* and *natural language processing. Machine learning* programs the computer to learn how to solve a problem on its own. Basically, this involves absorbing massive amounts of data, seeking patterns, and then predicting outcomes within a percentage of certainty. The computer uses *algorithms* to derive knowledge from data and interprets data for itself. *Algorithms* are automated instructions that tell a computer what to do. The algorithm manipulates data in a variety of ways, such as sorting,

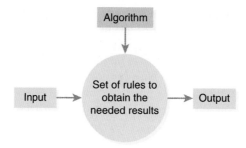

Figure 1-5 Definition of Algorithm

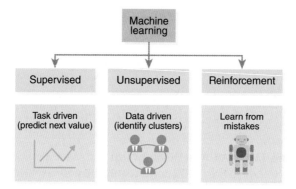

Figure 1-6 Types of Machine Learning

inserting, replacing, or searching for a data attribute. It solves problems when it carries out the instructions (**Figure 1-5**).

As more data are presented to the *machine learning* application, the computer learns from the data and corrects outputs. Machine learning can be *supervised* (task driven), *unsupervised* (data driven), or *reinforcement* (learning from mistakes) depending on the type of input data in the program and the type of outputs expected (**Figure 1-6**).

Another term encountered in AI is *deep learning*, which is a subset of machine learning. This computer approach involves networked algorithms called *neural networks* because the inspiration for their creation was how neurons are networked in our brain. In deep learning, algorithms called *nodes* fire the algorithm, process it as instructed, and pass its information to another node in the computer. A *deep learning* model can contain billions of nodes embedded in many layers (**Figure 1-7**).

Natural language processing (NLP) is another computer technology that allows computers to comprehend, recognize, interpret, and produce human language and speech. NLP is a tool that allows computers to comprehend, recognize, interpret, and produce human language and speech.

AI is also used to develop robotics applications that are used to assist humans in performing labor intensive tasks. **Box 1-2** summarizes the major technologies that make up AI: machine learning, neural networks in deep learning, natural language processing, and robotics.

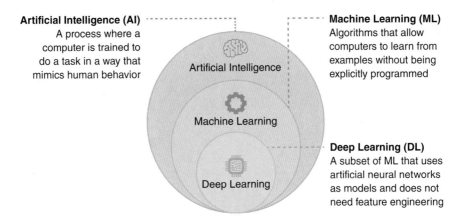

Artificial Intelligence (AI)
A process where a computer is trained to do a task in a way that mimics human behavior

Artificial Intelligence

Machine Learning (ML)
Algorithms that allow computers to learn from examples without being explicitly programmed

Machine Learning

Deep Learning (DL)
A subset of ML that uses artificial neural networks as models and does not need feature engineering

Deep Learning

Figure 1-7 Machine Learning and Deep Learning in Artificial Intelligence

AI systems work by ingesting large amounts of data, analyzing the data for correlations and patterns, and using these patterns to make predictions about future states. **Figure 1-8** uses the definitions and explanations previously provided to show the process of AI technology. Data is input and processed using algorithms to interpret outcomes. The outcomes are interpreted, adjusted, and reassessed to get the best results.

The impact of AI in medicine and health care continues to grow exponentially. AI technology holds significant potential to create more sophisticated and complex simulations that can help nurses develop critical thinking skills and prepare for real-world client care situations. A list of future AI technology predicted to impact nursing in the future is listed in **Box 1-3**.

The integration of AI in healthcare offers a combination of advantages and challenges. It is crucial for nurses to implement AI strategically and manage expectations intelligently to achieve the desired outcomes. Pros and cons of AI technologies are listed in **Box 1-4**.

Despite there being both positives and negatives associated with artificial intelligence in health care, AI will continue to be developed and used more widely in the future. Medical professionals are likely to rely on it even more for guidance and support, using it effectively to provide accurate and timely treatment to clients. To help make the best decisions about AI technology use, nurses should engage in all project development phases, from defining the problem to using the tool, to evaluating its impact. AI technology training should focus on why AI is needed, what drives the recommendations, and how it can inform client care. Nurses who understand the differences in using AI technology support, along with AI identified risk factors, are critical to the development and use of reliable solutions. Success in AI requires careful consideration of the most useful technology, engagement with the nurses who will actually use the tool, and nurse involvement in its implementation and evaluation. Artificial intelligence (AI) has the potential to make substantial progress toward the goal of making health care more personalized, predictive, preventative, and effective. We believe AI will continue its present path and ultimately become an established and effective tool for the healthcare sector.

Summary

This chapter introduces the Miller–Stoeckel Client Education Model. The model serves as the conceptual framework around which this text is organized and written. The four major concepts

Box 1-2 What Is Artificial Intelligence?

Machine Learning	Neural Networks	Natural Language Processing	Robotics
Using sample data to train computer programs to recognize patterns based on algorithms	Computer systems designed to imitate the neurons in a brain	The ability to understand speech as well as understand and analyze documents	Machine that can assist people without actual human involvement

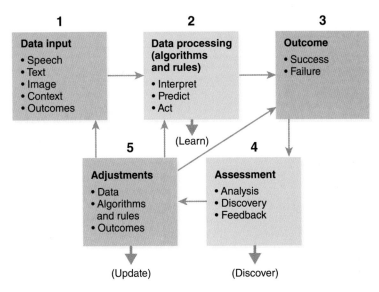

Figure 1-8 How AI Works

Box 1-3 Artificial Intelligence Applications in Nursing

Artificial Intelligence (AI) Applications in Nursing

- Illness detection and diagnosis
- Risk prediction for falls, sepsis, reactions, relapse, etc.
- Drug creation and development
- Medical imaging
- Managing medical records (EMR)
- Robotic virtual assisted care
- Monitoring health using wearables and personal devices
- Efficient staffing
- Digital health coaching
- Use of voice-assisted commands
- Gene editing

Data from Khan, B., Fatima, H., Qureshi, A., Kumar, S., Hanan, A., Hussain, J., & Abdullah, S. (2023). Drawbacks of artificial intelligence and their potential solutions in the healthcare sector. *Biomedical Materials & Devices*, (New York, N.Y.) 1–8. Advance online publication. https://doi.org/10.1007/s44174-023-00063-2

of Nurse as Educator, Client as Learner, Nurse–Client Relationship, and Client Education Outcomes were defined and explained, as were the four embedded concepts of Cultural Caring, Communication, Negotiation, and Collaboration.

The nature of the Nurse–Client Relationship involves the Nursing Process, the Teaching and Learning Process, Clinical Judgment, and EBNP. The model concludes with an examination of Client Education Outcomes that encompass Formative and Summative Evaluation. Finally, the future challenges and trends facing Nurses as Educators were discussed, including AI technology. In this section, we examined how health education can impact health, illness, and wellness in the local, national, and global health arenas. In the subsequent chapters of this book, we delve into greater depth about all aspects of providing health education.

Box 1-4 Pros and Cons of AI Technology

Pros of AI Technology	Cons of AI Technology
■ Ability to analyze data and improve diagnostics ■ Better accessible patient care ■ Reduced cost of care ■ Improved workload and reduced staff stress ■ Greater support with administrative tasks ■ Health monitoring and digital consultation ■ Increased information sharing ■ Improved research support ■ Enhanced decision making	■ Training complications for healthcare professionals ■ Use of robots leading to unemployment issues ■ Extensive changes in health care causing disruption ■ Need for human input and surveillance ■ Increase security risk from cyber attacks ■ Lack of consideration of social variables that affect treatment decisions ■ Inaccuracies due to mistakes and data collection errors ■ Algorithm development concerns ■ Ethical concerns

Exercises

Exercise I: Philosophy of Health Education

Purpose: Develop a philosophy of health education.

Directions: Working with a small group of colleagues, write your philosophy of health education. This will take time, thought, and discussion. Your philosophy statement should be about two to three pages in length. Include your beliefs about the following:

1. The value of health education as an aspect of comprehensive health care
2. Teaching and what it means
3. Learning and its place in the human experience
4. The role of the Nurse as Educator
5. The role of the Client as Learner
6. The relationship that should exist between the educator and the learner
7. The value of Client Education Outcomes

Exercise II: Apply the Miller–Stoeckel Client Education Model

Purpose: Gain experience using the model.

Directions: Select a client with whom you have worked who needs health education. Visualize how you could use the model to build a positive Nurse–Client Relationship and achieve the educational outcomes.

- How do you see your role as a nurse educator?
- How do you see your client as a learner?
- How can you use the nursing process to initiate and follow up with teaching your client?
- What teaching and learning principles can you use?

- How can you use clinical judgment to assess clients and design and implement client education?
- What research that is evidence-based supports your decisions?

Exercise III: Using the Stoeckel Wellness–Illness Continuum

Purpose: Self-analysis of wellness–illness state.
Directions: Chart and analyze your progress on the Stoeckel Wellness–Illness Continuum. Print a copy from the book to plot your score on, or write out your answers.

- Score each factor from 1 to 10: social, physiological, environmental, emotional, and health access.
- Make a summative statement about your overall health.
- Discuss in paragraph form how your personal beliefs, culture, and background affect your views of health, illness, and wellness.

Exercise IV: Ways to Promote Client Education

Purposes:

- Promote creative thinking.
- Raise consciousness regarding client education.

Directions: Form small groups and discuss the following situation. Take notes and prepare a report to be shared with the rest of your peers.

While carrying heavy patient care assignments and responsibilities, some nurses are managing to teach their clients in mutually satisfactory ways. What client teaching have you observed by your clinical instructors, supervisors, primary nurses, or other nursing personnel? What are you doing to promote client teaching? If you are not yet in the clinical area, seek out nurses in your school, hospital, or neighborhood and ask them what they are doing to promote health teaching. Draw on your experiences as a patient, client, relative, or observer. Upon reflection, summarize the nurse's role in client education.

References

Agency for Healthcare Research and Quality. (2002). *Systems to rate the strength of scientific evidence.* Summary, evidence report/technology assessment (No. 47, AHRQ Publication No. 02-E015). Rockville, MD: Author. Retrieved from http://www.thecre.com/pdf/ahrq-system-strength.pdf http://www.ahrq.gov/clinic/epcsums/strengthsum.htm

American Hospital Association. (1992). *A patient's bill of rights.* Retrieved from http://www.elcamino.edu/faculty/dcharman/RT%20106%20AHA%20%20Patient%20Bill%20of%20Rights.pdf

American Nurses Association. (1998). *Standards of clinical nursing practice* (2nd ed.). Washington, DC: Author.

Bastable, S. B., & Alt, M. F. (2014). Overview of education in health care. In S. B. Bastable (Ed.), *Nurse as educator: Principles of teaching and learning for nursing practice* (4th ed., pp. 3–30). Burlington, MA: Jones & Bartlett Learning.

Buchanan, C., Howitt, M. L., Wilson, R., Booth, R. G., Risling, T., & Bamford, M. (2021). Predicted Influences of artificial intelligence on nursing education: Scoping review. *JMIR Nursing, 4*(1), e23933. doi:10.2196/23933

Benner, P. (1984). *From novice to expert.* Menlo Park, CA: Addison-Wesley.

Bliss-Holtz, J. (2007). Evidence-based practice: A primer for action. *Issues in Comprehensive Pediatric Nursing, 30*(4), 165–182.

Breckon, D., Harvey, J., & Lancaster, R. (1998). *Community health education: Settings, roles, and skills for the 21st century.* Sudbury, MA: Jones and Bartlett.

Campinha-Bacote, J. (1998). *The process of cultural competence in the delivery of healthcare services* (3rd ed.). Cincinnati, OH: Transcultural C.A.R.E. Associates.

Castellanos S. (2018) What exactly is artificial intelligence. *The Wall Street Journal.* www.wsj.com/articles/what-exactly-is-artificial-intelligence-1544120887

Chitty, K. K., & Black, B. P. (2007). *Professional nursing: Concepts and challenges* (5th ed.). St. Louis, MO: Elsevier.

Davidhizar, R., & Cramer, C. (2002). The best thing about the hospitalization was that the nurses kept me well informed: Issues and strategies of client education. *Accident and Emergency Nursing, 10,* 149–154.

Donner, C. L., Levonian, C., & Slutsky, P. (2005). Move to the head of the class: Developing staff nurses as teachers. *Journal for Nurses in Staff Development, 21*(6), 277–283.

Esteva, A., Robicquet, A., Ramsundar, B., et al. (2019). A guide to deep learning in healthcare. *Nature Medicine, 25,* 24–9.

Fawcett, J. (2005). The structure of contemporary nursing knowledge. In *Contemporary nursing knowledge: Analysis and evaluation of nursing models and theories* (2nd ed., pp. 1–48). Philadelphia, PA: F. A. Davis.

Fernandes, F., Santos, P., Sá, L., & Neves, J. (2023) Contributions of artificial intelligence to decision making in nursing: A scoping review protocol. *Nursing Reports, 13*(1), 67–72. https://doi-org.dml.regis.edu/10.3390/nursrep13010007

Green, L. W., & Kreuter, M. (1991). *Health promotion planning: An educational and environmental approach.* Mountain View, CA: Mayfield.

Hall, A. (2001). Client education. In P. Potter & A. Perry (Eds.), *Fundamentals of nursing* (7th ed., pp. 328–347). St. Louis, MO: Mosby.

Khan, B., Fatima, H., Qureshi, A., Kumar, S., Hanan, A., Hussain, J., & Abdullah, S. (2023). Drawbacks of artificial intelligence and their potential solutions in the healthcare sector. *Biomedical Materials & Devices,* 1–8. Advance online publication. https://doi.org/10.1007/s44174-023-00063-2

Knowles, M. S. (1990). *The adult learner: A neglected species* (4th ed.). Houston, TX: Gulf.

Lin, S., (2022). A clinician's guide to artificial intelligence (AI): Why and how primary care should lead the health care AI revolution. *The Journal of the American Board of Family Medicine,* January, *35*(1) 175–184. https://doi.org/10.3122/jabfm.2022.01.210226

McFarland, G. K., & McFarland, E. A. (1997). *Nursing diagnoses and intervention, planning for patient care* (3rd ed.). St. Louis, MO: Mosby.

McGrow, K. (2019). Artificial intelligence. *Nursing, 49*(9), 46–49. https://doi.org/10.1097/01.NURSE.0000577716.57052.8d.

Melnyk, B. M., & Fineout-Overholt, E. (2004). *Evidence-based practice in nursing and healthcare: A guide to best practice.* Philadelphia, PA: Lippincott Williams & Wilkins.

Melnyk, B. M., & Fineout-Overholt, E. (2011). *Evidence-based practice in nursing and healthcare: A guide to best practice* (2nd ed.). Philadelphia, PA: Wolters Kluwer.

National League of Nursing Education. (1918). *Standard curriculum for schools of nursing.* Baltimore, MD: Waverly Press.

National League of Nursing Education. (1937). *A curriculum guide for schools of nursing.* New York, NY: Author.

Orlando, I. J. (1972). *The discipline and teaching of nursing process: An evaluative study.* New York, NY: G. P. Putman's Sons.

Ormrod, J. E. (2012). *Human learning* (6th ed.). Boston, MA: Pearson.

Pender, N. (2011). *The health promotion manual.* Retrieved from http://research2vrpractice.org/wp-content/uploads/2013/02/HEALTH_PROMOTION_MANUAL_Rev_5-2011.pdf

Peplau, H. E. (1952). *Interpersonal relations in nursing.* New York, NY: G. P. Putnam's Sons.

Potter, P., & Perry, A. (2009). *Fundamentals of nursing* (7th ed.). St. Louis, MO: Mosby.

Rankin, S. H., Stallings, K. D., & London, F. (2005). *Patient education in health and illness* (5th ed.). Philadelphia, PA: Lippincott Williams & Wilkins.

Redman, B. (2006). *The practice of patient education: A case study approach* (10th ed.). St. Louis, MO: Mosby Elsevier.

Rosenstock, I. (1974). Historical origins of the health belief model. *Health Education Monographs, 2*(4), 336–353.

Scheffer, B. K., & Rubenfeld, M. G. (2006). Critical thinking: A tool in search of a job. *Journal of Nursing Education, 45*(6), 195–196.

Tanner, C. (2005). What have we learned about critical thinking in nursing? *Journal of Nursing Education, 44*(2), 47–48.

Tanner, C. (2006). Thinking like a nurse: A research-based model of clinical judgment in nursing. *Journal of Nursing Education, 45*(6), 204–211.

The Joint Commission. (2009). *The Joint Commission 2009 requirements related to the provision of culturally competent patient-centered care critical access hospitals (CAH).* Retrieved from http://www.jointcommission.org/assets/1/6/2009_CLASRelatedStandardsCAH.pdf

U.S. Department of Health and Human Services. (2012). *Healthy People 2020.* Washington, DC: Author. Retrieved from http://www.healthypeople.gov/2020/default.aspx

Webster's All-In-One Dictionary and Thesaurus (2nd ed.). (2013). Springfield, MA: Federal Street Press.

World Health Organization. (1948). *Constitution of the World Health Organization.* Retrieved from http://www.who.int/governance/eb/who_constitution_en.pdf

World Health Organization. (2004). *About the World Health Organization.* Retrieved from http://www.who.int/suggestions/faq/en/index.html

Wurzbach, M. E. (2004). *Community health education and promotion: A guide to program design and evaluation* (2nd ed.). Sudbury, MA: Jones and Bartlett Publishers.

PART II

The Learning Process

CHAPTER 2

Thinking and Learning

OBJECTIVES

Upon completion of this chapter, you will be able to do the following:

- Apply the concepts of thinking and learning to the Miller–Stoeckel Client Education Model.
- Analyze definitions of thinking and learning and formulate your own definition.
- Differentiate among cognitive, affective, and psychomotor domains of learning by giving an example of each.
- Give examples of how you have engaged in the following ways of thinking in the context of health education: problem solving, critical thinking, creative thinking, intuition, reflection, fantasy, and reverie.
- Identify at least two ways to help clients as learners (individuals, families, groups and communities, and health team members) develop their thinking abilities.
- Describe the following styles and models of thinking and learning: Sternberg's thinking styles, Witkin and Goodenough's Cognitive-Style Dimensions, Kolb's Experiential Learning Model: Learning Cycle and Styles, and Gardner's Multiple Intelligences.
- Describe how to apply the thinking and learning styles to client education.

CHAPTER OUTLINE

Introduction

Thinking and learning form the basis for the teaching and learning process, which undergirds the nurse–client relationship in the Miller–Stoeckel Client Education Model. This chapter focuses on thinking and learning and how they impact your approach to teaching clients. Thinking and learning are purposeful activities with the goal of bringing about a necessary change. The teaching and learning process encourages clients to engage in activities that are necessary to acquire new knowledge and new skills, and to incorporate new attitudes. Clients as learners do this by modifying and reorganizing knowledge that is already in place or by acquiring new knowledge. Clients as learners need specific, new information or assistance in learning how to use known information to their best advantage. Nurses also need to engage in self-assessment of their individual thinking and learning styles (**Figure 2-1**).

This chapter introduces the broad domains of learning: cognitive, psychomotor, and affective. Next, we examine thinking and the many ways thinking is categorized. The nursing process and clinical judgment were discussed in the previous chapter; now we discuss problem solving, critical thinking, creative thinking, intuition, and reflection. The chapter concludes by examining how thinking translates into various styles of learning and the implications this has for health education.

Domains of Learning

Clients learn as total beings, with all their senses. When they learn, they have thoughts about learning, and they experience feelings about what they are doing, thinking, and learning. The doing, thinking, and feeling aspects of learning are clearly related, but they are not the same. When nurses help clients learn something, they select one or more domains in which clients need to focus most of their energy. The three domains that have received the most attention in educational literature are the **cognitive**, **affective**, and **psychomotor** domains (Bloom, Engelhart, Furst, Hill, & Krathwohl, 1956).

The learning domains have been separated for research and study purposes, but that separation is arbitrary. Human behavior includes components of each domain (Kretchmar, 2008). When providing health education to clients, the domains provide an organizational framework that is useful as you contemplate what clients need to learn and what should be taught. **Figure 2-2** illustrates the interactive, interdependent relationship among the three domains. The most effective

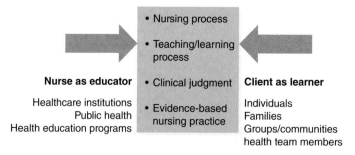

- Nursing process
- Teaching/learning process
- Clinical judgment
- Evidence-based nursing practice

Nurse as educator

Healthcare institutions
Public health
Health education programs

Client as learner

Individuals
Families
Groups/communities
health team members

Figure 2-1 Nurse–Client Relationship in the Miller–Stoeckel Client Education Model

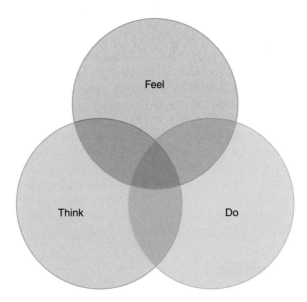

Figure 2-2 The Interacting Domains of Learning:
Cognitive (Think), Affective (Feel), and Psychomotor (Do)
Maximize Learning

learning occurs when all three domains are engaged in the learning process, as illustrated by the center triangle (Goulet & Owen-Smith, 2005).

Cognitive Domain

Cognitive learning is concerned with intellectual activities such as thinking, remembering, reasoning, and using language (The Merriam-Webster Dictionary, 2016). It involves judging, considering, believing, reflecting, and recalling. It also means using the mind to exercise judgment, draw inferences, arrive at conclusions, and make decisions (Miller & Babcock, 1996). The cognitive domain was the first domain developed by Bloom and colleagues in 1956. It has received the most attention in educational circles and enjoys the widest application to learning, in part because of the emphasis of Western cultures on reason over emotions (Kretchmar, 2008). Cognitive learning objectives are concrete and reflect this emphasis on reason. They are relatively easy to conceptualize, write, and measure.

Affective Domain

The affective domain deals with personal issues: attitudes, beliefs, behaviors, and emotions (Krathwohl, Bloom, & Masia, 1964). In the past, educators believed that the affective domain was an area of learning that was too complex and fraught with conflicts. Research in this area, however, is changing that perception, as educators realize the importance of integrating the affective domain into their teaching. Because the affective domain deals with personal issues such as attitudes, beliefs, behaviors, and emotions, it is increasingly integral to a comprehensive program of health education. Educational research indicates that there is a relationship between emotional intelligence and general intelligence in academic achievement with implications for health education. Learning objectives in the affective domain focus on influencing attitudes, motivating learners, developing respect, and clarifying values.

Attitudes are acquired by associating with others and participating in satisfying experiences. Clients are influenced by nurses' attitudes. Role modeling, for example, occurs when nurses work with clients. Nurses are constantly observed by clients, who are influenced by their behavior. Characteristics of kindness, fairness, compassion, honesty, punctuality, dependability, and competence are evident to clients as they observe nurses working. These characteristics help clients determine their perception of the quality of care they receive. Some examples of the way that nurses display their values are by treating clients with respect, such as providing privacy, adapting nursing interventions to their expressed concerns, and giving them undivided attention. It is important to include learning objectives in the affective domain as you provide health education for clients. Affective learning can also be facilitated by persuasion from other trusted authorities, such as parents, teachers, scientists, spiritual leaders, and valued colleagues with special expertise. Participating in group discussions and role playing also helps promote affective learning.

Psychomotor Domain

Psychomotor learning encompasses many physical procedures that individuals use in their activities of daily living and the complex physical activities required for work and recreation. It also includes learning physical skills and procedures applicable to healthcare delivery. Psychomotor learning requires that individuals acquire information and store it in memory. During the initial practice of a procedure, skills are shaped and learned until they become automatic (Marzano & Kendall, 2007). This type of learning is the most concrete, and it is the easiest to teach, observe, and measure. Clients form a mental image of how a skill is performed and then translate that image into external behavior. An example of psychomotor learning is performing an insulin injection. This type of learning is usually done best in a step-by-step fashion, from the simple to the complex. Nurses show clients how to perform the skill; then they guide them through return demonstrations. Nurses correct errors and reinforce correct responses. Practice is encouraged until both clients and nurses are satisfied with the clients' skills.

Thinking

Thinking is categorized in different ways. In this section, we look at definitions of thinking and ways of thinking engaged in by clients and nurses: problem solving, critical thinking, creative thinking, intuition, reflection, and other ways of thinking. The nursing process and clinical judgment, also ways of thinking, were discussed in the previous chapter. Each type of thinking has a distinct focus because they overlap, are complex, and cannot be confined to distinct categories. They are described separately for purposes of this discussion to highlight the particular focus of each type of thinking.

Definitions of Thinking

To think is an activity of the mind that is essential to living. It involves myriad processes such as observing, recalling, remembering, reasoning, drawing inferences, calculating likelihoods, reflecting, and deciding. It encompasses our knowledge, beliefs, opinions, and judgments. Thinking has a subjective quality in that all past experiences influence how we see the world. It includes our personal knowledge, our interpersonal relationships, and our role as nurses.

Ruggiero defined thinking as "any mental activity that helps formulate or solve a problem, make a decision, or fulfill a desire to understand. It is a searching for answers, a reaching for meaning" (2012, p. 4). It also involves such mental activities as wondering, imagining, inquiring, interpreting, evaluating, and judging. Thinking can be concrete, referring to physical materials or objects (What instructional materials do I need to teach this information?), or abstract, referring to a quality of something (What value do instructional materials have in learning?). Thoughts can be about the past (What worked best yesterday in teaching Ms. Jones about diabetes?), the present (How shall I best present this material on smoking cessation?), or the future (How shall I use client feedback to improve my teaching?).

Thinking is complex, multifaceted, dynamic, and it involves the creation of images (Halpern, 2014). For example, when you wonder if the intravenous solution is about to run out, you picture what the fluid level in the bottle looked like the last time you were in the room, and you think about the amount of time that has passed. In this sense, thinking is imagery accompanied by silent, internal speech.

Thinking is described as directed and nondirected or automatic (Halpern, 2014). Directed thinking is a conscious mental focus on a problem or issue with a desired outcome. It is purposeful and goal directed. Directed thinking has an evaluation component that considers the effectiveness of thinking outcomes; that is, if the decisions were effective. For example, you might ask yourself, "Did I make a good decision in this situation?" In contrast, nondirected or automatic thinking occurs as a result of routine habits, such as getting up in the morning, going to work or school, and so forth. Many aspects of life involve nondirected, automatic thinking.

Ways of Thinking

Nurse educators engage in a variety of ways of thinking while providing health education to clients and healthcare professionals. **Figure 2-3** illustrates some of these ways.

Problem Solving

The most common type of thinking is problem solving. Problem solving is a process of developing, testing, and evaluating a method for overcoming an obstacle by identifying a problem and finding the best alternative to solve it. Problem solving consists of these steps: identifying the problem, analyzing aspects of the problem, collecting pertinent information, hypothesizing about its cause or causes, generating possible solutions, trying out one of the hypotheses, and evaluating the results.

In the process of problem solving, individuals use critical thinking skills to understand and solve a problem. Sometimes a situation requires considerable thought and contemplation (Should I attend school full or part time?), and at other times it is relatively simple (What shall I do this weekend?). Problem solving is conscious, focused thinking over which individuals exert control.

Problem solving requires being open to new ways of thinking, reflection, and clinical judgment. Nurses use problem solving most effectively in working with clients, assisting them to think through their health problems, and finding workable, realistic, and appropriate solutions.

Critical Thinking

Critical thinking is a specific type of thinking that emphasizes rational cognitive processes and certain attitudes and values. The word *critical* often connotes negativity, whereas the intended meaning of the word is *analytic*. Ideas about critical thinking that are applicable to all disciplines

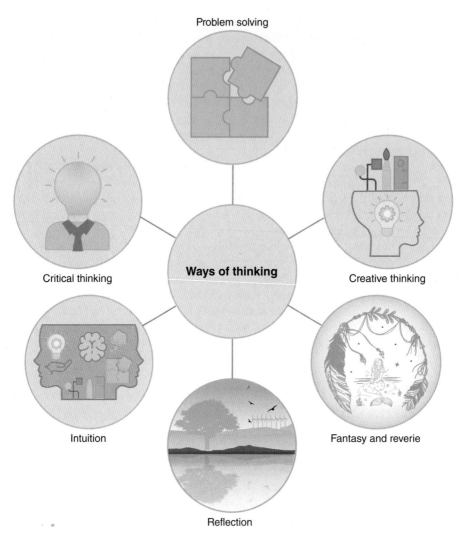

Figure 2-3 Ways of Thinking: Problem Solving, Critical Thinking, Creative Thinking, Intuition, Reflection, Fantasy & Reverie

Problem solving: © canbedone/Shutterstock; Creative thinking: © ImageFlow/Shutterstock; Fantasy & reverier: © Ironika/Shutterstock; Reflection: © martinho Smart/Shutterstock; Intuition: © AndryDj/Shutterstock; Critical Thinking: © Rawpixel.com/Shutterstock

come from educators in the fields of philosophy and education (Brookfield, 2012; Browne & Keeley, 2012; Halpern, 2014; McPeck, 1990; Paul, 1995; Ruggiero, 2012; Watson & Glaser, 1980). Their interest was in defining and identifying critical thinking processes applicable to everyday living. Common themes in these definitions include conscious awareness of one's thinking processes, such as acquiring knowledge and understanding. It involves examining assumptions and validating inferences, examining evidence, and searching for meaning and solutions through rational thinking processes. It is purposeful, directed toward solving problems and resolving issues. The definitions also address attitudes, values, and dispositions, for example, intellectual honesty, flexibility, and willingness to listen to other points of view. To be a critical thinker is to be analytic, reflect constructively, and evaluate fairly.

Nursing recognizes the importance of critical thinking in preparing practitioners (Kaddoura, 2013; Wallace & Moughrabi, 2016; Whiffin & Hasselder, 2013) and accepts critical thinking as an essential component of nursing practice and nursing education programs (Chan, 2013; Holland & Ulrich, 2016). However, the nursing profession continues to lack a widely accepted definition of critical thinking (Chan, 2013; Kaddoura, 2013; Victor-Chmil, 2013). Nurse educators accept rational, logical thinking as central features of critical thinking and recognize that critical thinking is different from clinical reasoning and clinical judgment. We agree with Victor-Chmil that these are distinct but interrelated concepts.

The most widely accepted definition of critical thinking comes from the research of Scheffer and Rubenfeld (2000). They conducted a study to define critical thinking in nursing with input from an international panel of nurse experts on critical thinking. They identified both cognitive and affective dimensions of critical thinking in nursing. Their consensus definition is as follows:

> Critical thinking in nursing is an essential component of professional accountability and quality nursing care. Critical thinkers in nursing exhibit these habits of the mind: confidence, contextual perspective, creativity, flexibility, inquisitiveness, intellectual integrity, intuition, open-mindedness, perseverance, and reflection. Critical thinkers in nursing practice the cognitive skills of analyzing, applying standards, discriminating, information seeking, logical reasoning, predicting and transforming knowledge. (p. 357)

Because of the research supporting this definition, we believe it best represents the meaning of critical thinking in nursing.

Creative Thinking

To create is to bring into being—to cause to exist (*The Merriam-Webster Dictionary*, 2016). It is the ability to go beyond current knowledge and think in a new way. Creative thinking has both a creative and a judgmental phase (Ruggiero, 2012). Individuals have creative thoughts and ideas and then proceed to judge them as they look for solutions to problems and answers to questions. This thinking moves back and forth between creating ideas and then judging them, the former being creative thinking and the latter being critical thinking. Halpern (2014) sees creativity as producing an unusual outcome while also being appropriate and useful to the situation. Thus creative thinking and critical thinking are intertwined.

Creative thinkers are curious, adventurous, resourceful, undaunted by the prospect of failure, and independent in the sense that they are willing to speak freely and do not need a lot of approval from others (Ruggiero, 2012). Creative thinkers tolerate ambiguity and uncertainty, adjust easily to new and changing situations, and freely abandon old assumptions when confronted with new evidence. Creative thinkers are willing to be different, to think outside the box. In problem solving, creative thinkers propose multiple options to consider that are appropriate to the context rather than immediately focusing on one option.

Santrock (2023) described the creative process as a five-step sequence, the first of which is *preparation*. In this step, a problem or issue arouses interest and curiosity. The next step is *incubation*, whereby individuals think about the problem and mull over ideas. The third step is *insight*, that moment when the pieces of the puzzle seem to fit together. The fourth step is *evaluation*, when individuals bring their judgment to bear on a tentative solution to determine if it is workable and realistic. The final step is *elaboration*, the most difficult step requiring the most time.

These steps move back and forth and do not follow a linear, sequential path. For example, insight and incubation can occur throughout each step, and evaluation is ongoing.

Intuition

Intuition is quick and ready insight, knowing things without conscious reasoning (*The Merriam-Webster Dictionary*, 2016). It is information that is not acquired by rational, analytic processes; rather, it occurs outside of conscious thought. Its source is from within the person and is based on life experiences and accumulated knowledge. It is the aha experience that occurs with sudden insight. For example, nurses sense something important about a client, often described as a gut feeling or a flash of insight, but they are unable to verbalize it or they verbalize it with difficulty. However, based on that insight, nurses adjust their teaching and care to be more suitable for the client.

Intuition was once thought to be characteristic of only expert nurses (Benner, 1984). However, intuition is now known to be used by nurses at all levels of expertise, including the novice (Ruth-Sahd & Hendy, 2005). The primary difference between novice and expert nurses is their knowledge, expertise, and years of experience. Those with greater knowledge, expertise, and experience bring more to assessment, intervention, and evaluation when working with clients (Faugier, 2005). Thus, intuition has somatic, affective, and cognitive components, but further research is needed to understand how these components are integrated (Hodgkinson, Langan-Fox, & Sadler-Smith, 2008). Your intuitive knowledge is important to take into consideration when making health education decisions. However, you should validate your intuitions through evidence-based research because many psychologists have found that spontaneous, intuitive approaches to solving problems are frequently wrong (Halpern, 2014).

Reflection

Reflection results from meditation (*The Merriam-Webster Dictionary*, 2016) and is an important aspect of thinking. The word *reflective* comes from the Latin word *reflectere*, meaning bending back, casting back, introspecting, and deliberating. Reflection helps to clarify thoughts and values and how they affect problem solving and decision making. It is important to reflect on health education activities and consider what is and is not effective. If nurses fail to reflect, it reduces the self-correction that comes with evaluating teaching effectiveness.

Reflective skepticism is an important aspect of critical thinking. Reflective skepticism requires thinking about the universal truth of statements rather than immediately accepting or rejecting them. Rather than accepting or rejecting statements at face value, reflective critical thinkers ask questions, analyze responses, reflect, and evaluate the merits of statements. This process is not cynical or dismissive of new ideas; rather, it is a process of analyzing and determining what to believe. Reflective skepticism requires reflecting on beliefs, assumptions, and intuitive responses to clarify thinking (Browne & Keeley, 2012).

Reflection is described as an important parameter of clinical judgment (Tanner, 2006). Saylor (1990) describes reflective thinking as essential for self-evaluation and improving clinical performance. Reflection is viewed overall as a form of systematic inquiry that is used as a means to improve practice or as a way to make sense of learning, evaluation, and promotion of learning. Reflection may be a solitary process or involve collective reflection with colleagues and teachers or interaction with theoretical literature.

Table 2-1 Reflective Practice Questions

Reflection Before Action	Reflection in Action	Reflection on Action
Anticipatory Reflection	*Evaluation in Action and Revision*	*Analysis of Past Actions and Rationale*
What do I want?	What is effective, and what needs to be different?	Why did I act as I did?
What outcome do I want?	What is the client's response?	What was the client outcome?
What is my plan?	What other options are available?	What actions did I take?
What is my rationale?	What is the plan revision?	Why did I respond as I did?

Three different aspects of reflective practice are *reflection before action*, *reflection in action*, and *reflection on action*. Reflection before action is anticipatory reflection involving the careful consideration of what to do and why to do it before engaging in action. The nurse develops a rationale for actions, organizes and prioritizes a vision for future action, and examines core beliefs and values. Reflection before action gives the nurse an opportunity to deliberate about possible alternatives, decide on a course of action, develop plans, and anticipate what the experience will be like for the nurse and the client.

Reflection in action refers to reflective thinking as one is doing the action. Reflection in action in health education refers to the nurse's thinking about the teaching and learning process while directly engaged in teaching. Reflection is usually stimulated by a problem that the nurse is facing. The process of analysis includes asking questions, such as how the problem was perceived, what action was taken, and why this course of action was chosen. The nurse evaluates how the client is responding in the situation and then takes the opportunity to adjust the interventions based on that assessment. During reflection in action the problem is restructured and approached differently. This enables the nurse to reshape what they are doing while doing it.

Reflection on action occurs after the experience has taken place. The nurse looks back on experiences to analyze learning that occurred in light of the client outcomes. It means recalling the client's response and the evidence of client learning. It means assessing the client's satisfaction with the interaction. The act of reflecting on action enables the nurse to spend time exploring why they personally acted in a certain way and what was happening. In so doing, the nurse engages in self-questioning and considers ideas about how activities and practices could be done differently. Reflection on action may involve colleagues who observe, engage in critical conversations, and help the nurse become aware of aspects of practice they have not thought about. **Table 2-1** summarizes reflective practice questions.

Other Ways of Thinking

Other ways of thinking include fantasy and reverie. Fantasy is the free play of creative imagination in the realm of the wild, visionary, or fancy (*The Merriam-Webster Dictionary*, 2016). It is a mental image, a capricious or whimsical idea or notion, a dramatic fiction characterized by highly fanciful or supernatural elements. Fantasy is useful in mentally working through difficult situations. For example, suppose you want to devote more time to teaching clients and anticipate that your supervisor will resist this idea. Fantasizing the supervisor's arguments helps you prepare to counter them.

Reverie, a synonym for daydream, is similar to fantasy and means dreamy thinking, imagining, or being lost in thought (*The Merriam-Webster Dictionary*, 2016). In general, reverie has a more meandering, less vivid quality to it than fantasy. An example of reverie occurs when a lecture is boring and learners' minds wander to something more engaging, like what they did last night or what they will do tonight. Fantasy, however, is more directed—for example, helping a client in labor to relax during contractions by focusing her mind on warm, soothing waves of water rushing over her body.

Reflecting on Your Thinking

Nurses are encouraged to become aware of their point of view and thinking processes. Thinking about thinking is called metacognition (Ruggiero, 2012). Nurses enhance their effectiveness when they reflect on the results of their thinking and decisions. For example, was a decision effective? Was there sufficient information on which to base good decisions? Were the inferences accurate? What were the underlying assumptions, and how did they affect problem solving? What influence did beliefs and values have on how the problem was framed and approached? Were the generalizations justified? When nurses internalize critical thinking skills, they are more effective in helping clients think more clearly.

How nurses think and go about their professional responsibilities are important insights. Although thinking per se is difficult to define, nurses will become skilled thinkers and increase their efficiency if they monitor their thought patterns. It is important to develop clear, analytic thinking habits. As nurses verbalize and critique their thoughts and practice clear thinking, they will develop confidence in their critical thinking skills (Miller & Babcock, 1996).

Promoting Thinking in Clients

The Miller–Stoeckel Client Education Model promotes thinking as an integral component of the teaching and learning process in the nurse–client relationship. Before nurses can promote critical thinking in clients, they need to be good listeners. Nurses in the educator role should listen to what clients say they want to learn. Frequently, clients know what they need to learn and will verbalize it if they think the nurse is interested. Listen to how clients view their illness, what they think caused their health problem, and what home remedies they have taken to treat it. This will give you multiple clues for situation-appropriate health education. If the clients are team members, listen to what they already know and want to learn, then make client education plans accordingly.

Just as important as listening is respecting clients and colleagues. Showing respect is fundamental for promoting critical thinking skills. Seeing life from the perspective of the other person creates a safe environment for that person to experiment with new thoughts and behaviors. As nurses go about their responsibilities, they serve as role models for critical thinking.

When assisting others in their thinking processes, nurses should note the client's frame of mind and readiness to entertain additional information and develop new insights. Remember that as an educator, nurses cannot completely change a client's thinking framework. Nurses can, however, promote small, incremental growth and expand clients' perceptions of their circumstances and options, and they can facilitate problem solving.

When clients share insightful information or engage in critical thinking, nurses should reinforce that behavior. Praise clients for their thinking processes and the decisions they make, when appropriate. Reinforce clients even when they question your procedure or teaching. Responses such as "I am glad you asked," "Let me think; that's a complex question," and "That is a good point" are ways to reinforce thinking.

When conversing with clients, it may be helpful to mirror their attitudes, rationalizations, and habitual ways of thinking and behaving. As you reflect your observations back to them, monitor their responses. Ask yourself how your comments are being received. Are your comments accepted or annoying clients? If you encounter resistance, stop your intervention and assess what is happening.

Nurses should ask questions as they teach. As clients answer, it tells you if your comments are understood. It also provides opportunities to stimulate thinking. For example, ask "If that is so, then how do you feel about . . .?" or "Will you explain . . .?" Another fruitful line of questioning that helps clients anticipate consequences is "What will you do if . . .?"

When teaching stress management, pain control, weight reduction, blood pressure control, and management of other stress-related diseases, make good use of the imaginative forms of thinking: fantasy and reverie. Nurses who specialize in counseling and psychotherapy make use of these strategies. A nurse used fantasy to help a client who was under stress to relax. The client found the sounds of surf soothing, so the nurse used this image and said, "Picture the waves of the ocean rolling over you. Flow with the waves. Listen to the surf. Smell the salty air. Feel the warm mist on your skin."

Role playing is based on recall and fantasy. It is an excellent diagnostic tool for discovering the client's way of thinking and approaching interpersonal problems. Role playing is also helpful to the client who is learning to be more assertive. When used by the nurse psychotherapist, role playing may take on more intensity, such as that encountered in gestalt exercises, sociodrama, and psychodrama.

The Socratic method uses creative questioning to enhance critical thinking skills. In Socratic teaching, the focus is on asking questions, not giving answers. Nurses model what it means to have an inquiring mind by continually exploring a subject by asking questions. Socrates described a true teacher as one who is the midwife to another person's discovery of truth. Socratic learning is joining in discussions with others, asking questions, thinking and reasoning clearly, and discovering answers (Paul, 1995). Questions elicit new ideas and make connections with previous knowledge and experiences. Questions expose the truth and bring unconscious beliefs to the surface of self-awareness.

Styles of Thinking and Learning

Learning styles refer to how individuals prefer to process information and learn. Styles develop from life experiences in the family, at school, and at work and result in preferred ways to learn. Consider how you learn best. Is it by reading a book, creating a mental image, watching a video, or hearing an explanation? Is it by working alone on a project or with a study group? Is it in a quiet environment or with music in the background?

While learning styles have been popular guides for teachers in education circles for many years, some question the validity of the research designs supporting the various learning styles.

They point out that the concept of learning styles was embraced before sufficient research was conducted. Regardless, knowing about and attending to clients' learning preferences (styles) will enhance the effectiveness of your teaching.

In this section, we examine ways that thinking and learning styles are conceptualized. Styles are unique to each person and should be taken into consideration when providing health education. Keep in mind that one style is not better than another; styles are simply characteristics that individuals bring to the situation. Also keep in mind that individuals may change their style preference depending on the demands of the learning situation. They are not confined to only one style. The nature of the material will also lend itself to a particular learning style. For example, teaching self-injection of insulin is best taught with a syringe, sponge, and vial rather than through lecture alone. It will also be affected by the learner's past experiences, cultural background, and physical abilities.

Sternberg's Thinking Styles

Robert J. Sternberg (1997) distinguished between thinking ability and thinking style. Style refers to how an individual uses the abilities they possess. Sternberg draws an analogy between how individuals think, which he called mental self-government and civil government. He uses the descriptive terms of the latter to describe his model of thinking styles. For example, *legislative individuals* are creative and prefer to decide for themselves what they will do and how they will do it. They like problems that are not already structured and prefer to create the framework themselves. They prefer to solve problems, apply rules to problems, apply lessons based on other people's work, and enforce rules. They tend to be nonconforming individuals.

Executive individuals like problems that have some structure so they can address problems within that structural framework. They like guidelines and prefer to follow directions. These individuals are usually successful as students and employees because they do as they are told and like being evaluated on that basis.

Judicial individuals like to oversee, analyze, and evaluate existing rules, procedures, and ideas. They like to critique, give opinions, and judge people and their work. These individuals prefer positions in which they can evaluate the effectiveness of programs, tasks, and human endeavors.

Sternberg distinguishes between global versus local individuals. Global thinkers see the forest rather than the trees; that is, they prefer to deal with relatively large and abstract issues, whereas local thinkers are more pragmatic, preferring to focus on details. Sternberg also distinguishes between the thinking of internal individuals, who tend to be introverted, task oriented, and prefer to work alone, and external individuals, who tend to be extroverted, outgoing, and people oriented. Individuals have a profile of thinking styles and may use more than one.

Witkin and Goodenough's Cognitive-Style Dimensions

Field preference is another way to conceptualize how individuals learn and process information. Developed by Herman Witkin and Donald Goodenough, it is a bipolar continuum with traits of field dependence and independence at opposite ends. Field refers to how individuals perceive their surroundings. It is important to view field dependence and independence as relative dimensions, not fixed ones. Although individuals favor a particular cognitive style, no one is exclusively one way or the other. The cognitive style dimensions are value neutral; each has qualities that are adaptive in particular circumstances (Witkin & Goodenough, 1981). Knowledge of these dimensions is useful for nurses as educators in planning health education activities.

Field-dependent and field-independent individuals have different perceptual and intellectual qualities (Cassidy, 2004; Claxton & Murrell, 1987; Garity, 1985; Noble, Miller, & Heckman, 2008; Witkin & Goodenough, 1981). Individuals who are relatively *field dependent* rely on an external frame of reference rather than imposing their own. They see the whole situation and its context rather than focusing on the smaller aspects. They are sensitive to their surroundings and open to external sources of information. They show more social behaviors, which contribute to effective interpersonal relationships. They pay attention to social cues in the environment by look-ing at others' faces and listening to verbal messages to sense what others are thinking and feeling.

In a learning situation, field-dependent learners prefer the spectator role and are influenced by authority figures. They like structure, guidance, and clearly defined learning goals provided by the educator. They are motivated by extrinsic rewards rather than intrinsic ones. They enjoy inter-action with other learners and prefer to cooperate and collaborate. They are sensitive to criticism; when they talk they refer more to others and less to themselves. They are holistic in their approach to problem solving but are often unable to see the smaller components of larger problems, thereby making them less efficient.

Individuals who are relatively *field independent* are more autonomous and have a strong sense of self and differentiation from others. By having an internal frame of reference, they grasp the whole situation and its component parts. They are self-reliant, intrinsically motivated, and have their own learning goals. They are less sensitive to the social environment and less inclined to conform to group pressure.

In a learning situation, field-independent learners prefer to structure their own learning and study strategies. They are analytic, interested in abstract and theoretical concepts, and question opinions, ideas, and hypotheses. In learning situations, they are able impose their own structure. They are less affected by criticism and make more I statements. They tend to be better at problem solving. **Table 2-2** summarizes these characteristics.

Kolb's Experiential Learning Model: Learning Cycle and Styles

Many educators believe that education, work, and personal development are closely linked in a process of learning called experiential learning. They believe that learning is an ongoing, con-tinuous process that occurs as individuals adapt to their social and physical environment. The emphasis of experiential learning is on the learning process itself, rather than on the behavioral outcomes; it is grounded in experiences as the individual adapts to the world (Kolb, 1984).

Based on this philosophy, David Kolb (1981, 1984) proposed an experiential learning model that has a four-stage cycle with four adaptive learning modes: *concrete experience*, *reflective observation*, *abstract conceptualization*, and *active experimentation* (**Figure 2-4**).

The experiential learning model describes the learning cycle—that is, how experience trans-lates into concepts that guide the choice of new experiences. Entry into the cycle begins with concrete experience (CE) followed by reflection and observation (RO). The third stage is abstract conceptualization (AC), which becomes the basis for ideas and theories that guide future behav-ior. In the fourth stage, active experimentation (AE), the individual tests the implications of new concepts and theories in different and more complex situations. By experimenting and applying new learning, individuals again engage in CEs, and so the cycle continues. As the knowledge base expands, the learning experiences become increasingly complex. Based on heredity, past experi-ences, and the demands of the present environment, individuals develop a unique, preferred style of learning. Based on his learning cycle, Kolb (1981) identified four learning styles: **converger**,

Table 2-2 Field Preference Characteristics

Field-Dependent Individuals	Field-Independent Individuals
External frame of reference	Internal frame of reference
See the whole situation	See both whole and parts of a situation
Sensitive to surroundings	Less sensitive to surroundings
Open to external sources of information	Strong sense of autonomy
Social and people oriented	Impersonal orientation to others
Attend to social cues	Less sensitive to social environment
Prefer the spectator role	Prefer active learner role; self-reliant
Influenced by authority figures	Analytic, test opinions and ideas
Prefer structure and guidance	Enjoy abstract and theoretical concepts
Prefer clear learning objectives	Set own learning goals
Motivated by extrinsic rewards	Structure own learning
Prefer group work and discussions	Intrinsically motivated
Sensitive to criticism	Less sensitive to criticism

Figure 2-4 The Experiential Learning Model

Data from Friere, P. (1970). *Pedagogy of the oppressed.* New York, NY: Continuum; Kolb, D. (1984). *Experiential learning: Experience as the source of learning and development.* Englewood Cliffs, NJ: Prentice-Hall.

which combines AC and AE; **diverger**, which combines CE and RO; **assimilator**, which combines AC and RO; and **accommodator**, which combines CE and AE. Their strengths are shown in **Table 2-3**.

Teaching strategies can be employed that are suitable for the different learning modes (Burris, Kitchel, Molina, Vincent, & Warner, 2008). For example, clients who favor CE benefit from small-group discussion, specific examples, practical exercises, and role playing. Clients who favor RO benefit from creative problem solving, personal journals, discussion groups, and thought

Table 2-3 Kolb's Learning Styles

Learning Style	Strength
Converger (AC and AE)	■ Applies practical application of ideas ■ Focuses on specific problems ■ Is relatively unemotional ■ Prefers dealing with things rather than people ■ Has a tendency to narrow interests ■ Specializes in physical sciences
Diverger (CE and RO)	■ Has good imaginative ability, generates ideas ■ Sees multiple perspectives ■ Is interested in people; emotional ■ Has broad cultural interests ■ Specializes in the arts and humanities
Assimilator (AC and RO)	■ Creates theoretical models ■ Reasons inductively, logically sound theories ■ Is interested in abstract concepts ■ Has less interest in people ■ Focuses less on practical use of theories ■ Specializes in basic sciences and math
Accommodators (CE and AE)	■ Likes to do things (plans, experiments, new experiences); willing to take risks ■ Adapts well to specific immediate circumstances ■ Solves problems intuitively, trial and error ■ Relies on others for information rather than self ■ Likes people; sometimes impatient ■ Specializes in technical or practical fields, such as business

Data from Kolb, D. A. (1981). Learning styles and disciplinary differences. In A. W. Chickering & Associates (Eds.), *The modern American college* (pp. 232–255). San Francisco, CA: Jossey-Bass; Kolb, D. A. (1984). *Experiential learning*. Englewood Cliffs, NJ: Prentice Hall.

questions. Clients who favor AC benefit from hearing lectures, analogies, and questioning. Clients who favor AE benefit from case studies, projects, and psychomotor activities.

Gardner's Multiple Intelligences

The study of intelligence originated when the French government commissioned Alfred Binet to develop a measure of intelligence. In 1904, Binet produced the first measure that assessed a broad range of skills and performances. The findings were reduced to a single score, called the intelligence quotient or IQ (Slavin, 2015). IQ testing of school children was widely adopted in the United States. It is often used as a tool to place students in ability groups or tracks in the educational system.

Howard Gardner, professor of cognition and education at Harvard Graduate School of Education, is critical of quantifying actual or potential intelligence by using a single number expressed as the IQ score. In the early 1980s, Gardner began looking for other ways to measure intelligence and developed the theory of multiple intelligences (Gardner, 1983). He has a pluralistic view of intelligence and believes that all humans possess these intelligences in varying degrees, with several of them working together. Where people differ is in the degree to which they possess the intelligences and the unique combinations in which they appear in each individual (Gardner, 2011).

Gardner defined intelligence as a biopsychological potential "to process certain kinds of information in certain kinds of ways" (2006, p. 64) and "the ability to solve problems, or to fashion products, that are valued in one or more cultural or community settings" (1993, p. 7). The phrase *fashion products* includes things such as writing a symphony, creating a painting, staging a play, building up and managing an organization, and carrying out an experiment.

Gardner's theory of multiple intelligences (2011), also called frames of mind, includes six autonomous intellectual competencies or strengths. He has attempted to capture those intelligences valued by human cultures and states that his list is neither fixed nor exhaustive. The intelligences are relatively independent of one another but are combined in a variety of ways by different individuals and cultures. Each type of intelligence is important and has equal status with the others. Because these intelligences are pertinent to health education, they are described here. The first two are highly valued in Western societies (*linguistic* and *logical mathematical*) because much academic testing and employment is based on verbal and mathematical skill. The next two intelligences are associated with the arts (*spatial* and *musical*). The next intelligence, *bodily kinesthetic*, involves psychomotor skills and physical movement. The last intelligence (*personal*) combines two aspects: intrapersonal and interpersonal.

In most individuals, the intelligences work together to solve problems. Most professions and vocations involve several intelligences working together to be successful. Most individuals possess several intelligences, although they may be able to process information better in one area than another. In terms of health education, a person may have difficulty learning in one area but be successful in another, so it is reasonable to try a variety of teaching strategies to help clients grasp the health information. A discussion of Gardner's (2011) multiple intelligences is provided in the following sections.

Linguistic Intelligence

People with this intelligence are sensitive to sounds, rhythms, and meanings of words, and they have a facility with words. They are interested in language and are sensitive to its different functions. They like to read, write, and tell stories. Linguistic intelligence is universal and constant across cultures. Poets, orators, and journalists possess this intelligence.

Logical Mathematical Intelligence

People with this intelligence have the ability to discern logical or numerical patterns and are skilled at handling long chains of reasoning. These people have a passion for abstraction and ideas that are characteristic of scientific thinking. In gifted individuals, the process of problem solving is often rapid, and frequently a solution is found before it is articulated. Mathematicians and scientists possess this intelligence.

Spatial Intelligence

People with this intelligence rely on the sense of sight, whereas people with visual impairments rely on tactile ability to achieve spatial understanding. These individuals have the ability to see things accurately in their environment. They are also able to create mental images, visualize objects, and re-create past visual experiences at will. They like to design and create things. Sculptors, architects, navigators, inventors, and land surveyors possess this intelligence.

Musical Intelligence

People with this intelligence can produce and appreciate rhythm, pitch, timbre, and the many forms of musical expression. Music is integral to life. This intelligence emerges earliest in life. Composers and musical artists possess this intelligence.

Bodily Kinesthetic Intelligence

People with this intelligence have the ability to control their bodily movements to express an emotion (dancer), play a game (athlete), or create a new product (inventor). They like physical activities and have the ability to skillfully use body cues and motions for expression, handling objects, and achieving goal-directed purposes. Athletes, actors, craftspeople, and surgeons possess this intelligence.

Personal Intelligences

This intelligence has two aspects: It looks inward toward the self (intrapersonal), and it looks outward to the relationship with others (interpersonal). Neither aspect can develop without the other, nor are they characterized by the culture in which they develop. Intrapersonal intelligence involves knowing one's self and one's feelings and emotions. It is awareness of how this knowledge guides one's behavior. It is looking inward to the self. People with this intelligence focus inwardly on their feelings, talents, interests, and so forth. They are able to discriminate among their emotions, label them, and use them to understand and guide their behavior. It is the most private intelligence. They like to work alone and follow their interests. Persons with in-depth self-knowledge possess this intelligence.

Interpersonal intelligence involves one's relationship to others—one's interactions with family, colleagues, and community. It is the ability to observe the behavior of others in terms of their moods, feelings, motivations, and intentions. It is looking outward from the self. People with this intelligence have the ability to understand others through social interactions. They notice differences in moods, motivations, and intentions. This allows them to understand and work with others. They have many friends and like to talk to others. Helping professionals (nurses, doctors, therapists) and gifted salespersons possess this intelligence.

Multiple intelligences theory is a challenging view of learning because of the many ways that intelligence is expressed in different individuals. People learn differently and cannot be so easily assigned or confined to categories. **Table 2-4** offers some suggestions for how nurses as educators can work with clients who appear to fit this theory. To determine what kind of learners clients are, ask them how they best learn.

Sensory-Based Learning Styles

A common model for assessing learning styles is based on sensory input, such as auditory, visual, kinesthetic, and tactile. Visual learners prefer to see what needs to be learned in terms of pictures, movies, models, diagrams, and watching demonstrations. Auditory learners prefer to hear explanations from an instructor or from audio books and Kindle books/tablets. Kinesthetic and tactile learners prefer physical involvement as a way to learn. This can be physical activity and movement, such as learning new exercises and proper body mechanics. It can also include hands-on activities, such as learning how to bathe a newborn or change a dressing. The final style

Table 2-4 Multiple Intelligence and Teaching Strategies

Intelligence Type	Learns By	Teaching Strategies
Linguistics	Reading, writing, talking	Use handouts, pamphlets; encourage client to verbalize or write about experiences; encourage client to keep a journal if appropriate; discussion
Logical mathematical	Reasoning, computing, problem solving	Use case examples; ask questions; identify problems to solve ("how would you handle . . ."); encourage critical thinking in pondering solutions
Spatial	Forming mental images	Draw pictures, especially helpful with children; mind mapping, visualizations are helpful
Musical	Listening to music	Background music; comfortable learning environment; use rhythm or songs to aid memorization
Bodily kinesthetic	Touching, moving	Handle and manipulate equipment; develop skills
Personal	Sharing with others	Interpersonal individuals form groups to discuss common health problems or develop projects; group activities
	Working alone	Intrapersonal individuals use programmed instructional software; computer-assisted instruction; self-paced learning; individual learning projects

Data from Holland, F. (2007). Bringing the body to life: Using multiple intelligence theory in the classroom. *SportEX Dynamics, 14*, 6–8; Miller, M. A., & Babcock, D. E. (1996). *Critical thinking applied to nursing.* St. Louis, MO: Mosby.

is multisensory learners, who learn in all of these ways—for example, videos, slide shows with audio, and active participation in demonstrations. In reality, learning is rarely confined to one sensory mode. Individuals learn through all their senses even though they may favor one particular style over another (Reid, 1987; Vaseghi, Ramezani, & Gholami, 2012).

Implications for Health Education

How does knowing about thinking and learning styles and models help nurses as educators? It is not possible to give clients a battery of tests to determine thinking and learning styles, so talk with clients and get a sense of how they learn. For example, do they become informed by reading, watching videos, talking with a professional, taking classes, or observing others performing (Chang & Kelly, 2007)? Ask if they have hobbies and what they enjoy doing in their spare time to gather clues to their thinking and learning styles. As you work with clients, be especially observant to note what is and is not effective in helping them learn. In working with clients in a nurse-managed center, Kessler and Alverson (2003) found that 82% of clients surveyed preferred hands-on instruction, 63% preferred reading, and 59% preferred listening.

Nurses also have a preferred style of thinking and learning and tend to teach in ways that are consistent with these. Being aware of this adds to teaching effectiveness. Rassool and Rawaf (2007) found that undergraduate nursing students preferred the reflector learning style. Noble and colleagues (2008) found that nursing students were more field dependent than students in other health-related disciplines. D'Amore, James, and Mitchell (2012) found that first-year nursing students preferred Kolb's diverger and assimilating learning styles. When the clients' thinking and learning styles fit with the learning setting, the task at hand, and the teacher's preferred style, clients thrive. When clients' thinking and learning styles do not fit with these factors, clients may have difficulty grasping the health message (Dunn, 1983; Sternberg, 1997). Clients are best served by having abundant reading materials (books and pamphlets), pictures, videos, interactive instructional materials, demonstrations, and resource persons available. Many choices allow clients to select among the learning options that best suit their own thinking and learning styles because no single option is best for everyone (Moran, Kornhaber, & Gardner, 2006).

Summary

This chapter introduced thinking and learning processes that undergird the nurse–client relationship of the Miller–Stoeckel Client Education Model. It stressed how that knowledge increases the effectiveness of nurses as educators in working with clients. The three domains of learning—cognitive, affective, and psychomotor—provide a framework for developing learning objectives. The cognitive domain involves intellectual activities, the affective domain deals with attitudes and values, and the psychomotor domain involves learning motor skills. Thinking underlies these domains, and a summary of ways of thinking was discussed. In addition to nursing process and clinical judgment, these ways include problem solving, critical thinking, creative thinking, intuition, reflection, fantasy, and reverie. It is important to understand your own thinking and how to promote thinking in clients.

This chapter also examined several styles and models of thinking and learning, including Sternberg's thinking styles, Witkin and Goodenough's Cognitive-Style Dimensions, Kolb's Experiential Learning Model, Gardner's Multiple Intelligences, and the sensory-based learning style. Each view of learning provides insight into the nurse–client relationship and how nurses as educators can best promote learning.

Exercises

Exercise I: Learning Domains

Purpose: Distinguish among cognitive, affective, and psychomotor learning domains.
Directions: Working alone, examine the learning objectives for the course you are taking. Place each objective into one of the learning domains. Then form small groups and compare your answers. Was each learning objective categorized correctly?

Exercise II: Affective Domain

Purpose: Examine the affective domain in teaching and learning.
Directions: Reflect on a client situation in which the client's point of view, attitudes, and beliefs were different from your own. Journal about the following questions:

1. What was the difference between your point of view, attitudes, and beliefs and those of the client?

2. Did the difference affect how you felt about the client?
3. How did you respond to the client when you became aware of the differences?
4. Do you think the client was aware that your point of view, attitudes, and beliefs differed from theirs?
5. What effect did it have on the care you delivered?

Exercise III: Thinking

Purpose: Examine the various factors that influence your thinking.
Directions: Divide into small groups and discuss the following:

1. Identify factors that influence your present thinking. Consider your parents, siblings, close friends, schools attended, religion, music, and the media.
2. Under what circumstances do you do your best thinking? Consider factors such as noise level, time of day, and activity you may be engaged in, such as driving, gardening, sports, or watching TV. Why is this so?

Exercise IV: Ways of Thinking

Purpose: Examine the ways of thinking presented in this chapter.
Directions: Divide into small groups and discuss the following:

1. Share examples of how you have used these ways of thinking: problem solving, critical thinking, creative thinking, intuition, reflection, fantasy, and reverie.
2. Share examples of observing these ways of thinking in others (classmates and clients).
3. Identify ways you can stimulate thinking with your clients.

Exercise V: Critical Thinking

Purpose: Examine the impact of different frames of reference.
Directions: Divide into groups of four or five. Discuss the following situation and answer the questions. Then rejoin the larger group and compare your group's answers with the answers of other groups. How were your answers alike? Different? Discuss why the differences occurred.

A 23-year-old woman had given birth to her second child and subsequently experienced kidney failure. On her 5th day of peritoneal dialysis, the client asked the nurse what the doctors left in her body that they were trying to wash out. She understood neither what the treatment was nor why it was necessary. Had she not asked the question, her misperceptions would never have been known. Pretend you are the nurse in this situation and answer the following questions:

1. Restate the problem from the client's perspective and from the nurse's perspective.
2. How is the nurse's frame of reference different from the client's?
3. What is the significance of this situation?
4. What is the nurse's goal in this situation? What is the nurse trying to achieve?
5. What assumptions has the client made? What assumptions has the nurse made?
6. What evidence does the client have? What evidence does the nurse have?
7. How has the client interpreted the evidence? How has the nurse interpreted the evidence?
8. What inference, or inferences, did the nurse make?
9. What value judgments did the nurse make?
10. What are the implications of this situation for the client? What are the implications of this situation for the nurse?

Exercise VI: Creative Thinking

Purpose: Conceptualize your creative thinking.
Directions: Divide into small groups and have each participant draw a picture of how they think.

1. Is your thinking scattered and free associating? Is your thinking goal directed and focused? Do ideas pop into your thinking when you are thinking about something else?
2. Compare your drawings with those of your group members. How similar and how different are they?
3. How did this exercise help you understand your thinking? Did it give you insight into how others think?

Exercise VII: Creative Thinking

Purpose: Generate creative solutions that are both novel and appropriate to the situation.
Directions: Divide into small groups of three to four. Have each participant describe a recent clinical situation with a client that required problem solving. Before stating how each problem was solved, have each group member describe how they would have handled the problem. Finally, share how the participant solved it. Discuss the following:

1. How were the solutions alike? How were the solutions different?
2. Which solution was the most novel?
3. Were the solutions appropriate (useful)? Were some more appropriate (useful) than others?

Exercise VIII: Intuition

Purpose: Examine intuition in teaching and learning.
Directions: A client was due to be discharged and needed instruction on how to change a dressing. When the nurse talked with the client, the client was distracted and busy collecting her possessions for discharge. The nurse had a hunch that the client was concerned about something else rather than learning how to change a dressing. How would you handle this situation? What is the appropriate use of intuition in this situation? Is there a difference between how you and others in your class would handle this situation?

Exercise IX: Learning Style

Purpose: Reflect on your partner's learning style in class.
Directions: Divide into groups of two and ask each other the following questions:

1. When you want to learn something, how do you go about it? Consider visual (movies, pictures, videos, TV), auditory (lectures, discussions, DVDs, audio books), kinesthetic and tactile (hands-on, demonstrations, games, trips, experiments), and multisensory modalities.
2. Under what circumstance do you learn best (group, individual, structured, unstructured)?
3. What environmental conditions help or hinder your learning (quiet, music, lighting, study area, snacks)?
4. What kinds of information are easiest and most difficult for you to learn?
5. Which of the thinking and learning styles in this chapter apply to your responses?

References

Benner, P. (1984). *From novice to expert*. Menlo Park, NY: Addison-Wesley.

Bloom, B. S., Engelhart, M. D., Furst, E. J., Hill, W. H., & Krathwohl, D. R. (Eds.). (1956). *Taxonomy of educational objectives: The classification of educational goals. Handbook I: Cognitive domain*. New York, NY: David McKay.

Brookfield, S. D. (2012). *Teaching for critical thinking: Tools and techniques to help students question their assumptions*. San Francisco, CA: Jossey-Bass.

Browne, M. N., & Keeley, S. M. (2012). *Asking the right questions: A guide to critical thinking* (10th ed.). Upper Saddle River, NJ: Prentice Hall.

Burris, S., Kitchel, T., Molina, Q., Vincent, S., & Warner, W. (2008). *The language of learning styles* (Research report). Alexandria, VA: Association for Career and Technical Education.

Cassidy, S. (2004). Learning styles: An overview of theories, models, and measures. *Educational Psychology*, 24(4), 419–444.

Chan, Z. C. Y. (2013). A systematic review of critical thinking in nursing education. *Nurse Education Today*, 33(3), 236–240.

Chang, M., & Kelly, A. E. (2007). Patient education: Addressing cultural diversity and health literacy issues. *Urological Nursing*, 27(5), 411–417.

Claxton, C. S., & Murrell, P. H. (1987). *Learning styles: Implications for improving educational practices* (ASHE-ERIC Higher Education Report No. 4). Washington, DC: Association for the Study of Higher Education.

D'Amore, A., James, S., & Mitchell, E. K. L. (2012). Learning styles of first-year undergraduate nursing and midwifery students: A cross-sectional survey utilising the Kolb Learning Style Inventory. *Nursing Education Today*, 32(5), 506–515.

Dunn, R. (1983). Can students identify their own learning styles? *Educational Leadership*, 40(5), 60–62.

Faugier, J. (2005). Basic instincts. *Nursing Standard*, 19(24), 14–15.

Gardner, H. (1983). *Frames of mind*. New York, NY: Basic Books.

Gardner, H. (1993). *Multiple intelligences: The theory in practice*. New York, NY: Basic Books.

Gardner, H. (2006). *Multiple intelligences: New horizons*. New York, NY: Basic Books.

Gardner, H. (2011). *Frames of mind: The theory of multiple intelligences*. New York, NY: Basic Books.

Garity, J. (1985). Learning styles basis for creative teaching and learning. *Nurse Educator*, 10(2), 12–16.

Goulet, C., & Owen-Smith, P. (2005). Cognitive-affective learning in physical therapy education: From implicit to explicit. *Journal of Physical Therapy Education*, 19(3), 67–72.

Halpern, D. F. (2014). *Thought and knowledge: An introduction to critical thinking* (5th ed.). New York, NY: Psychology Press.

Hodgkinson, G. P., Langan-Fox, J., & Sadler-Smith, E. (2008). Intuition: A fundamental bridging construct in the behavioural sciences. *British Journal of Psychology*, 99, 1–27.

Holland, C. & Ulrich, D. (2016). Critical thinking cards: An innovative teaching strategy to bridge classroom knowledge with clinical decision making. *Teaching and Learning in Nursing*, 11(3), 108–112.

Holland, F. (2007). Bringing the body to life: Using multiple intelligence theory in the classroom. *SportEX Dynamics*, 14, 6–8.

Kaddoura, M. (2013). New graduate nurses' perceived definition of critical thinking during their first nursing experience. *Educational Research Quarterly*, 36(3), 3–21.

Kessler, T. A., & Alverson, E. (2003). Health concerns and learning styles of underserved and uninsured clients at a nurse managed center. *Journal of Community Health Nursing*, 20(2), 81–92.

Kolb, D. A. (1981). Learning styles and disciplinary differences. In A. W. Chickering & Associates (Eds.), *The modern American college* (pp. 232–255). San Francisco, CA: Jossey-Bass.

Kolb, D. A. (1984). *Experiential learning*. Englewood Cliffs, NJ: Prentice Hall.

Krathwohl, D. R., Bloom, B. S., & Masia, B. B. (1964). *Taxonomy of educational objectives: The classification of educational goals. Handbook II: Affective domain*. New York, NY: David McKay.

Kretchmar, J. (2008). *The affective domain. EBSCO research starters*. Ipswich, MA: EBSCO.

Marzano, R. J., & Kendall, J. S. (2007). *The new taxonomy of educational objectives* (2nd ed.). Thousand Oaks, CA: Corwin Press.

McPeck, J. (1990). *Teaching critical thinking*. New York, NY: Routledge.

Miller, M. A., & Babcock, D. E. (1996). *Critical thinking applied to nursing*. St. Louis, MO: Mosby.

Moran, S., Kornhaber, M., & Gardner, H. (2006). Orchestrating multiple intelligences. *Educational Leadership*, 64(1), 22–29.

Noble, K. A., Miller, S. M., & Heckman, J. (2008). The cognitive style of nursing students: Educational implications for teaching and learning. *Journal of Nursing Education*, 47(6), 245–253.

Paul, R. (1995). *Critical thinking: What every person needs to survive in a rapidly changing world*. Rohnert Park, CA: Foundation for Critical Thinking.

Rassool, G. H., & Rawaf, S. (2007). Learning style preferences of undergraduate nursing students. *Nursing Standard*, *21*(32), 35–41.

Reid, M. J. (1987). The learning style preferences of ESL students. *TESO Quarterly*, *21*(1), 87–111.

Ruggiero, V. R. (2012). *The art of thinking* (10th ed.). New York, NY: Pearson Education.

Ruth-Sahd, L., & Hendy, H. M. (2005). Predictors of novice nurses' use of intuition to guide patient care decisions. *Journal of Nursing Education*, *44*(10), 450–458.

Santrock, J. W. (2023). *A topical approach to life-span development* (11th ed.). New York, NY: McGraw-Hill LLC.

Saylor, C. R. (1990). Reflection and professional education: Art, science, and competency. *Nurse Educator*, *15*(2), 8–11.

Scheffer, B. K., & Rubenfeld, M. G. (2000). A consensus statement on critical thinking in nursing. *Journal of Nursing Education*, *39*(8), 352–359.

Slavin, R. E. (2015). *Educational psychology theory and practice* (11th ed.). Boston, MA: Pearson Education, Inc.

Sternberg, R. J. (1997). *Thinking styles*. Cambridge, United Kingdom: Cambridge University Press.

Tanner, C. A. (2006). Thinking like a nurse: A research-based model of clinical judgment in nursing. *Journal of Nursing Education*, *45*(6), 204–211.

The Merriam-Webster Dictionary (7th ed.). (2016). Springfield, MA: Merriam-Webster, Inc.

Vaseghi, R., Ramezani, A. F., & Gholami, R. (2012). Language learning style preferences: A theoretical and empirical study. *Advances in Asian Social Science*, *2*(2), 441–451.

Victor-Chmil, J. (2013). Critical thinking versus clinical reasoning versus clinical judgment: Differential diagnosis. *Nurse Educator*, *39*(1), 34–36.

Wallace, D. & Moughrabi, W. (2015). The efficacy of simulation debriefing in developing critical thinking in accelerated baccalaureate nursing students. *Journal of Nursing Education and Practice*, *6*(5), 13–18.

Watson, G., & Glaser, E. M. (1980). *Watson-Glaser critical thinking appraisal manual*. New York, NY: Harcourt Brace Jovanovich.

Whiffin, C. J., & Hasselder, A. (2013). Making the link between critical appraisal, thinking and analysis. *British Journal of Nursing*, *22*(14), 831–834.

Witkin, H. A., & Goodenough, D. R. (1981). *Cognitive styles: Essence and origins*. New York, NY: International Universities Press.

CHAPTER 3

Theories and Principles of Learning

OBJECTIVES

Upon completion of this chapter, you will be able to do the following:

- Apply the following learning theories to selected teaching–learning situations: behaviorism (stimulus–response and operant conditioning), cognitivism (gestalt, constructivism, and information processing), and social cognitive theory.
- Apply principles of learning in selected client education situations.
- Describe how theories and principles of learning enhance the teaching and learning process in the nurse–client relationship.

CHAPTER OUTLINE

Introduction
Value of Theory
Theories of Learning
Behavioral Views of Learning
- Stimulus-Response
- Operant Conditioning
- Propositions of Behavioral Theory
- Implications for Health Education
Cognitive Views of Learning
- Gestalt View of Learning
- Implications for Health Education
- Constructivism View of Learning
- Implications for Health Education
- Information Processing View of Learning
- Implications for Health Education
Social Cognitive View of Learning
- Implications for Health Education
Principles of Learning
- Focusing Intensifies Learning
- Repetition Enhances Learning
- Learner Control Increases Learning

- Active Participation Is Necessary for Learning
- Learning Styles Vary
- Organization Promotes Learning
- Association Is Necessary to Learning
- Imitation Is a Method of Learning
- Motivation Strengthens Learning
- Spacing New Material Facilitates Learning
- Recency Influences Retention
- Primacy Affects Retention
- Arousal Influences Attention
- Accurate and Prompt Feedback Enhances Learning
- Application of New Learning in a Variety of Contexts Broadens the Generalization of That Learning
- The Learner's Biologic, Psychologic, Sociologic, and Cultural Realities Shape the Learner's Perception of the Learning Experience
Summary
Exercises
References

Introduction

The teaching and learning process as a component of the nurse–client relationship in the Miller–Stoeckel Client Education Model involves understanding theories and principles of learning and how they enhance client education (**Figure 3-1**). This chapter begins by introducing the value of theory and how theories help us understand observations and experiences. We examine the learning theories of **behaviorism**, **cognitivism**, and **social cognitive theory** and how each conceptualizes how people learn.

For each theory, you will learn how to apply theory and principles to working with clients as learners in a health education context. This knowledge is applied to situations in which nurses are the primary educators and clients are the primary learners.

Value of Theory

Theory is a way to explain some observed phenomenon. Expressed as abstract thoughts or general subject principles, theories help make sense of the world and research findings (*The Merriam-Webster Dictionary*, 2016). Theories provide the framework to view the process of learning, the progress of learners, and nurses' role as educators. Although theories help to understand learning, no single theory explains everything about a subject.

Nurses are often pragmatic and eclectic thinkers. They tend to freely select ideas from diverse sources and conclude that something is good if it works. For example, when you observe something, you try to make sense of it by fitting it into your mental and experiential framework. This is most effective when you know something about what is observed and have had experience with it. When you observe things that are outside your framework—that is, things for which you have neither an explanation nor experience—you become curious and begin to seek answers. Current emphasis on using evidence-based research leads us to look to the current literature for studies that answer questions. This search for answers is the foundation of theory development. Theory helps make sense of what you observe; it is a way to view relationships among observed phenomena. **Box 3-1** identifies how theory is useful.

Theories of Learning

Learning theories provide the theoretical framework to understand how people learn. We want to know how people acquire new knowledge, develop skills, modify attitudes and values, and

Figure 3-1 Nurse–Client Relationship in the Miller–Stoeckel Client Education Model

---

Box 3-1 Reasons for Theories

You need a theory when you:

■ Confront a new situation and what you already know does not apply to that situation
■ Want to increase your understanding of something relatively familiar
■ Face a familiar situation, but what you already know does not work
■ Wish to teach what you know to a colleague or client
■ Question the validity of a cherished belief
■ Explore new hypotheses
■ Observe events for which you can find no explanation

---

learn new behaviors. We know that learning is a dynamic, lifelong process that is unique to each individual.

In the context of health education, knowing about learning theories is a way to understand how people learn. Theory-based teaching is an effective way to organize your thinking and conceptualize what you want to convey to clients and team members. Clients experiencing health problems may need to learn new ways to maintain their health or deal with illness or disability. This is the time when clients are motivated to learn about their changing health status. Team members may also need to learn about new illnesses and new procedures. This need for continuing education falls under the nurse's purview as an educator.

Definitions of learning vary. Common to most definitions is the notion that a change occurs in the learner's *behavior, attitudes,* or *skills* (Merriam, Caffarella, & Baumgartner, 2007). The behavioral change is both observable and relatively permanent (Olson & Hergenhahn, 2013). Broadly speaking, learning theories fall into two camps: behaviorism and cognitivism (Ormrod, 2016). **Behaviorism** focuses on tangible, observable behaviors, such as learning to give an injection, changing dietary practices, and safely bathing an infant. **Cognitivism** focuses on the thought processes as humans learn; for example, seeing a relationship between food intake and blood glucose levels, using memory tricks to recall health instructions, and gaining insight into one's own behavior. Because there are many learning theories within these two camps and different ways to group them, for purposes of this discussion we will look at two theories of behaviorism (*stimulus–response* and *operant conditioning*), three theories of cognitivism (*gestalt, constructivism* and *information processing*), and **social cognitive theory**.

Behavioral Views of Learning

Behavioral learning theories were among the first to be developed and were the first to be used in the U.S. educational system. They continue to be pervasive. Some assumptions that have historically supported behavioral research and theories follow (Ormrod, 2020).

● Humans and animals learn in similar ways; consequently, early researchers studied rats and pigeons and applied that to human learning.
● Studying stimuli and response objectifies the learning processes.
● Internal processes, such as thoughts, motives, and emotions, are unimportant in understanding learning because they are not observable. Later behaviorists stated that motivation and the strength of the stimulus–response associations were important.
● Learning involves changing behavior.

- Organisms are born as blank slates with learning occurring after birth.
- Learning is largely the result of environmental events that condition behavior.
- The most useful theories explain behavior with as few learning principles as possible.

Learning for the behaviorist is focused on an observable change in the learner's behavior and is not concerned with the internal thought processes of the learner. The learner as a research subject is described as an organism rather than a person or human being. Behaviorists believe that the learner's behavior is shaped by elements in the environment that either precede the behavior (stimulus) or the consequences that follow it. These preceding events can precipitate the behavior, and the events that follow can have positive or negative consequences on the behavior. These events must occur closely in time so that a bond is formed, which is called the principle of contiguity (Olson & Hergenhahn, 2013). An example of a preceding event is a nurse approaching a child with a clearly visible syringe, intending to vaccinate him. The sight of the syringe frightens the child, who anticipates pain, starts crying, and clings to his mother for protection. Thereafter, the child may be frightened of syringes until he matures and learns differently. An example of a reinforcing event is a smile and hug from the child's mother that assures him he is safe and well. The child knows he can find solace and protection from his mother and will seek her out in future frightening situations.

Behavioral theories today encompass a number of individual theories and continue to be widely applied in understanding how people learn. We review the stimulus–response theories of Pavlov, Thorndike, and Guthrie, as well as Skinner's operant conditioning.

Stimulus-Response

Stimulus–response theories have their origins in the 19th century with Ivan Pavlov (1849–1936) and Edward Lee Thorndike (1874–1949), who studied how animals and humans learn. Pavlov was a Russian physiologist who is famous for discovering the principle of classical conditioning in his work with a hungry dog. He discovered that when meat powder was placed in a dog's mouth, the dog automatically salivated (unconditioned stimulus). When a bell was sounded simultaneously with the offering of meat powder, the bell (conditioned stimulus) became paired with the dog's salivation. Eventually the bell by itself stimulated the dog to salivate. If the bell was presented often enough without the accompanying meat powder, the dog eventually stopped salivating. This phenomenon was called *extinction*. Pavlov's experiment is commonly known as classical conditioning (Ormrod, 2020).

Thorndike did extensive pioneering research in learning, and his work is considered the first modern theory of learning. He noted that the most characteristic method of learning for both animals and humans was trial and error, also called connectionism or the stimulus–response theory of learning. The organism confronts a problem and selects a response most likely to lead to the goal. Much random behavior occurs until the goal is met. On each successive trial, the random behavior decreases and the goal-directed behavior increases. This forms the basis for the principle of positive reinforcement that Thorndike called the *Law of Effect*. It means that the organism remembers responses that had satisfying effects, which strengthens the connection. If the responses were unsatisfying, the strength of the connection decreases. Thorndike formulated two other laws, the Law of Exercise and the Law of Readiness. The *Law of Exercise* states that repeated use of meaningful connections results in substantial learning, whereas lack of connections inhibits learning. The *Law of Readiness* states that learning is enhanced when the organism is ready for the connection; otherwise, it is inhibited (Olson & Hergenhahn, 2013).

Edwin Ray Guthrie (1886–1959) built on the work of Thorndike and Pavlov. Guthrie felt that the rules they proposed were unnecessarily complicated; he proposed one law of learning, the Law of Contiguity (Olson & Hergenhahn, 2013). He wrote, "A combination of stimuli which has accompanied a movement will on its recurrence tend to be followed by that movement" (Guthrie, 1935, 1952, p. 23). In other words, events that occur together in time tend to be paired. If, for example, a person did something in a given situation, they tend to repeat the action when faced with that situation again. Guthrie proclaimed, as do behaviorists today, that a science of psychology must be based on a study of what is observable: behaviors, bodily changes, or data that can be detected by an observer or a measuring device. All data are admissible except introspection, which can be reported only by the person. Later, Guthrie revised his theory to recognize the many stimuli to which the organism is exposed and that associations cannot be formed with all of them. The organism responds selectively to only a small number of stimuli, and those are the ones that become associated with the response. What captures the organism's attention becomes important along with the association that is formed.

Operant Conditioning

Burrhus Frederic Skinner (1904–1990) is probably the most familiar of the behaviorists in the United States. He is famous for his Skinner box, an experimenter-controlled cage in which the behavior of animals (rats and pigeons) was studied. Skinner acknowledges two kinds of learning. The first is *respondent behavior*, which occurs in response to a known stimulus, such as a knee jerk in response to an examiner's hammer. The second type of learning, which Skinner believes is more important in human behavior, is an *operant response*, which refers to the consequences of behavior. When a response is reinforced, whether random or planned, the behavior tends to be repeated; when the consequences are unpleasant, the behavior tends to be suppressed (Slavin, 2015). This statement is a simple way to explain operant learning. Most human behavior is the result of operant learning, according to Skinner.

Propositions of Behavioral Theory

The propositions of behavioral theory as they are understood today are as follows (Olson & Hergenhahn, 2013; Slavin, 2015):

1. Behavior that is followed by reinforcement tends to strengthen the behavior. After being taught how to transfer from a bed to a chair, a client is given smiles and verbal encouragement from the nurse. Praise reinforces the client's behavior and increases the likelihood of further attempts to transfer.
2. Behavior followed by punishment tends to be suppressed. For example, a young man is compliant with his father's commands because he knows that his father will react negatively to his behavior. The son complies because he has learned that rebellion or questioning will result in punishment.
3. Behavior followed by the removal of a negative stimulus tends to increase in strength. Deep breathing relieves tension during an asthma attack and thus decreases the severity of the attack. When clients experience how proper breathing makes a difference, they are motivated to continue this type of breathing.
4. Behavior that tends to recur is in some way being reinforced or is reinforcing itself. An infant crawls and gets into things because it is fun and satisfies the infant's curiosity. Overeating under stressful conditions is reinforcing when it relieves anxiety.

5. A behavior may serve to reinforce or strengthen another behavior. Some individuals can be persuaded to act appropriately for something they value. For example, a client can be given something in exchange for sitting quietly.

6. Irregular and inconsistent reinforcement of a behavior strengthens the continuance of that behavior. Parents who try to resist an uncooperative child's demands but who eventually give in are inadvertently strengthening the behavior with the most powerful method known: intermittent reinforcement.

7. Immediate and consistent reinforcement of a behavior strengthens that behavior most rapidly. A baby at the breast or bottle soon learns that sucking satisfies hunger.

8. Rewards that are specific to and desired by the learner are more powerful than general or routine rewards. A teenage client may respond well to compliments from the nurse, whereas another client may respond better to matching wits with the nurse.

9. Rewards and punishments that are clearly connected to the behavior are more powerful than vague or inconsistent responses. A client who moves in certain ways after surgery quickly learns that certain motions produce pain, so those movements are avoided. This principle helps explain why eating disorders are so difficult to change. The pleasure or relief that the overeater experiences outweighs the hazards because the pleasure is more immediate and the hazards are more remote. The effects of overeating do not show up on the body or the scale for days, and the health hazards may not become evident for many years. The connection between overeating and health issues is vague and inconsistent because other variables, such as genetics and exercise, are thought to add to or reduce the health risks.

10. Behavior that receives no response and meets no biologic need tends to extinguish. Children bring home new words that they hear while playing. Some of the words may include language the family does not sanction. Children who experience no response when they try out the new vocabulary tend to lose interest in those words.

Behavior modification is the application of learning theory to modify a behavior by changing the stimulus that elicits it or by changing the consequences that follow it. Classical conditioning emphasizes that whatever came before a behavior (antecedent event) influences that behavior (responding behavior). Operant conditioning stresses that a behavior is influenced by the response that follows. A behavior that is followed by a negative response or no response at all will diminish, whereas a behavior followed by a positive consequence will increase. When both of these theories are applied together, behavior is seen as a result of an antecedent event, and that behavior is further influenced by the consequences that follow it. This is illustrated in **Figure 3-2**.

Implications for Health Education

To increase a desirable behavior, the educator changes the antecedent event to one that is more likely to evoke the desired behavior or reinforces the desired behavior when it occurs or does both actions. An example of controlling antecedent behavior is to advise a client who is learning weight control to shop on a full stomach and use a shopping list. The antecedent event of a full stomach and a shopping list prepared in advance influences shoppers' behavior in the desired direction: wise shopping for wholesome food.

Using behavioral principles, the nurse identifies a client's desired behavior and then creates an environment that stimulates the client to comply by producing this desired response. When the desired behavior occurs, the nurse reinforces it. Immediate reinforcement increases the likelihood that the behavior will recur. Over time, the nurse moves from reinforcing the behavior every time it occurs to an intermittent reinforcement schedule. This gives the new behavior more stability.

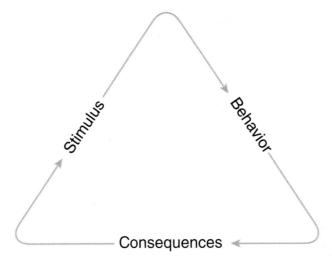

Figure 3-2 Stimulus-Behavior-Consequences. To change a behavior, you can change the stimulus that elicits it and/or the consequences that follow it.

Educators have discovered that punishment is not a long-term solution to undesirable behavior. Punishment may indeed suppress it, but if the behavior is meeting some need, that behavior is likely to return as soon as the threat is removed. Another possible consequence of punishment is an erratic and unpredictable response. The most effective way to eliminate an undesirable behavior is to find out what need the behavior is meeting and reinforce a more desirable method of meeting that need. The example used previously was an uncooperative child. It could be applied just as easily to an uncooperative client of any age. Solutions to this problem include frequent, pleasant, and predictable attention by nurses along with encouragement and assistance.

Cognitive Views of Learning

Cognitivism (also known as cognitive psychology) is the predominant theoretical perspective for studying human learning today. Its focus is on the cognitive processes; that is, "how people perceive, interpret, remember and in other ways think about environmental events" (Ormrod, 2012, p. 141). Whereas behaviorism focuses on observable behavioral changes, cognitivism expands the understanding of learning to include internal mental processes unique to each person, such as perception, insight, and meaning (Olson & Hergenhahn, 2013; Ormrod, 2020). Some underlying assumptions that support the cognitive view of learning follow (Ormrod, 2020).

- Some human learning is unique and differs from how animals learn.
- Learning is a mental activity and may not result in overt behavioral changes.
- People exert some control over their learning and actively participate in learning.
- Knowledge is organized and connected to the person's knowledge, beliefs, attitudes, and emotions.
- Unobservable mental processes can often be reasonably inferred by observable behavior.

Cognitive views of learning encompass several perspectives. In this section, we focus on *gestalt, constructivism,* and *information processing theory*.

Gestalt View of Learning

Three German psychologists, Max Wertheimer (1880–1943), Wolfgang Köhler (1887–1967), and Kurt Koffka (1886–1941), departed from behaviorism and are considered the founders of Gestalt psychology. Later, another German Gestalt psychologist, Kurt Lewin (1890–1947), developed a field theory of human learning. These psychologists insisted that behavior was much more than a conditioned response and that perception and memory can be studied by introspection in addition to external observation. Further, they posit that humans selectively perceive and react to complex patterns of stimuli as wholes, not as disconnected parts. It is the total pattern of stimuli that determines what a person perceives and learns (Olson & Hergenhahn, 2013; Ormrod, 2020).

Gestalt is a German word that means "the configuration or pattern" (Olson & Hergenhahn, 2013, p. 240), the whole or totality. In the field of gestalt psychology the concept means that the whole is more than merely the sum of its parts. Gestalt psychologists hold that psychological phenomena are irreducible wholes that cannot be derived just from analysis of their parts. If the totality of a particular perception is dissected, the meaning is lost. The focus is on understanding human sensation and perception and their meaning to the person. It melds past experiences, current environment, thoughts, feelings, motivations, and needs into an irreducible whole.

Lewin stated that each individual exists in an environment known as a field or life space, affected by many forces. *Life space* is a psychological field unique to each individual and includes things to which the person reacts; for example, material objects, people, private thoughts, tensions, and goals. He proposed that behavior is the interplay of these forces in the life space at the moment in which the behavior occurs. Analysis begins with examining the environment as a whole. Lewin made it clear that the environment as interpreted by the individual did not necessarily correspond with reality. Learning occurs as a result of a change in individual psychological interpretations or changes in the internal needs or motivations of the individual (Knowles, Holton, & Swanson, 2005; Olson & Hergenhahn, 2013).

Perception refers to the act of becoming aware of something by the use of any of the senses. To perceive means to take notice of, observe, detect, become aware of in one's mind, achieve understanding of, or apprehend. Perception refers to the portion of the world that is grasped mentally through sight, hearing, touch, taste, and smell (*The Merriam-Webster Dictionary*, 2016). Perception can vary among individuals and may be different from the reality of the situation.

Our perception of any object is affected by the context in which we become aware of it. Clients who are in an unfamiliar hospital and in pain will perceive your messages differently than clients who greet you in their homes. Team members who just heard about another reduction in work force and feel overloaded with responsibilities will perceive your messages differently than those who feel in control of their circumstances. Our perceptions of events are affected by life experiences and interests.

Gestalt and cognitive field theories of learning take into account both the learner and the learning context and all of the individual's experiences and perceptions. In many circumstances, individuals' perceptions are dissimilar, and other possible perceptions are not easily seen. Even individuals who experience the same event at the same time may have different perceptions of that event. Because of the tendency to assume that others perceive events the same way you do, you may be unaware that clients may see events differently.

Implications for Health Education

Nurses frequently deal with clients who are undergoing life transitions, such as birth, death, parenthood, or divorce. They also deal with clients who experience alterations in personal integrity, such as physical assault, accidental loss of sight or limb, loss of a way of life, or surgical removal of an organ. Such transitions can force clients into reconstructing and reorganizing their perceptions of themselves and reality (Edelman, Kudzma, & Mandle, 2014; Selder, 1989). When clients struggle with questions such as Who am I? and What is life about? they are going through the process of accommodation.

The following is an example of the use of gestalt psychology in teaching children. The nurse involved with doing preoperative teaching of young children arranges for the children and their parents to come to the day surgery area for a visit. While the children are in the unit, they see a video portraying surgery from a child's perspective. The video tells them the following:

> You wear green pajamas with a hat and socks to match. You get a shot (ouch) that makes you sleepy, and you ride on a table with wheels. The ceiling and people look funny when you ride flat. When you wake up, you will be sore, but you will get more shots that will make the soreness go away.

After the video, the children are led to a room with pieces of equipment, drapes, and surgical clothing that they are invited to play with. Dolls set up with various kinds of medical equipment (without real needles) are also within reach so that children can handle and play "operation." The nurse observes the children and listens to their conversations, using their responses as clues to what further teaching might be needed.

The main goal of the gestalt psychology perspective is to promote understanding and insight. Nurses as educators assess the client's perceptions and design a learning situation that will stimulate interest and understanding. Nurses organize the learning situation to fit the client's developmental stage, previous experiences, and learning ability.

Constructivism View of Learning

The constructivism view of learning has its roots in the work of Jean Piaget (1896–1980). Piaget, a Swiss psychologist, focused his detailed studies on the thinking process of children (1972). He conducted one-on-one interactions during which he presented various stimuli to infants and children. He then observed and recorded their responses. The responses led him to believe that thinking and learning are active processes, not merely passive or trial-and-error responses to stimuli as behaviorists believe. As the children grew old enough to speak, Piaget spoke with the children as he conducted the experiments. He concluded that intellectual development is a gradual process that evolves over time.

Learning is a transactional process in which individuals gain further understanding, new insights, or more developed cognitive structures through interaction. Two ways of learning that Piaget identified were *assimilation* and *accommodation*. Assimilation is a way of learning in which new ideas are incorporated by association with known ideas, concepts, and memories. Individuals may assimilate new ideas into their current beliefs. If the knowledge is different from what they already know, they may respond with the intellectual process known as accommodation, which is more difficult than assimilation. When accommodating new ideas, individuals give up former beliefs or substantially change their frame of reference, or they do both. Accommodation may also occur after a person has assimilated so many new concepts that the concepts can no longer be contained in the person's old cognitive structure. A paradigm shift occurs in the aftermath of an accumulation process (Santrock, 2023; Olson & Hergenhahn, 2013). **Figure 3-3** illustrates assimilation and accommodation.

Constructivism as a view of learning is gaining in popularity. It is an active learner-centered process whereby people construct, discover, and transform knowledge, thereby learning. This

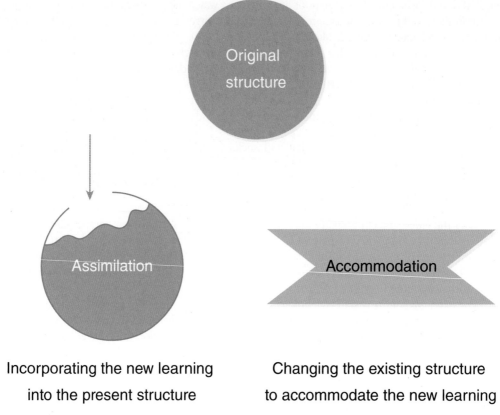

Incorporating the new learning
into the present structure

Changing the existing structure
to accommodate the new learning

Figure 3-3 Assimilation and Accommodation

view contrasts with the traditional educational model where learning is the passive transmission of knowledge from the teacher to the learner. Based on the learner's present reservoir of knowledge, past experiences, and unique style of learning, they actively attempt to make sense of learning. The principles of constructivism are (WGU, 2020):

- Knowledge is constructed built upon previous knowledge, experiences, beliefs, and insights.
- People learn to learn as they learn.
- Learning is an active process involving sensory input and active engagement.
- Learning is a social activity.
- Learning is contextual, connected to things already known and believed.
- Knowledge is personal.
- Learning exists in the mind.
- Motivation is key to learning.

The person in this view of learning actively examines and organizes learning in an attempt to make sense of it according to their personal unique learning style, their current knowledge and previous experiences. This view of learning is known as *individual constructivism*. The person is acquiring knowledge and working it into their mental framework rather than passively acquiring it from an external source. This view is applicable in working with a client as they gain new knowledge and skill and to a team member gaining new knowledge and skill. Learning can also occur in groups as nurses work collaboratively together to solve nursing care problems. It also applies to clients who are taught in groups. This is known as *social constructivism* (Ormrod, 2020).

Implications for Health Education

The role of nurse educator in Constructivism is as a facilitator of learning. It recognizes the uniqueness and individuality that clients and team members bring to the learning situation. The nurse educator focuses on what the person desires to learn, how they best learn, ideas they have for learning and proceeds from there. For example, if a client needs to learn self-care in the home, then focus on how they will manage there. Challenge the client to think through the equipment they will need and how they will handle their care in that setting. The client is thereby constructing their personal knowledge in self-care (individual constructivism).

If clients share a common issue such as managing diabetes or new baby care, form a group that addresses their needs. As a group, they can identify common concerns and share how they handle each one. They can compare strategies and share ideas for handling their challenges. This strategy is also effective for team members who need to update their nursing knowledge and skills. Meeting as a group allows them to share common challenges and solutions. Clients and team members are constructing their personal knowledge framework adapted to their unique needs (social constructivism).

Information Processing View of Learning

Another view of human learning is a sophisticated form of information processing. This view of learning was inspired by advances in computer science by theorists who hypothesized that human minds perform mental operations like computers. Slavin (2015) described a model of information processing proposed by Atkinson and Shiffrin as a model of information processing with three components focusing on how individuals register sensory information taken in from the environment (**sensory register**), how they process information (**working memory**) and how that information is stored and retrieved (**long-term memory**) (Slavin, 2015).

The first component of the information processing model is the sensory register, which receives large amounts of information from the five senses: sight, hearing, touch, smell, and taste. This component decides whether or not to notice or register an external sensory bit of information, such as an odor, flavor, touch, sound, or visual stimulus. It also decides whether or not to register sensory information that is internal; for example, an itch, a chill, a peristaltic wave, a headache, or a memory. Individuals' interpretations of sensory information is influenced by many factors, such as past experiences, knowledge, motivation, culture, gender, and so forth. The information is quickly lost if it is given no further attention. Individuals must pay attention to the sensory information if it is to be retained. People retain less if they are bombarded with too many diverse stimuli at one time (Slavin, 2015).

The second component of the information processing model is working memory, also called short-term memory. Here the individual pays attention to sensory information. Working memory holds thoughts a person is conscious of having at any given moment. The storage capacity of working memory appears limited in most individuals and holds approximately five to seven thoughts. As if they were bowling pins, ideas in the mind can be crowded out by the introduction of more items. These thoughts can be related to what the person is feeling, doing, or thinking at the moment, or they can be related to thoughts retrieved from storage in long-term memory that are associated with current stimuli. In this component, the mind processes the information by organizing it for storage, or associating it with other information, or discarding it. When the person stops thinking about the sensory information, it disappears from working memory.

For example, a nurse admits a small child for surgery who is tightly clutching a teddy bear. While observing the child's color, breathing ability, alertness, and the parent–child interaction, the nurse remembers a teddy bear from years ago or that of a daughter or son. Such recollections make the nurse more sensitive to the child at hand. If too many memories impinge on the nurse's consciousness, the memories may detract from the nurse's ability to note and track client data. Another example is a charge nurse giving instructions to a health team member at the change of shift. The team member is struggling with personal issues, including concerns about her teenager's behavior. Her personal concerns are crowding the space that might store the instructions she is receiving from the charge nurse.

The third component of the information processing model is long-term memory, in which an infinite amount of information is stored for a prolonged period of time. Long-term memory is thought to have a large capacity, provided it has not been damaged by pathology. Stored in long-term memory are images and thoughts about past experiences (episodic memory); facts, knowledge, general information that we have learned, and problem-solving and learning strategies (semantic memory); and procedural knowledge, such as how to do things like giving an injection, riding a bike, and general living skills (procedural memory) (Squire, Knowlton, & Musen, 1993).

Implications for Health Education

The nurse's job as an educator, from an information processing point of view, is to provide the client with new information. It is important to divide learning into steps that are compatible with the client's health, intelligence, and previous learning experiences. The nurse assists the client in acknowledging current beliefs that enhance or inhibit learning. The new information is then translated into a message that the client is able to process. This involves capturing the client's attention through teaching strategies and teaching materials. Selecting attractive, colorful materials with sufficient emphasis on fonts and type size helps clients attend to the message.

The information processing model is particularly useful for teaching skills online, such as procedures that must be done in an ordered sequence. As educators, nurses assess educational needs and choose online resources to facilitate learning. This is a useful teaching strategy for individuals who are self-directed, visual, and experienced with computers. Nurses give feedback through discussion forums, email, or phone calls.

In using the information processing model, it is important for nurses to avoid overloading clients with too much information, especially if the information is new. If a lot of information must be communicated in a short period of time, try grouping the information in categories that make sense. For example, if you are teaching a client who has been newly diagnosed with diabetes, it would be helpful to create groupings of information to aid the client's memory. Grouping information for clients with diabetes includes dietary information, exercise routine, injection procedure and supplies, and signs and symptoms of hyperglycemia and hypoglycemia. Having printed information about each group also facilitates learning. Clients who have concerns should be given written instructions to read at home that serve as memory aids. Booklets with illustrations are helpful.

If the client in the preceding example had diabetes for many years and was well informed about the disease, your approach would be different. Assess where the client has gaps in knowledge and provide appropriate instruction. The goal is to complement what the client already knows and facilitate learning where it is needed.

Social Cognitive View of Learning

In the 1960s and 1970s, a new view of learning emerged based on research by Albert Bandura, emeritus professor at Stanford University. His theory is an outgrowth of the behavioral theories of learning that he believed lacked a complete explanation for learning. He incorporated many contributions from cognitive theorists into what is now referred to as observational learning. Bandura believes that people are neither driven by inner forces nor automatically shaped by external forces; rather, they are creative, active participants in shaping their lives. In other words, people are proactive rather than reactive; they have some control over how they live their lives (Bandura, 1986, 2001). General principles that support the social cognitive view of learning follow (Ormrod, 2020; Slavin, 2015).

- People learn through a process of modeling and observing others' behavior.
- People learn vicariously from others' successes and failures.
- Learning may or may not result in an observable change of behavior.
- Cognition is important in learning such as awareness, attention, expectations, and retention.
- People can actively exert control over their actions and environments.

Bandura's theory of observational learning involves four phases and processes: *attention*, *retention*, *reproduction*, and *motivation* (Bandura, 1986; Olsen & Hergenhahn, 2013). The first phase, attention, occurs when the individual actively pays attention to the behavior of the model. Models that are similar to the observer in terms of age and gender—and who are respected, competent, powerful, and attractive—are attended to more often. Heroes in various age groups act as models for people of their age groups.

In the second phase, retention, the individual must have an opportunity to practice imitating the behavior of the model. For observation learning to be useful, what is learned must be remembered for future use. Learning can be stored verbally in words or in the form of mental pictures or images of modeled behaviors (imagined). When needed, learning is retrieved, rehearsed, and used long after it is observed.

In the third phase, reproduction, the individual tries to match the behavior of the model. This depends on the person's ability to actually perform what has been learned. Some individuals may be unable to perform or retain information because of age-related developmental immaturity, illness, or injury.

In the fourth phase, motivation, the individual finds satisfying reasons to imitate the behavior of the model. Motivation has two aspects: (1) the expectation that acting like the model in certain situations will result in reinforcement similar to that received by the model; and (2) it serves to motivate a person to use (perform) what has been learned. A teacher's smile and verbal reinforcement are important here.

Bandura's social cognitive theory states that people learn from observing others in a social setting. By observing others, people acquire knowledge and skills, learn social rules and norms, and develop beliefs and attitudes. They observe which behaviors are useful, appropriate, and valued by society and which are not. Social cognitive theory posits that people learn most efficiently from observing others' behavior and less from the consequences of behavior (Skinner's view). In other words, this theory states that people learn primarily by observing the successes and failures of others (Santrock, 2023; Slavin, 2015). It is important to distinguish between learning by observation and the act of imitation. Learning may or may not include imitating the observed behavior.

Models and *modeling behavior* are important concepts. A model can be anything that conveys information; for example, a person, film, television program, picture, or instructions. Models

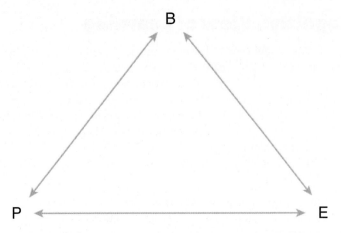

Figure 3-4 Reciprocal determinism. Behavior is the result of the bidirectional interaction of three classes of behavioral determinants: cognitive and personal factors (P), environmental events (E), and behavior (B), called reciprocal determinism.

Data from Bandura, A. (1986). *Social foundations of thought and action: A social cognitive theory*. Englewood Cliffs, NJ: Prentice-Hall.

convey messages about behavior. Bandura believes that behavior is the result of the bidirectional interaction of three classes of behavioral determinants: *cognitive and personal factors*, *environmental events*, and *behavior*. The interaction is reciprocal in that each operates interactively as determinants of the other. Behavior is a result of the interacting determinants and cannot be understood by viewing them in isolation. The strength of the influence of each determinant on behavior varies according to the situation. **Figure 3-4** illustrates this reciprocal relationship, which Bandura calls reciprocal determinism (Bandura, 1986; Olson & Hergenhahn, 2013).

The nurse as educator wittingly or unwittingly teaches clients and health team members by their behavior. This example helps to explain some cognitive factors in social learning. Emily, a new nurse, observes Nurse X assisting a physician during a diagnostic procedure. Nurse X is poorly prepared to assist the physician and does not have knowledge of the procedure or the physician's requirements and needs. Consequently, both Nurse X and the physician are unhappy at the conclusion of the procedure. The next day, Emily observes Nurse Y assist a physician with the same procedure. Nurse Y is prepared, organized, and familiar with the physician's requirements and needs. The outcome is better, and the physician thanks Nurse Y for her preparedness and efficiency. Later, Emily seeks out her supervisor, and together they discuss both situations. They identify what was effective and what was ineffective behavior of each nurse's performance. In this example, Emily observes both positive and negative modeling and is able to see the differences. Emily verbally rehearses her responsibilities with her supervisor. Six months later, Emily is assigned to assist a physician with the same diagnostic procedure. She mentally rehearses her role and responsibilities. The procedure goes smoothly, and the participants are satisfied. This shows how modeling can produce successful performance. From this example, the following components of social cognitive learning theory are illustrated (Bandura, 1986; Ormrod, 2020):

- Emily's learning was a mental activity; she learned by observing. She paid attention to what each nurse was doing and made a mental note of what was ineffective (Nurse X) and what was effective (Nurse Y). She learned by observing each nurse and mentally rehearsing effective behavior (*vicarious learning*).

- Although Emily did not have an opportunity to immediately imitate Nurse Y's behavior, her learning was verbal when she discussed her observations with her supervisor. Together they reviewed what she learned through observation.
- Emily had no opportunity to immediately imitate the desired assisting behavior; however, 6 months later she remembered what she learned and was able to imitate the behavior (*delayed modeling*).
- Emily was aware of how unhappy both Nurse X and the physician were at the conclusion of the procedure. Observing their unhappiness, Emily experienced vicarious punishment (*response–punishment contingency*) and did not want to experience the same outcome.
- Emily was aware of how pleased Nurse Y and the physician were at the conclusion of the procedure. Observing their satisfaction and the physician's compliments with her supervisor's positive input, Emily experienced vicarious reinforcement (*response–reinforcement contingency*), and she desired that outcome for herself.
- Emily felt confident and believed in her ability to successfully perform the behavior (*self-efficacy expectation*). Subsequently, when she was in the assisting role again, she fulfilled her expectations of herself and rewarded herself with a mental pat on the back.

Implications for Health Education

Role modeling is a form of observational learning. Nurses learn by observing their professional colleagues. In the same way, clients learn by observing nurses. Clients observe nurses and other healthcare providers and regard them as experts. If they model good health practices, that behavior sends an important message to clients; the converse is also true. Nurses who are overweight or smoke have little credibility when it comes to teaching clients about weight reduction or smoking cessation. The old adage is true: What we do is a stronger message than what we say, regardless of how sincerely we present the message. If nurses are to be effective educators, they must model good health practices and behaviors (Rush, Kee, & Rice, 2005; Spencer, 2007).

Bandura's modeling phases and processes are important when teaching clients by demonstrating a desired action and having them return the demonstration. By observing you performing, clients and health team members can mimic your performance while they are under your supervision. This gives you an opportunity to guide, correct, and provide positive reinforcement as indicated.

Table 3-1 summarizes the views of learning discussed in this chapter. Each view has advantages and disadvantages, depending on the type of intended learning and on the learner and teacher interaction. When selecting a view, ask yourself the following questions: What is the purpose of the learning? Who initiates the learning? Who evaluates whether or not the learning has been effective?

Educator responsibilities vary, depending on the learning view used. In each view, the teacher's role is that of director (behaviorism); designer (gestaltism); facilitator (constructivism), programmer (information processing); or model (social cognitive). The main goal of the learner in each view is to change behavior (behaviorism); understand (gestaltism); learn as they learn (constructivism), register, retain, and recall information (information processing); and observe and imitate (social cognitive). Table 3-1 compares these concepts.

Principles of Learning

Principles are the foundation or general laws of teaching and learning derived from research based on consistently observed phenomena. Learning principles are formulations that are generally true

Table 3-1 Views Regarding Thinking, Learning, Teacher, and Learner

Views of	Thinking	Learning	Teacher	Learner
Behaviorist	Covert trial and error	Change in behavior	Directs	Complies
Gestaltist	Knows, perceives	Understands, gains insight	Designs	Participates
Constructivism	Constructs knowledge	Learns as they learn	Facilitator	Active engagement
Processor	Processes information	Registers, retains, recalls	Programs	Inputs, outputs
Social cognitivist	Observes, mentally processes	Attends, retains, performs	Models	Imitates

Box 3-2 Principles of Learning

- Focusing
- Repetition
- Learner control
- Active participation
- Individual styles
- Organization
- Association
- Imitation
- Motivation
- Spacing
- Recency
- Primacy
- Arousal
- Accurate and prompt feedback
- Application
- Personal history

and applicable to multiple learning situations (Ormrod, 2020). These principles, summarized in **Box 3-2**, are derived from informal research and feedback from more than 800 registered nurses over 15 years who were taught clinical teaching methods in a baccalaureate registered nurse program by authors Babcock and Miller (1994). These principles of learning are widely applicable to health education.

Focusing Intensifies Learning

Individuals vary in ways that help them learn. Some learners depend on eye contact with the teacher; they focus on the teacher's verbalizations and body language. Others make images in their mind of what is being presented. Kinesthetic learners are people who learn through the awareness of body position. Some learners write images on paper or write notes to stay actively involved.

While studying, some learners listen to music to help them concentrate. Others want minimal auditory and visual distractions. Some learners have rituals that help them focus. Examples of rituals include meditation, organizing materials, and preparing a snack. Most learners enhance their ability to retain and recall information by developing a pattern that provides for physical comfort, a heightened level of arousal, and a clear mind.

Repetition Enhances Learning

Repeating information and applying it in different situations and contexts helps to remember it. Sustained practice enforces learning. This is true for memorizing facts and mastering psychomotor skills.

Learner Control Increases Learning

Learners do better when they feel in control of the learning process, and they are more likely to choose learning methods that worked for them in the past. Past experience demonstrates that nurses are successful adult learners who can verbalize what is needed to master new information and skills. Most nurses take responsibility for their learning and do better when educators acknowledge this in both actions and words. This same principle applies to learners of any age. Older learners generally need more time to absorb new information. They are successful when they are in control of both the pace and the increments of learning.

Active Participation Is Necessary for Learning

Learning is an active process. Most people find that the more they are able to involve themselves in learning, the more they are able to learn. Participation in learning means having input into the learning process, including the time, place, pace, and increments of learning.

Learning Styles Vary

Some learners find it easier to comprehend verbal discourse, while others comprehend visual cues more easily. Still others seek hands-on experience to grasp the meaning of concepts. Many find that a combination of verbal, visual, auditory, and kinesthetic experiences is most effective. Be aware of your preferred learning style because it is the style you are most likely to use when you teach. Assess your clients' learning styles so you can plan an approach to enhance learning. The skill in facilitating learning is to find an effective match between the clients' learning styles and your teaching approach.

Organization Promotes Learning

Learners often highlight readings, summarize paragraphs, explain their assignments to others, and ask questions. These are ways of actively organizing learning materials. This personal intellectual activity makes the information meaningful and easier to retain. Methods of organization vary, but to be most effective, materials should be organized in a way that fits both the content and the learner. A cognitive task, such as learning historical facts, is facilitated by using chronology. Learning of psychomotor skills is enhanced by teaching from the simple to the complex. Affective learning frequently is best organized around the principle of low- to high-risk behaviors from the learner's point of view.

Association Is Necessary to Learning

To retain any new information or skill, learners must be able to associate the new learning with phenomena that are already within their repertoire of experience. Association provides relevance to learners.

Imitation Is a Method of Learning

Imitating is particularly useful for mastering psychomotor skills, but attitudes and beliefs can also be incorporated if learners observe a respected role model.

Motivation Strengthens Learning

It is easier for learners to grasp facts, learn new skills, and change attitudes when they anticipate gaining benefits from the effort. Past success and the expectation of future success are powerful motivating forces. Educators should perform a needs assessment to understand what motivates clients and use this knowledge to create an atmosphere that sustains motivation and builds confidence.

Spacing New Material Facilitates Learning

It is wiser for educators to present small amounts of new material incrementally rather than larger amounts at one time. Learners should be encouraged to read instructional materials to give them exposure to information over time so they have a more thorough understanding. This also provides an opportunity to ask questions of the educators.

Recency Influences Retention

The more recently learners have been exposed to information or have practiced a skill, the greater the possibility they will recall it correctly. Retention is the ability to repeat information or grasp or hold on to information or a skill.

Primacy Affects Retention

People tend to learn the first few items best; this concept is referred to as primacy. Learners pay more attention to and devote more energy to items presented first. The human mind is capable of retaining a limited number (five to seven) of new bits of information at one time. When these new bits of information have been associated with other more solidly retained memories, learners are better able to grasp and retain other sets of facts.

Arousal Influences Attention

Arousal is affected by novelty. The human mind is attracted to change and glitches in patterns. Other sources of stimuli besides novelty include sensory intensity, emotional arousal, and other sources of tension. A certain amount of tension enhances learners' ability to focus. This tension is caused by fear, anger, anxiety, curiosity, and amusement. When tense, a client's neurochemistry changes. Chemicals are released that improve circulation, provide sugar to the brain and muscles, and enhance visual acuity. Clients vary in how much tension is ideal for them. This is illustrated in **Figure 3-5**. For example, too much tension interferes with learning, whereas a moderate level

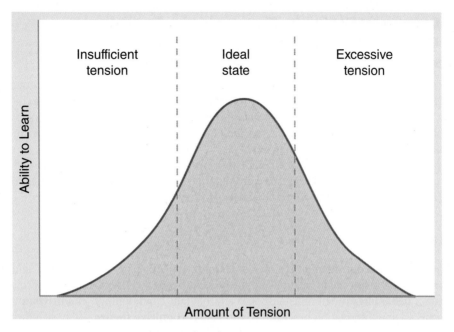

Figure 3-5 Arousal and learning: A moderate amount of tension enhances learning. Too little tension fails to engage a learner's attention. Too much tension interferes with learning.

of tension is motivating (Cassady & Johnson, 2002; Stephenson, 2006). With too much tension, clients may become immobilized or restless and engage in behavior that further obstructs learning. Fear of punishment, such as job loss, usually impedes learning and interferes with the ability to apply learning to new situations.

Accurate and Prompt Feedback Enhances Learning

Learners need to know how well they are meeting learning objectives. Self-assessments are helpful; consider how frequently newspapers and magazines publish self-scoring tests and questionnaires. Clients want to know how their attitudes and level of knowledge compare with others. Feedback is necessary for clients and educators to determine if learning occurred. Prompt feedback reinforces desired behaviors and gives clients feelings of satisfaction when they are successful. Even when correction is necessary, feedback can reduce tension because learners know what is learned and what is still to be mastered.

Application of New Learning in a Variety of Contexts Broadens the Generalization of That Learning

Application of knowledge helps to broaden and generalize learning. An example is practicing walking with a crutch in a lab setting and then applying the skill in actual practice settings, such as walking up and down steps. Exposure to a particular concept, attitude, or skill in varying situations assists learners to retain new material and develop the ability to apply the material in a wider variety of situations.

The Learner's Biologic, Psychologic, Sociologic, and Cultural Realities Shape the Learner's Perception of the Learning Experience

Health affects energy level and the ability to concentrate. Self-esteem and previous experiences with learning affect the willingness to risk, tolerance for temporary failure, and expectations of success. If clients are at a developmental level in which memorization and concrete processing are necessary, educators must respect that. Nurses as educators need to listen and be observant of the signs that learners are handling all they can.

Societal norms and learners' previous experiences with healthcare institutions affect the ability to learn. Clients' attitudes toward learning, their beliefs about personal responsibility for health, and the learning climate are all influenced by their culture.

Summary

This chapter examined prominent theories of learning as they relate to the teaching and learning process of the nurse–client relationship in the Miller–Stoeckel Client Education Model. The theories are **behaviorism** (stimulus–response and operant conditioning), **cognitivism** (gestalt, constructivism and information processing), and **social cognitive theory**. With each theory, application was made to how nurses as educators could apply that information in a clinical setting when working with clients as learners. Selecting which theory works best for clients and what is taught is your job as the educator. The chapter concluded with a discussion of principles of learning that are broadly applicable in a wide variety of health education situations.

Exercises

Exercise I: Integrating Learning Theories and Principles

Purpose: Apply learning theories and principles in preparation for client education.
Directions: Divide into groups and choose which assignment your group will prepare.

Group Assignment A

What learning theories and principles would you apply in each of the following situations? Act out one of the following scenes.

1. You are going to teach home safety and accident prevention to an older client after hip replacement surgery before she goes home.
2. As a nurse working in the gynecology clinic, you are to teach breast self-examination to a group of people in the waiting room.
3. As a public health nurse, you are to teach a group of young parents at a day-care center about behavior modification using the propositions of behavioral theory. The objective is to translate the most important concepts into plain English and give practical examples.

Group Assignment B

You are a group of nurse entrepreneurs who have been granted an interview with a TV station program producer. Select two members to collaborate in playing the role of station program producer.

1. Your task is to talk the TV producer into buying your television program package. Prepare the following information:
   a. Identify the target audience. Who are the viewers? Are they in school? If so, which grade level? Are they at the work site? If so, which one? Why did you choose this audience?
   b. What population trends make your program feasible?
   c. Suggest how often your program should be shown. Daily? Monthly? What day? What hour? Provide your rationale.
   d. List the topics you would cover with your target audience.
   e. Identify the sponsors you would approach.
2. Place yourself in the role of the producer. Identify questions and concerns you have. Consider issues such as profit; market acceptability; risk; controversy; sensitivities of various cultural, ethnic, and age groups; and timeliness. Present these concerns to the nurse entrepreneurs.

Group Assignment C

Conduct the following activities on your regular television health program:

1. Your first guest is a self-styled fitness expert or nutritionist who is very popular but whose scientific base you question. Conduct the interview in a way that will promote critical thinking in your audience.
2. Create a commercial break in which you do the following:
   a. Market nurses as health educators, consultants, and care providers
   b. Advertise a health product or system with which you would like to be associated
3. Interview a nurse colleague about the changing trends in health care and what that means for the average citizen.

Exercise II: Compare and Contrast Learning Theories

Purpose: Examine behaviorism, cognitivism, and social cognitive theories.
Directions: Divide into small groups of four to five and discuss the theories of learning described in this chapter. Discuss the following questions:

1. How are the theories alike?
2. How are they different?
3. What is the difference between learning, teaching, and health education?
4. Do people think like computers?
5. How have computers influenced your way of thinking?

Exercise III: Reflecting on Self-Learning

Purpose: Reflect on how you learn.
Directions: Form dyads with someone in the class whom you have not worked with before. Take a few minutes and reflect individually on how you learn, then share this with your partner. Is your learning consistent with the principles of constructivism? Listen to how your partner learns. Compare the ways your learning is alike and different.

Exercise IV: Information Processing and Memory

Purpose: Contemplate on the information processing model.
Directions: Form small groups of three or four; then do the following:

1. For 5 to 10 minutes, think alone about how you memorize lists and new information.
2. Discuss your thoughts and memory aids with others in your group and compare how your memorization strategies are alike and different.
3. Did you learn new strategies that will help you in the future?

Exercise V: Role Modeling

Purpose: Reflect on role models and role modeling.
Direction: Reflect on the following for 5 to 10 minutes, then form small groups and discuss your responses:

1. Who are your present role models in your social life? Who are your present role models in your role as a student?
2. What have you observed them doing that has helped you?
3. What have you observed them doing that you wish to avoid?
4. In what ways are you a role model to others?

References

Babcock, D. E., & Miller, M. A. (1994). *Client education: Theory and practice*. St. Louis, MO: Mosby.

Bandura, A. (1986). *Social foundations of thought and action: A social cognitive theory*. Englewood Cliffs, NJ: Prentice Hall.

Bandura, A. (2001). Social cognitive theory: An agentic perspective. *Annual Review of Psychology, 52*, 1–26.

Cassady, J. C., & Johnson, R. E. (2002). Cognitive test anxiety and academic performance. *Contemporary Educational Psychology, 27*(2), 270–295.

Edelman, C. L., Kudzma, E. C., & Mandle, C. L. (2014). *Health promotion throughout the life span* (8th ed.). St. Louis, MO: Elsevier Mosby.

Guthrie, E. R. (1935). *The psychology of learning*. New York, NY: Harper & Row.

Guthrie, E. R. (1952). *The psychology of learning* (rev. ed.). New York, NY: Harper & Row.

Knowles, M. S., Holton, E. F., III, & Swanson, R. A. (2005). *The adult learner* (6th ed.). Burlington, MA: Elsevier.

Merriam, S. B., Caffarella, R. S., & Baumgartner, L. M. (2007). *Learning in adulthood* (3rd ed.). San Francisco, CA: Jossey-Bass.

Olson, M. H., & Hergenhahn, B. R. (2013). *An introduction to theories of learning* (9th ed.). Upper Saddle River, NJ: Pearson Prentice Hall.

Ormrod, J. E. (2012). *Human learning* (6th ed.). Boston, MA: Pearson.

Ormrod, J. E. (2016). *Human learning* (7th ed.). Boston, MA: Pearson.

Ormrod, J. E. (2020). *Human learning* (8th ed.). New York: NY: Pearson.

Piaget, J. (1972). Intellectual evolution from adolescence to adulthood. *Human Development, 15*(1), 1–12.

Rush, K. L., Kee, C. C., & Rice, M. (2005). Nurses as imperfect role models for health promotion. *Western Journal of Nursing Research, 27*(2), 166–187.

Santrock, J. W. (2023). *A topical approach to life-span development* (11th ed.). Boston, MA: McGraw-Hill.

Selder, F. (1989). Life transition theory: The resolution of uncertainty. *Nursing and Health Care, 10*(8), 437–451.

Slavin, R. E. (2015). *Educational psychology theory and practice* (11th ed.). Boston, MA: Pearson Education, Inc.

Spencer, C. (2007). Should nurses model healthy behaviour? *Kai Tiaki Nursing New Zealand, 13*(7), 14–15.

Squire, L. R., Knowlton, B., & Musen, G. (1993). The structure and organization of memory. *Annual Review of Psychology, 44*, 453–495.

Stephenson, P. I. (2006). Before the teaching begins: Managing patient anxiety prior to providing education. *Clinical Journal of Oncology Nursing, 10*(2), 241–245.

The Merriam-Webster Dictionary (7th ed.). (2016). Springfield, MA: Merriam-Webster, Inc.

Western Governors University. (May 27, 2020). What Is constructivism? Retrieved July 13, 2023, from WGU.edu/blog/what-constructivism2005.html

PART III

Assessment for Health Education

CHAPTER 4

Learner and Setting Assessment

OBJECTIVES

Upon completion of this chapter, you will be able to do the following:

- Describe how the psychological factors of perception, motivation, and emotional status affect teaching and learning.
- Describe how the biological factors of health status, developmental stages, and physical challenges affect teaching and learning.
- Describe how the social factors of culture, socioeconomic status, and generational differences affect teaching and learning.
- Describe how the intellectual factors of educational background, willingness to learn, and background knowledge affect teaching and learning.
- Describe how the environmental factors of types of settings and physical and emotional atmosphere affect teaching and learning.

CHAPTER OUTLINE

Introduction
Psychological Factors
- Perception
- Motivation
- Emotional Status
Biological Factors
- Health Status
- Developmental Stages
- Physical Challenges
    - Hearing Impairment
    - Vision Impairment
    - Speech Impairment
    - Communication Challenges
Social Factors
- Culture/Support System
- Socioeconomic Status
- Generational Differences

Intellectual Factors
- Educational Level
- Willingness to Learn
- Background Knowledge
    - Assessing Recall and Understanding (Knowledge)
    - Assessing Analysis, Critical Thinking, and Performance (Skills)
    - Assessing Attitudes and Values (Attitudes)
Environmental Factors
- Types of Settings
    - Hospital
    - Long-Term Care and Assisted Living Facilities
    - Private Home
    - School
    - Work Site
    - Community

Introduction

In this chapter, we examine factors to consider when assessing the client and the learning environment in preparation for health education. Assessment, the first phase of the nursing process, is an essential step before developing the client education plan. A thorough learner assessment helps the nurse as educator build an effective nurse–client relationship in the Miller–Stoeckel Client Education Model. The client may not always be at an optimum point for learning, but through assessment, the nurse educator adjusts the client education plan to meet the needs of the client at whatever level they present. Client assessment is ongoing and informs the nurse educator of the psychological, biological, social, intellectual, and environmental factors that influence clients' learning needs. **Table 4-1** illustrates what comprises client assessment in preparation for health education. Each factor is examined in depth.

Psychological Factors

Assessment of psychological factors is critical in preparing a client education plan. Psychological factors to consider include perception, motivation, and emotional status. Each has a distinct focus and influences the client's ability to learn.

Perception

Perception is an active process of creating meaning by selecting, organizing, and interpreting people, objects, events, situations, and activities (Kanu, 2009). Perception plays an important

Table 4-1 Learner Assessment Factors

Psychological Factors	▪ Perception ▪ Motivation ▪ Emotional status
Biological Factors	▪ Health status ▪ Developmental stages ▪ Physical challenges
Social Factors	▪ Culture/support system ▪ Socioeconomic status ▪ Generational differences
Intellectual Factors	▪ Educational level ▪ Willingness to learn ▪ Background knowledge
Environmental Factors	▪ Types of settings ▪ Physical and emotional atmosphere

role in learning. Each person experiences and interprets the world differently and it is difficult for the nurse to know how each learner perceives people and situations. A good place to begin in understanding perception is with the self. As a nurse educator you have a "perceived self" that is a reflection of the person you believe yourself to be through self-examination. This includes your appearance, intelligence, abilities, and social skills. It is important to self-reflect about your perceived self, including your biases and perceptions drawn from past experiences. Your public image is your "presenting self." This is the socially approved image that you nurture for yourself and that clients witness. It includes the verbal and nonverbal ways you maintain your image to others. Managed impressions help us to accomplish our personal goals. It is important to be aware of the image you present as an educator to your clients and become aware of others' perceptions of you. Seek feedback. It is difficult to be objective about our own behavior so feedback from others is critical to our understanding of self-perceptions. Be aware that your client also has a perceived and presenting self.

As educators, we hold perceptions of our clients. Making perceptions clear to others is an important part of effective communication and mutual understanding. Clarifying your perceptions and noting differences are important for effective communication. We need to ask ourselves:

- What if our perceptions are inaccurate?
- What if there is more to the story of a person than what meets the eye?
- How can we develop skills to improve our ability to overcome common perceptual tendencies and situational factors?

Perception checking is a good tool to help you understand others accurately instead of jumping to conclusions or assuming that your first interpretation is the correct one (Kanu, 2009). This reduces defensiveness in the client by asking for clarification when there is a need. It also preserves face for both educator and client and prevents misunderstandings.

Perception checking involves either indirect or direct checking. **Indirect perception checking** is seeking additional information to confirm or refute interpretation of client behavior through passive means such as observing and listening. As a nurse educator, you want to consciously focus on feedback you are receiving when interacting with the client. Notice as much detail as possible while keeping a holistic view. It is important not to rush to judgment based on a few bits of information.

Direct perception checking is asking for verbal confirmation from the client about an interpretation about themselves. The three parts to direct perception checking (Kanu, 2009) are:

- Description of the behavior noticed,
- Two possible interpretations of the behavior, and
- Request for clarification about how to interpret the behavior.

Description of the behavior is stating what you observe about the client in a nonjudgmental manner based on facts rather than assumptions. For example, "I notice that you haven't attended the teaching session this week." This carefully worded approach avoids making conclusions about the behavior and states clearly what you observed, keeping in mind that first impressions are not always accurate.

Next, the educator would offer *two interpretations for the behavior* that shows interest in the client. For example, "I am not sure if you are having transportation issues" or "You're not feeling well." The intent is to show empathy and a willingness to hear the client's viewpoint. It is important to remember that clients from different cultural backgrounds do not always share the same meaning of events, objects, and behaviors.

Finally, there is the *request for clarification*. You might ask "What is going on?" This is done in a nonaccusatory manner to check the accuracy of your perceptions. Be aware of nonverbal behavior as you speak with the client. Using perception checking skills helps the nurse educator understand how clients experience the world to avoid misinterpreting their behavior.

Assessment of learners involves being aware of your personal perceptions and those of the client. Failures in communication frequently occur because people have inaccurate perceptions of each other or are unaware their perceptions are inaccurate. The skill of perception checking can avert this problem and contribute to a more accurate assessment in preparation for learning (Kanu, 2009), as self-perception affects the ability to learn.

Motivation

It is important to assess learners' motivation to receive health education. Motivation refers to "the reasons underlying behavior" (Guay et al., 2010, p. 712). Motivation to learn and behave comes from the behavioral, humanistic, cognitive, and social theories discussed in the previous chapter. Ryan and Deci (2000) describe motives for learning as intrinsic and extrinsic. *Intrinsic motivation* comes from within the client or from factors inherent in the task being performed. For example, clients who love exercising are intrinsically motivated to walk daily as it is enjoyable and rewarding. Strategies for promoting intrinsic motivation include arousing interest in the subject matter, encouraging curiosity, pursuing interesting presentation methods, and helping clients set their own learning goals. Other strategies such as giving client choices, demonstrating usefulness of content, and collaborating also encourage intrinsic motivation.

Extrinsic motivation comes from sources external to the client and the task. It can come through praise, recognition, or a system of rewards. For example, for clients who do not enjoy exercising, the recognition by peers of their improved appearance may prompt them to exercise more often. As educators, we hope to promote intrinsic motivation in our clients. It is only when behaviors are internally directed and valued by the client that sustained changes are possible. And, when healthy behaviors are sustained over time, better health outcomes are possible.

Franken (2002) identified two types of motivation: avoidant and approach. The *avoidant type* causes people to choose certain behaviors in order to avoid something. In contrast, the *approach type* causes people to be driven by want or need. For example, if a client wants to lose weight, they may choose the avoidance approach by avoiding fatty foods. The client realizes avoiding high-calorie foods can result in weight loss. However, in the approach type of motivation, the client may choose to exercise more, realizing that burning extra calories will result in weight loss. People may use a combination of avoidant and approach strategies to achieve a desired outcome.

Abraham Maslow's hierarchy of needs theory is another perspective on motivation (Maslow, 1954, 1987). His theory has been widely adopted in nursing education. He states that each person has basic needs (food, shelter, love, etc.) that must be met before learning can occur. If the basic needs are not attended to first, learning may be delayed or impossible to achieve. See **Table 4-2** for an illustration of how these needs apply to health education.

While researchers use different frameworks for thinking about motivation, they essentially agree on the major elements that learners need to have to be motivated. These are:

- Competence or self-efficacy (the belief that the client is capable of doing something)
- Autonomy/control (client's ability to set appropriate goals and see a correlation between effort and outcome)
- Interest/value (client's vested interest in the task and a feeling that its value is worth the effort to complete it)

Table 4-2 Maslow's Hierarchy of Needs and Motivation to Learn

Maslow's Hierarchy of Needs	Application to Health Education
Physiologic needs (oxygen, food, hydration, warmth, exercise, and sleep)	Clients who are tired, hungry, in pain, or critically ill have little motivation to focus on health education. Postpone teaching until a more appropriate time.
Safety and security needs	Clients who do not feel safe and secure are not open to health education. Inform them about routines and procedures.
Love and belonging needs	Clients who do not feel accepted by the healthcare team are not open to health education. Accept and welcome them to health education opportunities.
Self-esteem needs (feeling respected, valued, and appreciated)	Clients who do not feel respected, valued, or appreciated are not receptive to health education. Listen and appreciate their viewpoint and address their learning needs.
Self-actualization (achieving one's potential)	Clients who focus on lower-level needs will not achieve their full potential. Help them achieve their full potential by focusing on higher-level needs to improve their lives.

- Relatedness (the client's need to feel part of a family or group and exhibit behavior appropriate to that group) (Murray, 2011; Pintrich, 2003; Ryan & Deci, 2000)

These dimensions of motivation are shown in **Table 4-3**.

Motivation can be gauged through *motivational interviewing*, as it allows the client and educator to gain awareness of their situation. The interview is nonconfrontational and helps the client see the full scope of their situation (Lundahl, Kunz, Brownell, Tollefson, & Burk 2010). The nurses' support and empathy helps the client see that they have the ability to make changes for themselves. Through this process, the nurse can determine whether the client has the internal motivation needed to succeed. The four key principles of motivational interviewing are (Bray, Catley, Voelker, Liston, & Williams 2013):

- Resisting the "righting reflex"
- Understanding the client's motivation
- Listening to the client
- Empowering the client

In the traditional educator–client encounter, the nurse takes responsibility for providing information and coming up with a solution to the client's problems. This approach assumes the nurse is "right" and may prevent meaningful two-way communication and understanding of motivation. *Resisting the "righting reflex"* by affirming the client's interest or efforts is the first principle of motivational interviewing. This approach builds a trusting relationship. Once trust is established, then the client can openly express what causes resistance to learning. The nurse educator can then acknowledge the resistance and explore options.

The second principle of motivational interviewing is to *understand the client's motivations*. The nurse uses open-ended questions and reflective listening to get information about clients' values, attitudes, and beliefs. The nurse can then further clarify by asking the motivation ruler question:

Table 4-3 Dimensions of Motivation

Dimensions	Indicators
Competence (*Am I capable?*)	The client believes they have the *ability* to complete the task, which supports self-efficacy.
Control/autonomy (*Can I control it?*)	The client feels in *control* by seeing a direct link between their actions and an outcome. The client can choose a style of *avoidance or approach* and set their own goals.
Interest/value (*Does it interest me? Is it worth the effort?*)	The client has some interest in the task or sees the value of completing it. The client is *intrinsically or extrinsically* motivated.
Relatedness (*What do others think?*)	Completing the task brings the client *social rewards* such as a sense of belonging to their family or peer group or *approval* from a person of social importance to the client.

Data from Bandura, A. (1986). *Social foundations of thought and action: A social cognitive theory.* Englewood Cliffs, NJ: Prentice Hall; Murray, A. (2011). Montessori elementary philosophy reflects current motivation theories. *Montessori Life, 23*(1), 22–33; Pender, N. (2011). *The health promotion model manual.* Retrieved from https://deepblue.lib.umich.edu/bitstream/handle/2027.42/85350/HEALTH_PROMOTION_MANUAL_Rev_5-2011.pdf; Pintrich, P. R. (2003). A motivational science perspective on the role of student motivation in learning and teaching contexts. *Journal of Educational Psychology, 95*(4), 667–686; Ryan, R. M., & Deci, E. L. (2000). Self-determination theory and the facilitation of intrinsic motivation, social development, and well-being. *American Psychologist, 55*(1), 68–78; Seifert, T. L. (2004). Understanding student motivation. *Educational Research, 46*(2), 137–149.

"On a scale of 1 to 10, with 10 being completely motivated and 1 being no motivation at all, how motivated are you?" When the client identifies their self-rated motivation, the educator can further clarify by asking, "What gives you this level of motivation?" and "How could you increase your motivation?" This approach can also be used to explore their level of interest and confidence in learning new behavior.

The third principle of motivational interviewing is *listening to the client*. When the nurse educator asks open-ended questions and actively listens to the client's response, this relays an expression of empathy and acceptance. Reflective listening or reflecting back what the client says allows the nurse to "get it right." This process of open-ended questioning and reflective listening shifts the encounter to a client-centered focus.

The final step in motivational interviewing is to *empower the client*. The nurse educator shows they believe the client is capable of learning and changing. Since it is the client, not the nurse, who must initiate behavior change, supporting self-efficacy effectively shifts "ownership" of the solution to the client. The client must want to learn for teaching to be effective. If the client is not motivated to learn, the nurse should make the effort to discuss their interests and concerns to improve the chances of the client education plan being successful (Lundahl et al., 2010).

Emotional Status

Emotions have an impact on client learning and can influence the ability to accurately process information. Clients learn and perform more successfully when they feel secure, happy, and excited about the subject matter. Emotions such as anger, anxiety, and sadness have the potential to interfere with the clients' ability to attend to the task at hand (Pekrun Götz, Frenzel, Barchfeld, & Perry, 2011). Anxiety is an emotion characterized by feelings of tension, worried thoughts, and physical changes such as increased blood pressure. Clients with anxiety may have recurring intrusive thoughts or concerns and may avoid situations out of worry (American Psychological Association, 2017).

Nurse educators should assess clients' anxiety levels, especially before new information is presented (Stephenson, 2006). Mild anxiety can be useful by making the person more alert to their environment. As attention and awareness are stimulated, concentration is enhanced. A client who is moderately anxious will likely be attentive to information that will help them manage their condition. Unfortunately, once anxiety escalates to moderate levels, concentration becomes compromised. If the client is in a state of crisis with a high level of anxiety, delay teaching until the crisis is over. Severe or panic anxiety is detrimental to learning and should be managed before health education begins (Stephenson, 2006).

Acknowledging anxiety and correcting client misconceptions can alleviate concerns and improve clients' ability to concentrate. Having the nurse educator talk about positive and negative feelings is one way to help clients learn how to deal appropriately with emotions. A goal of the nurse educator is to determine if the client's anxiety could interfere with the educational goal. A general assessment includes assessing the following:

- Behavioral cues: verbal and nonverbal
- Current stressors: physical, financial, and social
- Support systems
- Prior coping mechanisms
- Expectations or prior experiences with client education.

Anxiety measurement tools are useful to gauge the client's level of anxiety (Ashton & Oermann, 2014). These tools include:

- Mini-Assessment for Screening for Anxiety or Depression
- State-Trait Anxiety Inventory
- Hospital Anxiety and Depression Scale
- Psychosocial Vital Signs (PVS)

Our focus here is on the last tool, psychosocial vital signs (PVSs). It is a reliable assessment tool that combines the measurement of a client's psychological experiences with the nurse's observations of anxiety and human responses as part of a holistic view of the client's health status (Spade & Mulhall, 2010; Spade, Fitzsimmons, & Houser, 2015). Each client completes a self-report of their perceptions on a 1-to-10 scale in four areas: client's perception of the situation, client's sense of support, client's coping ability, and client's anxiety level. Nurse observations include the anxiety level measured as mild, moderate, severe, or panic, and observations of human responses, including cognitive, affective, spiritual, behavioral, and physical. This assessment tool engages clients through effective communication in a "collaborative patient centered relationship" (p. e150).

Regardless of the number on the PVS scale, the nurse must observe a client's level of anxiety. Even if a client states they are calm but you observe behavior or thinking that is at a higher level of anxiety, the client will have difficulty learning. A client with an anxiety level of severe or panic will be incapable of learning. These instances require the nurse to use therapeutic communication skills to facilitate clear thinking and delay health education to a more appropriate time. The PVS tool is shown in **Figure 4-1**.

Psychosocial Vital Signs Assessment Tool

| Name: |
| Date: |

Patient Self-Reporting [Scale: 1-10]

1. **Perception (P)** – Person's thinking about a situation.

   10   "What are your thoughts about your health situation and all it involves?"

   "On a scale from 1-10, how would you rate this health situation? One is positive/best & 10 is negative/worst?"

   1   Pt. Rating: ____

2. **Support (S)** – Person's sense of support from people who care.

   10   "Who is there for you right now?" "Who can you depend on to give you some support during this?"

   "How would you rate your sense of support? Is it a 1, everyone you need; is it a 10, meaning you have *no one*?"

   1   Pt. Rating: ____

3. **Coping (C)** – Person's sense of being able to cope with the situation.

   10   "How are you dealing with this?" Or, "How are you able to cope with this?"

   "From easiest to most difficult (1-10), how would you rate this health situation?"

   1   Pt. Rating: ____

4. **Anxiety (A)** – Person's feelings about the situation.

   10   "How are you feeling about all this?" Or, "How is this situation affecting you?"

   "From feeling calm to terrified, how would you rate yourself on a scale with calm being 1 and terrified being 10?"

   1   Pt. Rating: ____

Clinician Observation of Anxiety *[Scale: 1-4]

Anxiety Level	Thinking	Focus	Speech	Behavior	Physiology
4 Panic	• Impaired thinking	• Cannot be directed	• Incoherent • Shouting or Mute	• Aggressive or very withdrawn • Poor coordination • Terrified expression	• Hyperventilating • Dizziness • Heart Palpitations • Hypotension
3 Severe	• Cannot concentrate	• Focus on *specific* detail(s) • Cannot be redirected to *bigger picture*	• Rapid, loud or mute	• Persistent foot/finger tapping/leg swinging • Cannot relax • Startles easily	• Short of breath • Diaphoretic • Urinary urgency • Rapid heart rate
2 Moderate	• Poor concentration	• Easily directed & focused • May be in denial	• States is "nervous" and/or "upset"	• Fidgeting • Trembling lips	• Dry mouth • Pulse increasing
1 Mild	• Alert • Concentrates • Motivated		• Speaks clearly, normal rate/volume		• Heart rate & blood pressure sl. elevated

Summary: Patient Ratings & Clinician Observation of Anxiety Level = PVS: P___ S ___ C ___ Ax ___ *[   ]

Clinician Observation of Human Responses (Narrative Descriptors)

Cognitive/Thinking: Logical, goal-directed, clear, realistic understanding of situation, poor concentration, confused, denial, illogical, loose associations, hallucinations, "worried," suicidal or homicidal thoughts

Affective/Emotions: Feels calm, feeling capable or confident ("I think I can get though this."), uneasy, "nervous," labile, "upset," flat affect, guilt, shame, numb, sad, frustrated, angry, helpless, fearful, terror

Spiritual: Hopeful, "at peace," agony or anguish, speaks of losing purpose/meaning ("no reason to live"), hopeless, "abandoned/alone"

Behavioral: Sociable, calm, cooperative, fidgeting, restless, startles easily, vigilant, pacing, rapid speech, loud, hostile, aggressive, withdrawn

Physical: Vital signs WNL, adequate sleep, elevated VS, dilated pupils, SOB, N/V, diarrhea, insomnia, hypersomnia, loss of appetite, urinary urgency/frequency

PVS Assessment Tool: A baseline assessment of psychosocial variables of health: psychometric measurement of patient/client self-reporting, clinician observation, & narrative descriptors of human responses.
Copyright © 2015 C. M. Spade. Reprinted with permission.

Figure 4-1 Psychosocial Vital Signs

Biological Factors

Biological factors to assess include the client's health status, developmental stages, and physical challenges. The physical challenges include hearing impairments, vision impairments, speech impairment, and communication challenges that impact the development of the client education plan.

Health Status

Health status is the impact of disease as reported by the client. The range of disease manifestations include symptoms, functional limitation, and quality of life (Rumsfeld, 2002). Review the Stoeckel Wellness–Illness Functional Continuum in the first chapter, which plots the degrees of wellness and illness as reported by the client. This gives a picture of how the client perceives their state of health.

Many clients have multiple and complex illnesses. Factors that affect physical comfort such as pain, fatigue, anxiety, or fear can affect a client's ability and motivation to learn. The nurse educator needs to know this information as it interferes with learning. While clients may adjust well to the constraints imposed by illness, many find that illness causes them to lose the ability to perform a range of activities. Preteaching assessment should include a review of the client's health history, medication data, vital signs, physical assessment, and physical abilities. It is particularly important to assess clients' understanding of their condition, diagnoses, treatments, and expectations of self-care. See **Table 4-4**.

Developmental Stages

An individual's age and developmental stage significantly influence the ability to learn. At each stage throughout life there are major factors to consider when providing health education. These factors include the physical, cognitive, and psychosocial developmental stages, which are milestones of normal progression throughout the life cycle. Knowledge of development—including intellectual, psychosocial, and physiologic age—is necessary before selecting appropriate teaching strategies. Delayed development in any of these areas should be considered.

Children have limited past experience; adults learn more quickly because they are able to build upon previous knowledge. Chronological age is used to assess whether the developmental stage is as would be expected. Actual chronological age is only a relative indicator of someone's developmental stage and should not be taken in isolation to determine ability to learn (Ohio State University College of Medicine, 2017). Review the development stages in the chapters on the child, adult, and older learners.

Timing of teaching is also important because clients may not possess the necessary prerequisite skills and abilities to take advantage of new information and experiences. By supporting each stage in the developmental cycle, nurse educators ensure that clients are given care and help to reach their fullest potential. Developmentally appropriate teaching provides meaningful experiences at the optimal time so that clients can move to the next stage.

Physical Challenges

To assess clients accurately, you must be skilled at both verbal and nonverbal communication. It facilitates health education or hinders it. Words convey a variety of meanings and can be

Table 4-4 **Learner Health Status Assessment Tool**

Health Status Assessment	Client Response
Name	
Age	
Diagnosis ■ Understanding of the diagnosis ■ Explanation/acceptance of diagnosis	
Past medical history	
Present medical provider ■ Financial and insurance status	
Current physical abilities ■ Vital signs ■ Physical examination	
Medications taken ■ How much, when, and for how long ■ Food and drug interactions ■ Action of the medication ■ Side effects ■ Special considerations for mixing and administering; ability to read labels ■ Storage, expiration, disposal ■ Use of complementary alternative medications; recreational drugs	
Medical equipment and supplies ■ Safe use of equipment	
Diet and nutrition	
Pain management	
Personal care, hygiene, activities of daily living	
Exercise and other health interests	

misinterpreted, especially by members of different cultural groups. Never assume that all clients from one ethnic group hold the same beliefs. Nurses can overcome these problems by asking clients how they interpret the health message. Nonverbal communication (body cues, tone of voice, facial expression, and space between communicants) sends a message. Nurses who answer clients' or team members' questions, but appear to be in a hurry, will stifle communication (Horowitz, 2014).

Communication difficulties become challenges for nurses to overcome as they provide health education. The sources of these challenges come from clients as well as nurses (Pohl, 1981). This section addresses hearing, vision, and speech impairments as well as common communication problems affecting teaching and learning and suggests solutions.

Hearing Impairment

Approximately 17% of American adults (36 million) report some degree of hearing loss. Hearing loss increases with age. According to the National Institute on Deafness and Other Communication Disorders (2013), 18% of American adults aged 45–64 years, 30% of adults aged 65–74 years, and 47% of adults aged 75 years and older have hearing loss. The prevalence of hearing trouble is defined as a little trouble, a lot of trouble, or deaf. Clients with long-standing hearing deficits tell nurses what modes of communication work best for them. During the initial assessment, nurses can identify various ways that clients communicate. Clients or family members can provide this information, but family members should not be used as interpreters if confidentiality is a concern (Lieu, Sadler, Fullerton, & Stohlmann, 2007). To quickly assess a client's hearing, talk to the client in a normal tone of voice and note their reaction. If the client answers appropriately, you will know the client's hearing is sufficient for teaching and learning. Another assessment strategy is to cover your mouth and ask a question, again in a normal tone of voice. A client with a hearing impairment will not hear to answer you.

Check to see if the client wears a hearing aid. If so, make sure it is turned on and that the batteries are working. Creating other means of sound augmentation, such as cupping your hands around the client's ears or using the stethoscope in reverse, are other options.

When working with clients who have hearing loss, position yourself close on the same level as the client, and face the client so that person knows you are communicating with them. The client should be able to see your face and read your lips. Avoid standing in an area with a background glare because that interferes with the client's ability to read your lips. Remember to enunciate clearly and slowly. Clients who are proficient lip readers discern less than half of what you say and depend on the context and guesses to determine your meaning (Lieu et al., 2007).

Clients who use American Sign Language (ASL) require the assistance of a qualified sign language interpreter. This is considered a reasonable accommodation that healthcare institutions are required to offer under the Americans with Disabilities Act. Communication tools, such as flash cards, pencils and pads, and a laptop computer, are all helpful to clients who know how to write and have the strength to do so. If you are using writing, remember to choose simple words and phrases and write legibly (Lieu et al., 2007). The most important thing is to find a way to elicit responses that help you assess the client's hearing abilities and comprehension.

Vision Impairment

According to the Centers for Disease Control and Prevention (CDC) (2014), approximately 14 million people aged 12 years and older have a visual impairment, and 80% of those problems could be corrected to good vision with refractive lenses. The prevalence of visual impairment increases with age, particularly among those aged 40 years and older, based on 2010 census figures (U.S. Census Bureau, 2012). The most common problems in this age group are cataracts, refractive errors, diabetic retinopathy, glaucoma, and age-related macular degeneration. The number of people with visual impairments is expected to increase due to the increasing incidence of diabetes and other chronic diseases in the rapidly aging U.S. population (Prevent Blindness America, 2012).

As clients live longer and visual impairment becomes more common, it is an important consideration for nurses providing health education. To quickly assess a client's vision, provide a magazine or newspaper and have the client read a paragraph out loud. As the client does so, note the distance between the paper and the client's face. Holding the paper more than 14 inches away may indicate presbyopia or hyperopia. This will give you a sense of the client's visual capabilities and how to adapt your client education plan.

People who have been blind for some time develop other senses, particularly hearing, to compensate. Their acute hearing makes being shouted at a painful experience, and it does not aid their comprehension. Clients who are blind are unable to make use of body language or lip reading. If you are accustomed to expressing yourself with your hands and shaking your head, be aware that such clues are unavailable to blind clients. We recommend that you learn to use more verbal descriptions and psychomotor learning strategies that might not be necessary with a sighted client.

Blind people can often discern if a door is open or closed by the sound in a room. A door half-way ajar, however, can be deceiving and dangerous. We recommend that you close doors or open them all the way. It is also courteous to announce your presence and your purpose; for example, "My name is Fred Jones, and I'm your nurse for today. I'm going to teach you about . . ., then later we'll review. . . . Tell me what you are most interested in learning."

Speech Impairment

Speech problems impact clients who have a pathologic impairment in their ability to communicate. The type of impairment is related to the location and type of brain lesion. There are other forms of speech impairment related to a psychological etiology, but our reference here is to clients with brain pathology resulting in dysphasia, which is impairment of speech consisting of lack of coordination and failure to arrange words in the proper order. If a client has a form of dysphasia as an aftermath of stroke, consult with a psychologist and neurologist to determine the best way to deal with the speech impairment. One client may understand your words and not be able to answer. Another may not understand your words but can interpret your pantomime, drawings, flash cards, or objects. Shouting is not helpful in communicating with clients who are speech impaired.

Communication Challenges

The final communication problem we address is the one that nurses might inadvertently create. Mumbling, using technical jargon, or talking when you should be listening interferes with effective communication. Learn to recognize signs of poor client communication: confused facial expression, lack of attention, and questions that indicate a lack of understanding.

Suggestions to reduce this barrier include the art of active listening and observing. Listening includes not only hearing what the client is saying and the tone with which it is said, but also observing body language. It is developing a sensitivity to the spoken and unspoken meaning of the client's communication. Listening is an active, not a passive, process. Listening is an essential skill required of effective nurses in the educator role. Nurses may not agree with everything a client or team member says, but it is important to listen and respect the individual. Give complete attention to the learner and do not be preoccupied with your own thoughts. As educators, it is easy to think we should do the talking, but it is just as important to listen (Stuart, 2005).

As you listen, learn from the client's story and experience with the health problem. The problem may manifest in a manner that is not entirely consistent with the textbook description, which is called a variant of normal. Learn how the health problem is affecting the client's activities of daily living, and consider ways that you can help improve the client's adjustment and reaction. As a practicing nurse, you will be exposed to a broad range of human adaptations to health problems.

Social Factors

Social factors are important to assess in preparation of a client education plan. In this section, we discuss tools to assess clients' culture/support system, socioeconomic status, and generational differences.

Culture/Support System

Culture is a framework that a person uses in viewing the world, including health and the need for care. Culture shapes self-concept and influences perception of health teaching. Successful client education plans are congruent with client and family cultural values (Price & Cordell, 1994). Some cultures value education that will improve their condition while others view change or new practices as threatening. Nurses need to learn as much as possible about clients' cultural beliefs. An approach that focuses on inquiry, reflection, and analysis throughout the assessment process is helpful for acknowledging that culture is a critical factor that influences health beliefs and practices (Bonder, Martin, & Miracle, 2001).

The basic premise of the *cultural assessment* is that clients have a right to their cultural beliefs, values, and practices. These factors should be understood, respected, and considered when giving culturally competent care. Data obtained from a cultural assessment will help the client and nurse formulate a mutually acceptable, culturally responsive client education plan.

Cultural assessment begins by determining the client's understanding of their illness in the context of their unique culture. Remember that the client's personal interpretation of the illness experience is more significant than your view of the illness. The client's concept of the illness and its cause will help the nurse assess and prioritize learning needs and incorporate cultural beliefs into the client education plan (Chang & Kelly, 2007).

Another important aspect of cultural assessment is to determine how embedded the client is in their culture. Cultural embeddedness refers to the degree of alignment with the culture of origin. The extent of the client's cultural embeddedness has a major influence on healthcare teaching. Once assessment is done, cultural negotiation can take place in terms of agreeing on an education plan that is acceptable to both the client and nurse. The goal of cultural negotiation is to join Western and non-Western beliefs in a way that helps the client achieve a healthy outcome. Nurse educators should teach from a position of mutual understanding and collaboration rather than trying to impose traditional Western medical practices that are unlikely to be effective.

Assessment of cultural beliefs includes the client's perception of health, illness and treatment, family support, communication, behaviors, expression of pain, folk beliefs, and past experience with care and language. By asking the client and family questions about these issues, you can obtain valuable information needed for the client education plan. See **Box 4-1**.

The family comprises the social support context in which response to teaching occurs. Each person has a unique family background with certain cultural values that may have an effect on how teaching and learning is perceived. Family members are the client's support system and a vital link to helping clients learn.

The Joint Commission (2013) describes the family as the person or persons who plays a significant role in the individual's life, including persons not legally related to the individual. *Family* is defined here as any person who plays an important role in the client's life. How a family functions influences the health of its members and how individuals react to illness. Families must be included in the teaching process.

Box 4-1 Cultural Assessment of the Learner

- Do you identify with a particular ethnic or cultural group?
- Are you an immigrant or first- or second-generation citizen in this country?
- What do you believe is the cause of your health problem?
- What do you believe makes you healthy?
- What do you believe makes you sick?
- What remedies have you used to treat your health problems?
- What is your religious affiliation?
- Do you engage in any religious practices that you believe affect your health?
- Do you read and write in English, or do you prefer another language?
- What foods do you prefer, and what foods do you avoid?
- Do you have sufficient income (money) to meet your needs?
- Do you have family or friends who are available to support you if you need help?

The nurse as educator can help assess family style and structure by talking with the client and family and by observing their interaction. In particular, observe whom the client talks about most, who visits or accompanies the client, and the client's reaction to specific family members. **Table 4-5** is a way to begin assessing where the family is developmentally.

Information about family function, stress, transitions, and expectations can be invaluable in developing a client education plan that will be effective for both the client and family. You will be more effective if you are able to identify the family's interaction style and find ways to sustain and incorporate recommendations into it, rather than trying to impose a different pattern. A family's attitude and support, or lack of it, has a greater impact on the degree to which clients follow health advice than information presented by health professionals. The nurse educator can intervene in this type of situation by including the family members early in the teaching process to gain their understanding and support. The family may also influence the individual's beliefs about the severity of various illnesses and the benefits and costs of treatment. If family members fail to realize the importance of treatment, their attitudes may be a direct barrier to client adherence.

A rapid assessment tool called the *Family APGAR* was developed by Smilkstein (1978) to assess family function. This tool is composed of five questions that address *Adaptive Abilities*, *Partnership*, *Growth*, *Affection*, and *Resolve*. The following adaptation of the tool is intended to gain subjective information from clients to determine the level of support when learning new behaviors. See **Table 4-6**.

Socioeconomic Status

Nurses as educators need to consider socioeconomic factors when planning for health education because they have a significant impact on the health status of clients, especially underrepresented ethnic or racial groups. Socioeconomic factors include the client's living situation, financial status, health insurance or lack thereof, occupation or employment status, education, and the impact of these factors on the nature of the illness. Sufficient income affects the location and quality of housing, the level of education acquired, and occupational status. Clients' financial resources influence health status and health education. Middle- and high-income clients who are employed and have health insurance can purchase necessary services and supplies. A goal of Healthy People 2020 is to address health equity and disparities. Health equity is defined as the "attainment of the highest level of health for all

Table 4-5 Assessment of Family Basic Tasks

Family Life Stages and Tasks	Client Perspectives
Early married life ■ Establish a satisfying marriage	
Childbearing family (children from birth to 30 months) ■ Adjustment to parenthood ■ Encourage development of infants	
Preschool family (2.5–5 years) ■ Nurture children in growth-promoting ways	
School age family (5–13 years) ■ Socialize and educate children	
Family with teenagers (13–20 years) ■ Balance freedom with responsibility	
Launching family ■ Release young adults ■ Maintain supportive home base	
Middle-aged parents ■ Rekindle and rebuild the marriage relationship	
Aging family ■ Adjust to retirement and death of spouse	

Data from McKelvey, J. & Borgersen, M. (1990). Family development and the use of diabetes groups: Experience with a model approach. *Patient Education and Counseling, 16*(1), 61–67.

Table 4-6 Assessing Family Function

Assessment Items	Client's Responses
Adaptation: Describe your comfort level in asking help from your family to change behavior.	
Partnership: Describe your comfort level in communicating with your family about changing behavior.	
Growth: Describe your family's willingness to accept changes in your behavior.	
Affection: Describe your family's willingness to be supportive of your desire to change behavior.	
Resolve: Describe your comfort level in spending time with your family as you learn new behavior.	

Data from Smilkstein, G. (1978). The family APGAR: A proposal for family function test and its use by physicians. *Journal of Family Practice, 6*(6), 1231–1239.

people. Achieving health equity requires valuing everyone equally with focused and ongoing societal efforts to address avoidable inequalities, historical and contemporary injustices, and the elimination of health and healthcare disparities" (National Partnership for Action, 2011, para. 1). Health equity ensures that all people have access to health care regardless of their socioeconomic status, which is a goal of the Patient Protection and Affordable Care Act that passed in 2010 and was implemented in 2013.

Educational level has a profound impact on health status. The Centers for Disease Control and Prevention (CDC, 2012, https://www.cdc.gov/media/releases/2012/p0516_higher _education.html) reported a number of health differences between those with less than a high school education and those with a bachelor's degree or higher. Consider these examples:

- Obesity among boys and girls aged 2–19 years decreased as the educational level of the head of the household increased. Obesity of boys decreased from 24% to 11%; obesity of girls decreased from 22% to 7%.
- Among 25-year-old females, the obesity range decreased from 39–43% to 25% for those with more education.
- The range of adults aged 50–75 years of age who reported a colorectal test or procedure increased from 45% to 67% among those with more education.

Similar findings related to the level of education were reported for life expectancy, depression, smoking, and other health problems (National Center for Health Statistics, 2011).

Clients living alone need to be more independent in meeting their healthcare needs than clients living with supportive families and significant others. Clients living alone need realistic options that are suitable for their living situations. For example, a client living alone without neighbor or family support, who needs a dressing change, must be taught how to do this safely and independently. A client living with supportive family members may wish to have a family member learn how to do the dressing change. Clients experiencing homelessness and those living in shelters present additional health education challenges (Bassuk, Volk, & Olivet, 2010). A difference in health perception is illustrated when nursing students serving in a homeless shelter were puzzled when they observed a 5-year-old child rolling an apple around on the floor. When the student spoke with the child's mother, she explained that her child had never seen an apple before and thought it was a toy. Regardless of the living situation, health education must be appropriate to the client's actual situation. **Box 4-2** provides basic information needed to offer financially appropriate health suggestions.

Nurses as educators need to be more sensitive, creative, and adaptable in meeting the health education needs of clients with limited financial resources. Nurses should be aware that decreasing the number of prescriptions, not taking prescribed medications, and skipping doctor visits are common behaviors of clients with limited financial resources (Brown, 2008; Roberts-Grey, 2008). Part of your assessment is to verify whether clients are taking all their medications and teach them

---

Box 4-2 Rapid Socioeconomic Assessment Tool

- What is your occupation?
- Is your monthly income sufficient to meet your expenses?
- Do you have health insurance?
- Do you have unmet financial needs related to health care?

the importance of taking their medications as prescribed. A trusting nurse–client relationship will encourage the client to discuss their needs so the education can be appropriate.

In addition to socioeconomic factors affecting illness, clients' illnesses can impinge on their socioeconomic well-being. Individuals who are obese or suffering the effects of AIDS or hepatitis C may find that their diagnosis is a barrier to employment, social freedom, and other sources of socioeconomic support. Illnesses that family and friends perceive to be contagious can impinge on clients' socioeconomic well-being and lead to social isolation.

Generational Differences

Nurses as educators must consider the age of the client as an important assessment factor when preparing health education offerings to adult learners. It is important to be aware of potential factors that can impede or promote learning. When building a client education plan, it is helpful to consider fundamental generational differences beyond learners' control to choose effective teaching methods and strategies. **Table 4-7** examines the psychological and generational differences among the silent, baby boomer, generation X, millennial, born generation Z, and born generation Alpha generations. This is not intended to describe an individual, but rather to understand a cohort of learners.

Intellectual Factors

Intellectual factors are important to assess and include the client's educational level, willingness to learn, and current background knowledge. Background knowledge includes assessing recall and understanding (knowledge); assessing analysis, critical thinking, and performance (skills); and assessing attitudes and values (attitudes).

Educational Level

You will promote effective learning if you are aware of the client's intellectual ability, communicate respectfully, and avoid "talking down" to them. The term *intellect* refers to an understanding of the mental powers and mental capacity of a particular person. Success in school is generally closely related to the level of intellect. Clients with limited intelligence often encounter difficulty in understanding and following health teaching. This can be a result of a learning disability.

The nurse educator should also be cognizant of any change in mental capacity or impairment of decision-making ability (Church & Watts, 2007). Four abilities should be assessed (Tunzi, 2001):

- Ability to understand information about treatment
- Ability to understand how information applies to them personally
- Ability to reason with the information
- Ability to make a choice and express it

If an abrupt change in the mental functioning of older clients is noted, this may indicate the need to administer the Mini-Mental Status State Examination (MMSE) (Folstein, Folstein, & McHugh, 1975). Simple open-ended screening questions can also be used to detect reduced capacity. For example, "What is your treatment about?" and "Why is it difficult to manage your medications at home?" (Church & Watts, 2007).

Knowledge of the nature of the client's intellect is valuable preparation for teaching. The intellectual capacity of the individual is of prime importance in determining how to design the learning process. Factors that influence mastery of what has been taught may affect success of the

Table 4-7 Generational Differences

Years	Silent 1925–1945	Boomer 1946–1964	Generation X 1965–1980	Millennial 1981–2000	Born Generation Z 1997–2012	Born Generation Alpha 2010 and 2025
Other names	Veterans Traditionalists	Consciousness generation Me generation	Lost generation Latchkey Slacker generation	Generation Y Echo boom Generation next	Gen Z, The Realists, The Internet Generation, Zoomers	Gen alpha, mini millennials, "Gen C" or "Generation COVID"
Family life	Earliest to marry and have children Divorce common Large number of women entered the workforce	Religious and spiritually oriented Health conscious Defer childbirth until later in life Attentive to children; helicopter parents	Adult oriented at an early age Less parental supervision than earlier generations Little peer interaction in childhood Balance work and family	Children considered special and are eagerly anticipated Families with fewer children Balance work and family	Parenting style encourages realistic expectations. Form small families later in life that are more diverse and "untraditional." Favor balance in family life and work.	Alpha has spent more time at home with their parents as a result of the COVID-19 pandemic. First generation to grow up largely during the COVID-19 pandemic and the response to it. They are children of millennials and more likely to be only children.
Work	Many entered the helping professions Hard work is good Respect authority Sacrifice Duty before fun Adhere to the rules	Workaholics Career focused Work efficiently Personal fulfillment Desire quality Will question authority	First to seek balance between work and life Self-reliant Want structure and direction Skeptical Challenge others Work is a difficult challenge	Financially oriented More discretionary income than any previous group Multitasking Tolerant Goal oriented	Want a mentor not a boss. Willing to work harder than previous generations, Want job security, good benefits, clear expectations and a retirement plan. Technology immersed, used to diversity, flexible hours. Believe in social responsibility	They bring tech-savvy skills, entrepreneurial spirit, and drive for inclusiveness and sustainability to the workplace.

Learning preferences and interactive style	Like traditional structure Will not contradict instructor in public Do not like being singled out in discussions Prefer to practice alone May not ask questions in discussions May struggle with technology Prefer learning individually	Enjoy working creatively and independently Sensitive to criticism May have significant professional experience Like interaction, discussion, and group work May dislike authoritarian teachers Prefer learning as part of a team	Self-reliant Like frequent feedback May lack interpersonal skills Largest segment of online learners Often impatient but adaptable and informal Technologically capable Value autonomy Prefer an informal learning approach	Team oriented, like group work Multitask and technological experts Goal and achievement oriented Require more structure and mentoring Enjoy active learning Prefer participative learning	Have a short attention span, are savvy consumers, seek self-development, want self-expression, prefer collaboration and participative learning style. Want learning environments that flex their aptitude for self-reliance and their ability to self-educate. Prefer class discussion and working through problems as a group	Preference for visual and interactive learning. More likely to engage with educational content that is presented in an entertaining and interactive way. Tend to learn better through visual aids and hands-on experiences. They are comfortable with technology, prefer visual and interactive learning, value collaborative learning, benefit from personalized learning experiences, and have a lifelong learning mindset.
Communication style	Formal Memo	In person	Direct Immediate	Email Texting Voice mail	Use smartphones, apps/Snapchat/video, use images and symbols. Prefer instant messaging, face-to-face interaction or facetime. Have an 8-second attention span and have trained their brains to expect instant gratification.	Habitual use of social media, including sharing photographs, videos, or stories. Will be online from birth affected by the emerging use of artificial intelligence (AI) both through voice assistants like Siri or Alexa and natural language processing tools like ChatGPT.

(*continues*)

Table 4-7 Generational Differences

(continued)

Years	Silent 1925–1945	Boomer 1946–1964	Generation X 1965–1980	Millennial 1981–2000	Born Generation Z 1997–2012	Born Generation Alpha 2010 and 2025
Teaching strategies	Emphasize important points in the client education plan Use font large enough to see writing, and read handouts Fastest-growing group learning Encourage periodic movement while teaching	Give time to practice skills Use font large enough to see for older learners May not like role-playing exercises Enjoy most team projects Like being group leaders Like well-organized materials with headings	May resist group work outside of a formal class Give individual attention Prefer information in short lectures (15–20 minutes) Like working in small groups to review information Prefer graphics that are visually appealing and reflect the culture Want to have explanation for learning and skill acquisition	Present information and activities in steps Use up-to-date technology and resources Make learning relevant to real-life situations Encourage creativity and be creative in presentations Give supplemental reading and instructional materials	Prefer the use of mentors and peer experiences. Want to be actively engaged in their learning, not passive bystanders. Prefers digital textbooks so they can easily access them on devices, they use daily. They are proactive, independent, social/internet computer/app-based.	Literate in digital technology and cyberspace through the use of video calls, meetings, and remote classroom settings. Prefer visual and interactive learning. Teacher should be able to implement technology, support student relationships, be forward thinking, and embrace change.

Data from Baker College Effective Teaching and Learning Department. (2004). *Teaching across generations.* Retrieved from https://my.methodistcollege.edu/ICS/icsfs/teaching_across_generations_-_Baker_College.pdf?target=e083a9b8-f814-456a-8cb1-64c36a0bba4c; Parent Institute for Quality Education. (2023). *Generational Differences or Generational Strengths?* Retrieved from https://www.piqe.org/generational-differences-or-generational-strengths/

Pew Research Center. (May 14, 2020). *On the cusp of adulthood and facing an uncertain future: What we know about Gen Z so far.* https://www.pewresearch.org/social-trends/2020/05/14/on-the-cusp-of-adulthood-and-facing-an-uncertain-future-what-we-know-about-gen-z-so-far-2/. Accessed July 12, 2023.

client education plan. If the plan proceeds too rapidly and does not constantly evaluate the extent to which the content is grasped, the client may not successfully meet the learning outcomes.

Assessment of the *level of literacy* is essential in educating clients. Approximately 30 million people older than 16 years of age in the United States cannot read better than the average third grader, 14% read at or below the fifth-grade level, and 29% read at the eighth-grade level, according to ProLiteracy Worldwide (2014). Health literacy is a concern in working with clients who need supplemental written material but are unable to read at a level sufficient to understand. Health literacy has profound implications for nurses as educators while they communicate with clients and provide health education reading materials.

The vocabulary that clients use is, to some extent, a measure of their health literacy and educational level. Those with large vocabularies are more apt to comprehend what you are saying. Clients with less education are less likely to comprehend more abstract and technical language that you might inadvertently use. Concrete answers and examples are more likely to be meaningful to those with less education. A client's vocabulary impacts the type of health education materials you provide, such as booklets and pamphlets (Seligman et al., 2007).

As you interact with clients, assess their knowledge about health and illness. Such an assessment provides clues that can guide health education activities. The client's level of education is often related to knowledge about health and illness. In general, the higher the level of education, the more likely the client is to engage in health-promoting behaviors such as exercise, proper diet, and smoking cessation (National Center for Health Statistics, 2011).

Clients who research health problems may have comprehensive knowledge of their illnesses. Nurses report this phenomenon more often in this era of increased availability of information on the internet and the vast availability of materials and publications from libraries and healthcare providers. Clients are often articulate and well informed about the latest treatments for disease and are eager to collaborate with healthcare providers.

Health literacy of the client is important in health education. To assess health literacy, we are recommending a tool called the Newest Vital Sign (NVS), published by the American Academy of Physicians (AAP; Weiss et al., 2005) which can be accessed at the AAP website. The tool takes approximately 3 minutes to administer and involves clients reading a nutrition label and then answering six questions. Four or more correctly answered questions indicate adequate literacy. The tool is also available in Spanish.

Assessing health literacy is also a concern when teaching team members, not those who have years of formal educational preparation, but for team members in support roles such as nursing assistants. Team members may have limited knowledge of health and illness and often possess inaccurate information. They benefit from in-service activities that advance their understanding of their responsibilities. When preparing educational activities for team members, it is helpful to know what kind of theoretical and experiential preparation they have for their respective roles. This will help you plan educational activities that build on their current level of knowledge. If clients or team members are from a different culture or have limited English-speaking ability, this can affect their vocabulary and communication skills.

Health literacy and educational level are only approximations of what an individual client or team member can grasp. As educators, nurses must monitor the feedback from clients as they engage them in educational activities to determine their effectiveness. Also keep in mind that emotions may influence clients' ability to understand. For example, clients and their families have repeatedly stated to us that their anxiety level and other concerns interfered with their ability to comprehend material that would be quite understandable under normal circumstances.

Willingness to Learn

Assessing willingness to learn is a dimension of the intellectual factors. Willingness to learn is an aroused interest or expression of curiosity that occurs when the client makes a conscious choice to learn. It is manifest by listening to the client's concerns and the questions they ask. This may occur while the nurse is administering medications, performing nursing procedures, or delivering nursing care. It can be an unplanned opportunity when the client is open to informal health education, or it can occur during a deliberate encounter between educator and client. Willingness to learn is most intense when the client's life situation creates the desire or necessity to acquire new knowledge, attitudes, and skills. See **Table 4-8**.

Determining the *learning styles* of clients can assist the nurse educator in understanding clients' willingness to learn. Assessment of learning styles can be accomplished using the VARK method (Fleming & Mills, 1992). This method categorizes learning styles into Visual, Auditory, Reading/Writing, and Kinesthetic. Visual learners have a preference for seeing and thinking in pictures. Auditory learners have a preference for learning materials through listening. Some learners prefer reading and writing as a style of learning. Kinesthetic learners have a preference to experience, move, touch, and do. Asking your client their preferred learning style aids the nurse educator in preparing a client education plan that supports individual learning.

Background Knowledge

It is important for the nurse as educator to check the client's background knowledge and recall of information. Doing so is grounded in learning theories (Ausubel, Novak, & Hannesian, 1968; Dewey, 1938) and is supported by research on the learning process (Dochy, Segers, & Buehl, 1999; Fisher & Frey, 2009; Tobias, 1994). The theory of constructivism supports this view of learning and proposes that new knowledge is constructed from old (Brooks & Brooks, 1993). It holds that as nurse educators, it is essential we make connections among new information that

Table 4-8   Assessment of Willingness to Learn

Level 1	Client verbalizes no interest in health education and avoids the topic. Client holds the healthcare team responsible for their health. Client lacks physiologic or developmental abilities required for learning.
Level 2	Client verbalizes some interest in health education but is easily distracted and unable to stay on the topic. Client is willing to follow some healthcare team directions. Client has limited physiologic or development abilities.
Level 3	Client verbalizes more interest in health education and is able to stay on topic for brief periods of time. Client seeks and follows healthcare team directions. Client has the requisite physiologic or developmental skills.
Level 4	Client verbalizes great interest in health education and asks many questions. Client follows healthcare team directions and assumes responsibility for their own health. Client has full physiologic and developmental ability to learn.

is being presented and clients' prior experiences. Determining what clients already know allows you to do the following:

- Target specific knowledge gaps (Angelo & Cross, 1993).
- Become aware of the diverse backgrounds of your clients.
- Create a bridge between clients' previous knowledge and new material.
- Check for misconceptions that may hinder learning new material (Ambrose et al., 2010).

You can choose from a variety of methods to assess clients' background knowledge and skills. Some methods are direct measures of clients' capabilities, such as written tests. Other methods use indirect measures, such as clients' self-reports of what they know. The method of assessment will depend on what is to be learned. Classroom Assessment Techniques (CATs) are a set of specific activities that educators use to quickly gauge learners' comprehension (Angelo & Cross, 1993). They are used to assess individual or group understanding of the material, and with minor modifications they apply to teaching in healthcare settings.

The following sections are a sample of different background learning assessment techniques using Bloom's taxonomy categories of knowledge, skills, and attitudes. These techniques may be used with individuals or groups. The three main areas of background knowledge assessment include assessing recall and understanding (knowledge); assessing skills in analysis, critical thinking, and performance (skills); and assessing awareness of attitudes and values (attitudes).

Assessing Recall and Understanding (Knowledge)

Assessing recall and understanding of knowledge can be done in several ways. A primary approach to determining prior knowledge is through the Background Knowledge Probe. This consists of short, simple questions that can be administered either verbally or written and are usually referred to as a pretest. This approach is helpful in determining the most effective starting point for learning and the appropriate level to begin instruction. Constructing a pretest serves several purposes, including: (1) current knowledge status, (2) guidance for future activities, (3) means of comparison for posttest results, and (4) determination of whether prerequisite knowledge is achieved.

To prepare a pretest, determine what key ideas and concepts you are trying to teach. Establish learning outcomes and objectives. Review the client's record or the group's course outline to help with this step. Brainstorm 10 to 15 questions that would effectively assess prior knowledge based on the learning outcomes and objectives you reestablished. A simple strategy to use in preparing questions is to reword the learning outcomes or objectives as questions. Be sure to select a variety of types of questions (multiple choice, true–false, fill in the blank, etc.). Varying the types of questions will peak the clients' interest in learning the material. Base your types of questions on your assessment and the information being taught.

Another approach to assessing prior knowledge is a technique called muddiest point. Here the individual or group is asked to share either verbally or in writing what questions confuse them about the proposed topic. For example, in an initial meeting the nurse educator says: You have heard about the different treatment options for acne. What questions would you still like answered regarding these treatment options?

A memory matrix could also be used to help determine how clients recall content and organize information. A matrix is created with rows, columns, and empty cells. This strategy assesses the ability of the learner to recall content and display skill in organizing information. This method can be presented on a white board or with cardboard figures and pictures on a desk or table. A

Table 4-9 **Memory Matrix Example for Increasing Red Blood Cell Count**

Nutrients	Action	Amount	Foods	Medication
Iron				
Folic Acid				
B12				
Copper				
Vitamin A				

memory matrix example for a client with iron deficiency anemia who needs to increase their red blood cell count is shown in **Table 4-9**.

Assessing Analysis, Critical Thinking, and Performance (Skills)

Assessing skill in analysis, critical thinking, and performance is done through a variety of approaches, depending on what aspect of skill is being assessed. In the problem recognition task, clients are presented with examples of common problems and are asked to identify the particular type of problem in each example. Clients read or are told the scenario; then they identify the problem. A sample problem is presented below. Identify and explain Mrs. Simpson's problem.

> Margaret Simpson is an 86-year-old woman who has lived alone in her own home for the past 20 years. Her son and daughter both live in different states but have frequent telephone contact and yearly visits. They are concerned about their mother and believe it is time for her to move into an assisted living facility where she will receive regular meals and routine assistance with activities of daily living. This is a sensitive topic, and the children are having a difficult time persuading their mother to see the benefits of moving.

Critical thinking skills can also be assessed by the series of events chain (see **Figure 4-2**). This method describes states of something in a linear procedure or the goals, actions, and outcomes of a behavior. Clients can be assessed either individually or as a group. Key questions for this activity could include the following: What is the object, procedure, or initiating event? What are the stages or steps? How do they lead to one another? What is the final outcome? From the answers, prior knowledge can be assessed regarding the order of events.

Assessing performance skills can be achieved in a number of ways, including client demonstrations, and work samples. To demonstrate skills, clients are given scenarios and are asked to perform skills such as checking blood glucose levels. Abilities are assessed through direct observation. Skills can also be assessed through past performance and past documentation, such as medical records or nurses' notes.

Assessing Attitudes and Values (Attitudes)

Assessing clients' awareness of their attitudes and values can be accomplished using the opinion poll strategy. This approach provides anonymity for clients and allows the educator to understand their opinions. Examples of survey statements are as follows: (1) it is important to stop smoking, and (2) drinking five beers a day is a safe amount of alcohol.

Figure 4-2 Series
of Events Chain

Another strategy to determine values is through a self-confidence survey. This type of survey consists of a few simple questions aimed at getting a rough measure of the client's self-confidence in relation to a specific skill or ability. Examples of questions are as follows: How confident are you about breastfeeding your baby? Do you feel comfortable giving your baby medication for a high fever?

In addition to using tools to determine background knowledge, each health team member has valuable information about clients and their learning needs and abilities. Collaborating with others who care for the client gives you a better picture and helps you design more effective teaching strategies. Determining learning needs, and preferred learning style, are all requirements included in The Joint Commission standards for client and family education. The process of assessing needs begins when health team members identify a need for a client to learn new skills or acquire more information. If a client asks a question (What exactly will this operation involve? How will I handle this when I go home?), they are already identifying the information need. If you, rather than the client, identify the need, your job will be not only to deliver the information in such a way that the client is able to understand it, but also to demonstrate to the client why the information is important.

In some instances, there are differences between the client's and the nurse educator's view of the need to know. The educator may perceive the need for information when the client does not. For example, a nurse tries to give the client medication information during discharge teaching. The client's response is, "I don't need to know that. Whatever my doctor ordered is fine. I don't need to know the details." In this example, the best approach would be for the nurse to start with why the information is important and why it is necessary to know information before taking medication.

Do not be tempted to overlook background knowledge when teaching new information. To do so is to build on an unstable foundation. Background knowledge has a profound influence on clients' abilities to comprehend what they are taught and believe. Its effect can be observed directly by the clients' expressions of knowledge on the topic. The indirect effect can be determined by the clients' abilities to resolve problems. Determining background knowledge is a part of the learning needs assessment that influences the nurse educator's approach to developing the client education plan.

Environmental Factors

Environmental factors are important to assess because they impact teaching and learning. Here we address the various settings where nurses as educators work with clients. The settings include the hospital, long-term care and assisted-living facility, private home, school, worksite, and community. Also important is the physical and emotional atmosphere where teaching and learning occurs.

Types of Settings

The teaching and learning settings we consider here include the hospital, long-term care and assisted-living facility, private home, school, work site, and community. Each has unique characteristics that affect the way health education is delivered.

Hospital

The value of health education is supported by hospitals. Although the quantity and quality are frequently affected by policies and administrative support, the importance of health education in acute care settings is reflected in role expectations and job descriptions. The mission and philosophy of hospitals reflect the importance of client education. Hospital administrators are now required to meet The Joint Commission standards by providing necessary support and resources for patient teaching. Every hospital has an education department that focuses on client and staff education. They are responsible for discharge planning and case management for clients and competency training for staff. Hospitalized clients have teaching needs that revolve around acute illness and discharge planning. Some hospitals also offer classes for the community related to health promotion.

Long-Term Care and Assisted-Living Facilities

Long-term care facilities include nursing homes, assisted-living homes, and other facilities in which care is provided for clients over a prolonged period of time. Long-term care includes a wide range of services that are provided over an extended period of time to clients who need help to perform normal activities of daily living because of a variety of health problems. Services within long-term care include rehabilitative therapies, skilled nursing care, palliative care, and social services, as well as supervision and a wide range of supportive personal care provided by family caregivers or home-care agencies. Most long-term care and assisted-living facilities also have education departments.

The goals of long-term care include training to help clients adjust to or overcome limitations. Like hospitals, health education in long-term care and assisted-living facilities can occur individually or in groups. Effective educational programs can prevent minor illnesses or injuries from progressing to the point of needing professional intervention. Increased client awareness through education can also result in earlier detection of problems and timelier outpatient intervention, thus decreasing hospitalizations. Clients with chronic illnesses who have been empowered through health education programs generally have better coping skills and are usually less reliant on healthcare providers.

Assisted living facilities for the rapidly aging population are becoming more popular. They provide apartment-type living for those who need only selected services, which are individualized to the client. For example, some clients may take one or all meals a day in a central dining room. Others may need assistance only with bathing or dressing. General housekeeping laundry service is also available. If additional services are needed, such as checking on selected clients more frequently, that can be arranged.

Private Home

Many health problems are being treated at home as chronic illnesses increase in an aging population. Home care is a formal, government-regulated program of care that provides a range of services offered by different agencies and are delivered by a variety of healthcare professionals. Among clients aged 65 years and older, cancer was more common among males, and essential hypertension was more common among females. In this group, females were more likely to be aged 85 years and older, and men were more likely to receive home care as postacute care (CDC, 2012). Common chronic diseases that are prevalent in this age group include heart disease, cancer, chronic lower respiratory diseases, and stroke. Also increasing in frequency are Alzheimer's disease and diabetes mellitus (CDC, 2010). This shows the importance of addressing health education in private homes.

Home visits for older clients have been found to have direct benefits when measured in terms of morbidity and admission to long-term institutional care. Clients are discharged from acute care settings with increasingly complex treatment and learning needs. Families are expected to learn skills and information that, only a decade ago, were reserved for healthcare personnel. Home care visits are also made by community health nurses to parents with newborns to teach them proper baby care. The nurse also observes and assesses progress in child growth and development.

Clients often find it easier to learn in familiar surroundings. Remember that in the client's home you are a guest and are not in charge, as you are when the client is in a healthcare institution. During home care nursing, it will be easier for you to be realistic in your teaching because you can see the reality of the client's environment. Family dynamics that may enhance or impede recovery will be more evident in the home, which means you will likely be more realistic in teaching the family and the client.

School

School is an ideal site for health education because it is a focal point for reducing health risk behaviors and improving the health status of youth. Based on the potential to reach a large number of youth, schools are logical sites for interventions that help them develop skills, change health behaviors, and empower them to take responsibility for their own health. Some of the most effective health education efforts for youth incorporate peer support. Although most schools require health education, teachers are often not comfortable with sensitive subjects and need the contributions of school nurses in addressing certain topics.

If you are teaching a class, you will want to find out more information about the group of students. Ask about the culture of the classroom. What ages are the children? Are they accustomed to discipline and to giving polite attention? Are they able to sit and listen? What are their learning style preferences? What health education tools are already available? This is important information for the client education plan.

Schools are often good settings for teaching and learning with multiple audiovisual aids. Teaching disease prevention and providing anticipatory guidance are excellent topics. Nurses are informed role models to address today's concerns about how to avoid communicable diseases and substance abuse and teach behaviors that promote healthful living. Learn the age of the group you will speak to and address age-appropriate topics. Ideally, health education begins in grade school.

Work Site

Work-site settings are beneficial to managers, employees, and the community. Nurses in work-site settings are effective providers of health education. These educational programs provide an opportunity to support health while reducing healthcare costs, increasing worker productivity, and decreasing absenteeism. Interventions in the workplace may target behavioral change, the development of policies to facilitate a healthier and safer workplace, and environmental support to maintain behavioral changes.

Concerns that nurses in work-site settings can address include consultation about cost-effective insurance plans, infection and accident control, and health promotion and maintenance programs. These nurses can also conduct physical assessments, teach prevention to employees, provide screening services, produce health newsletters, and inform employers about major health hazards in the setting. The political system at the work site greatly affects the ability of the nurse as an educator to be effective. Self-help groups for alcoholism, smoking cessation, stress management, prevention of accidents, and safety precautions are all worthy topics for consideration.

Community

Health education in the community focuses on health problems identified as a priority by the public health department or other community agency responsible for community health planning. The focus of nurses as educators in public health is to provide direct care through a process of evaluation and assessment of the needs of individuals in the context of their population group. Regardless of the environment within the community where nurses work, the health education process can be used to establish partnerships with clients so nurses can provide education and counseling to promote self-management. Nurses as educators work with other care providers to plan, develop, and support systems and programs in the community that emphasize health promotion, disease prevention, and access to care.

Community assessment focuses on populations rather than individuals. Those individuals who make up a population share one or more personal or environmental characteristics. A population can be categorized as a population at risk or a population of interest (Keller, Strohschein, & Briske, 2008). A population at risk shares an identified risk factor or risk exposure that threatens its health. For example, all individuals who smoke are at risk for developing respiratory and cardiovascular health problems.

A population of interest may be basically healthy but could improve its health and prevent illness from developing. Examples include making home visits to new mothers to encourage breastfeeding or working with adolescents to prevent sexually transmitted diseases by offering programs in public schools. Other populations of interest may be needs-based, such as mothers and infants or cancer survivors; age-based groups, such as adolescents or older adults (65 years and older); gender-based groups, such as men or women; and ethnic groups, such as African American, Hispanic American, Asian American, and Native American.

Physical and Emotional Atmosphere

The teaching and learning environment is composed of the psychological environment and physical environment in which teaching and learning take place. It is the nurse's responsibility to establish this environment to maximize learning.

The conditions in which learning takes place are important. This includes the room, written materials, equipment, supplies, and other instructional materials. Whether in the hospital or at the home, the conditions for learning must be favorable and adequate if teaching is to produce the desired results. It is difficult to do a good job of teaching in a poor environment without adequate equipment and instructional materials.

The setting where learning occurs also contains a variety of events that influence learning. For some clients, a room full of interesting stimuli increases their excitement about the task, and for others, high levels of stimulation overextend their ability to attend to the task. As such, the context that best suits the learning goal should be identified and arranged. In a given setting, a particular event will trigger the client to answer a question, complete an analysis, perform a skill, or other type of engagement in learning. How best to provide instructional triggers so that the client successfully participates in the learning experience is identified by careful assessment.

Psychological Environment

As educators, nurses create the emotional tone for the learning environment. A positive, enthusiastic tone does much to make clients comfortable and helps to create a therapeutic environment. If the nurse is stressed, clients pick up on it and may assume that the stress is related to them. Conversely, if the nurse enjoys teaching and shows enthusiasm, that perception is conveyed as well.

Showing respect for learners and valuing their questions and input are all part of creating a positive teaching and learning environment. The nurse's attitude should be nonjudgmental. However, that does not mean the nurse agrees with or condones the client's beliefs and statements. Respect is accepting and valuing the client. The nurse has a responsibility to correct misinformation.

Physical Environment

As educators, nurses are responsible for assessing the physical environment and making it as conducive to learning as possible (Hall, 2013). The physical environment includes space; temperature; visual, auditory, and olfactory stimuli; equipment; resources; furniture arrangement; physical comfort; and sufficient time for learning.

Space is needed so you can display and get maximum use of your instructional materials. This is true whether you are speaking to an individual, a family, or a group in a living room or an auditorium. Examine the space for sight and sound barriers. Pillars will make it difficult for clients to see you. Poorly placed partitions may act as sound barriers that will prevent sound from getting through.

Temperatures that are too hot or too cold interfere with learning. Clients who are distracted by heat spend their time fanning themselves; if they are cold, they clutch their arms instead of listening to you.

Visual stimuli are distracting and interfere with vision. Do not place yourself in front of a sunny window. The glare behind you turns you into a shadowy figure. Your audience will be squinting and wanting to look elsewhere. Try to pick a spot where you can control the appearance of the learning situation. If you cannot control all the stimuli, look for ways to control the area in which you intend to teach. In the hospital, you may draw the curtain around the client's bed. One way to modify sound in a client's room is to hang a sign on the door that says, "Client teaching in progress. Please return in X minutes. Thank you."

If your client is a family, you may be able to cordon off a corner of the waiting room. In a dining area of an extended-care facility, you may be able to use moveable screens to provide privacy. Auditory stimuli may or may not be under your control. Choose a quiet place and turn off your cell phone. Olfactory stimuli are distracting and can be deflected by a fan. You could try cutting a lemon or putting a drop of cinnamon oil on a nearby heated surface, such as a light fixture, or use a room deodorizer.

The availability of equipment and teaching resources influence your options. Find out what equipment, expertise, and resources are available in the hospital or community to enhance

Table 4-10 Assessment of Learners' Emotional and Physical Environment

Description of the learner: ■ Age/gender ■ Culture	
Type of setting: ■ Hospital ■ Long-term care and assisted-living facilities ■ Private home ■ School ■ Work site ■ Community	
Emotional atmosphere: ■ Tone ■ Level of stimuli ■ Educator enthusiasm	
Physical environment: ■ Space ■ Temperature ■ Auditory effects ■ Olfactory effects ■ Equipment and resources ■ Room arrangements ■ Level of comfort ■ Time provided	

teaching. Observe where the electrical outlets are if you will need them, and arrange the room to allow access to the outlets.

Arrange furniture in a way that is conducive to learning. Be sure to take into account the learning objectives and teaching strategies. Do you plan to have the clients interact with one another? Do you wish a relative to see everything you are doing for the client? Do you plan to make a presentation to a group or have a guest lecturer? Nurses should be involved in designing the spaces where teaching occurs.

Physical comfort is an important variable in enhancing the teaching and learning environment. Teach clients after the morning routine when they are comfortable and relaxed. You will find that your clients learn better when they are sufficiently medicated to not be distracted by pain but are not too sleepy to pay attention. Lighting and temperature also affect comfort. You will want the lighting to be bright enough to allow lip readers to see your face but not so strong it creates glare.

Time is a factor to consider. Be sure you have sufficient time to teach. If time is limited, be selective about what you teach, focusing on only the most important topics. Do not make your teaching session too long. A mistake we have seen busy nurses make is trying to include too much information too quickly in the available time. **Table 4-10** is an evaluation tool to assist you. The second column is to record your pertinent observations.

Summary

This chapter addressed important learner assessment factors to consider when planning for health education with individuals, families, groups or communities, or health team members. Psychological factors to assess include perception, motivation, and emotional status. Biological factors to assess are health status, developmental stages, and physical challenges. Social factors to assess are the culture/support system, socioeconomic status, and generational differences. Intellectual factors to assess include educational level, willingness to learn, and background knowledge. And finally, the environmental factors to assess include the types of settings and the physical and emotional atmosphere.

Tools were provided to address each of the learner assessment factors. These tools will assist the nurse educator in gathering important information in anticipation of building an effective client education plan. Be aware that a client may *present at different levels of assessment*, which means that the nurse as educator will need to adjust the plan to accommodate needs at each stage or level. This makes the client education plan a constantly evolving tool to help the client reach the optimal outcome. A more extensive explanation of the client education plan will be covered in the Client Education Plan chapter.

Exercises

Exercise I: Perception in Assessment

Purpose: Demonstrate the skill of "direct perception checking" when working with a client who is not taking their medication.
Directions:

1. Describe the three parts of perception checking that are outlined in this chapter.
2. Give examples of how you would question the client using the three parts to interpret why the client is not taking their medication.
3. How does using perception checking help you effectively communicate with the client?

Exercise II: Assessing for Client Anxiety

Purpose: Apply the knowledge of how anxiety affects learning when working with a client that you suspect is anxious and is learning how to do self-injections of medication.
Directions:

1. State general areas to assess for anxiety before teaching.
2. Describe two tools used to assess levels of anxiety.
3. Give an example of how you would apply knowledge that the client is anxious when preparing a client education plan.

Exercise III: Assessing Family Support

Purpose: Examine how a client's family function affects learning in a client situation where you suspect there is spousal abuse.
Directions:

1. Describe the five areas of family function assessment you will use to gain information about the client's family interactions.

2. What findings in these five areas would cue you to dysfunction and the need for further preparation before teaching?
3. Give examples of how you would use family support information to impact your client education plan.

Exercise IV: Assessment of Willingness to Learn

Purpose: Apply assessment of willingness to learn.
Directions: Form small groups of three to four members and share in your groups responses to the questions related to personal experiences with willingness to learn.

1. Give an example where you were required to learn a health-related topic in which you had no interest.
2. Describe a situation where you had interest and were willing to learn about a health-related topic but were unable to physically engage in the behavior.
3. Describe what affects your willingness to learn about health and what influenced you to make a choice to learn.

Exercise V: Teaching and Learning Settings

Purpose: Assess the impact of teaching and learning settings on health education.
Directions: You are preparing to teach clients the importance of eating a healthy diet to include the food categories and daily nutritional requirements needed to maintain health. Discuss how your teaching approach will change in the following settings:

1. Hospital, convalescent, and nursing home
2. Client's private home
3. High school
4. Work site setting
5. Community setting

References

Ambrose, S. A., Bridges, M. W., DiPietro, M., Lovette, M. C., Norman, M. K., & Mayer, R. E. (2010). *How learning works: Seven research-based principles for smart teaching.* San Francisco, CA: Jossey-Bass.

American Psychological Association. (2017). *Anxiety.* Retrieved from http://www.apa.org/topics/anxiety/

Angelo, T. A., & Cross, K. P. (1993). *Classroom assessment techniques: A handbook for college teachers* (2nd ed.). San Francisco, CA: Jossey-Bass.

Ashton, K., & Oemann, M. (2014). Patient education in home care: Strategies for success. *Home Healthcare Nurse, 32*(5), 288–294.

Ausubel, D., Novak, J., & Hannesian, H. (1968). *Educational psychology: A cognitive view* (2nd ed.). New York, NY: Holt Rinehart & Winston.

Baker College Effective Teaching and Learning Department. (2004). *Teaching across generations.* Retrieved from http://www.mcc.edu/pdf/pdo/teaching_across_gen.pdf

Bandura, A. (1986). *Social foundations of thought and action: A social cognitive theory.* Englewood Cliffs, NJ: Prentice Hall.

Bassuk, E. L., Volk, K. T., & Olivet, J. (2010). A framework for developing supports and services for families experiencing homelessness. *The Open Health Services and Policy Journal, 3,* 34–40.

Bonder, B., Martin, L., Miracle, A. (2001). Achieving cultural competence: The challenge for clients and healthcare workers in a multicultural society. *Generations, 25,* 35–42.

Bray, K. K., Catley, D., Voelker, M. A., Liston, R., & Williams, K. B. (2013). Motivational interviewing in dental hygiene education: Curriculum modification and evaluation. *Journal of Dental Education, 77,* 1662–1669.

Brooks, J. G., & Brooks, M. G. (1993). *In search of understanding: The case for constructivist classrooms*. Alexandria, VA: Association for Supervision and Curriculum Development.

Brown, S. B. (2008). A dangerous bind for American workers. *Hospitals and Health Networks*, 82(11), 54.

Campbell, J., & Brooks, C. (2008). *Tools for effective teaching*. Retrieved from https://cache.trustedpartner.com/docs/library/000223/Transforming%20Behaviors%20Conference%20Materials/Effective%20Teaching%20Stategies_J%20Campbell_C%20Brooks_11_21_08.pdf

Centers for Disease Control and Prevention. (2010). *Deaths and mortality*. Retrieved from http://www.cdc.gov/nchs/fastats/deaths.htm

Centers for Disease Control and Prevention. (2012). *National home and hospice care survey*. Retrieved from http://www.cdc.gov/nchs/nhhcs.htm

Centers for Disease Control and Prevention. (2014). *Vision health initiative* (VHI). Retrieved from http://www.cdc.gov/visionhealth/

Chang, M., & Kelly, A. (2007). Patient education: Addressing cultural diversity and health literacy issues. *Urology Nursing*, 27(5), 411–417.

Church, M., & Watts, S. (2007). Assessment of mental capacity: A flow chart guide. *Psychiatric Bulletin*, 31, 304–307.

Dewey, J. (1938). *Experience and education*. New York, NY: Collier Books.

Dochy, F., Segers, M., & Buehl, M. (1999). The relation between assessment practices and outcomes of studies: The case of research on prior knowledge. *Review of Educational Research*, 69(2), 145–186.

Fisher, D., & Frey, N. (2009). *Background knowledge: The missing piece of the comprehension puzzle*. Portsmouth, NH: Heinemann.

Fleming, N. D., & Mills, C. (1992). Not another inventory, rather a catalyst for reflection. *To Improve the Academy*, 11, 137.

Folstein, M. G., Folstein, S. E., & McHugh, P. R. (1975). Mini-mental state. A practical method for grading the cognitive state of patients for the clinician. *Journal of Psychiatric Research*, 12, 189–198.

Franken, R. (2002). *Human motivation* (5th ed.). California: Wadsworth.

Guay, F., Chanal, J., Ratelle, C. F., Marsh, H. W., Larose, S., & Boivin, M. (2010). Intrinsic identified, and controlled types of motivation for school subjects in young elementary school children. *British Journal of Educational Psychology*, 80(4), 711–735.

Hall, A. M. (2013). Client education. In P. A. Potter, A. G. Perry, P. A. Stockert, & A. M. Hall (Eds.), *Fundamentals of nursing* (8th ed., pp. 328–347). St. Louis, MO: Mosby Elsevier.

Horowitz, J. A. (2014). The therapeutic relationship. In C. L. Edelman, E. C. Kudzma, & C. L. Mandle, (2014). *Health promotion throughout the lifespan* (8th ed.). St. Louis, MO: Elsevier.

Joint Commission, The. (2013). *Comprehensive accreditation manual for hospital*. Retrieved from https://www.jointcommission.org/assets/1/6/CAH13S1-Table_of_changes.pdf

Kanu, A. M. (2009). *Reflections in communication: An interdisciplinary approach*. Lanham, MD: University Press of America.

Keller, L. O., Strohschein, S., & Briske, L. (2008). Population-based public health nursing practice: The intervention wheel. In M. Stanhope & J. Lancaster (Eds.), *Public health nursing: Population-centered health care in the community* (7th ed., pp. 187–214). St. Louis, MO: Mosby Elsevier.

Lieu, C. C., Sadler, G. R., Fullerton, J. T., & Stohlmann, P. D. (2007). Communication strategies for nurses interacting with patients who are deaf. *Dermatology Nursing*, 19(6), 541–551.

Lundahl, B. W., Kunz, C., Brownell, C., Tollefson, D., & Burke, B. L. (2010). A meta-analysis of motivational interviewing: twenty-five years of empirical studies. *Research on Social Work Practice*, 20(2), 137–160.

Maslow, A. H. (1954). *Motivation and personality*. New York, NY: Harper & Row.

Maslow, A. H. (1987). *Motivation and personality* (3rd ed.). New York, NY: Harper & Row.

McKelvey, J., & Borgersen, M. (1990). Family development and the use of diabetes groups: Experience with a model approach. *Patient Education and Counseling*, 16(1), 61–67.

Murray, A. (2011). Montessori elementary philosophy reflects current motivation theories. *Montessori Life*, 23(1), 22–33.

National Center for Health Statistics. (2011). *Health, United States, 2011: With special feature on socioeconomic status and health*. Retrieved from http://www.cdc.gov/nchs/data/hus/hus11.pdf

National Institute on Deafness and Other Communication Disorders. (2013). *Health information*. Retrieved from http://www.nidcd.nih.gov/Pages/default.aspx

National Partnership for Action. (2011). *Health equity and disparities*. Retrieved from http://www.minorityhealth.hhs.gov/npa/templates/browse.aspx?lvl=1&lvlid=34

Ohio State University College of Medicine. (2017). *Getting your message across: Clear and effective health communication*. Retrieved from https://medicine.osu.edu/sitetool/sites/pdfs/ahecpublic/HL_Get_the_Message.pdf

Pekrun, R., Götz, T., Frenzel, A., Barchfeld, P., & Perry, R. P. (2011). Measuring emotions in students; learning and performance: The Achievement Emotions Questionnaire (AEQ). *Contemporary Educational Psychology*, 36(1), 36–48.

Pender, N. (2011). *The health promotion model manual*. Retrieved from https://deepblue.lib.umich.edu/bitstream /handle/2027.42/85350/HEALTH_PROMOTION_MANUAL_Rev_5-2011.pdf

Pew Research Center. (May 14, 2020). *On the cusp of adulthood and facing an uncertain future: What we know about Gen Z so far*. https://www.pewresearch.org/social-trends/2020/05/14/on-the-cusp-of-adulthood-and-facing-an -uncertain-future-what-we-know-about-gen-z-so-far-2/. Accessed July 12, 2023.

Pintrich, P. R. (2003). A motivational science perspective on the role of student motivation in learning and teaching contexts. *Journal of Educational Psychology*, *95*(4), 667–686.

Pohl, M. L. (1981). *The teaching function of the nursing practitioner*. Dubuque, IA: Wm. C. Brown.

Prevent Blindness America. (2012). *Vision problems in the U.S.* Retrieved from http://www.visionproblemsus.org/introduction .html

Price, J., & Cordell, B. (1994). Cultural diversity and patient teaching. *Journal of Continuing Educational Nursing*, *25*, 163–166.

ProLiteracy. (2014). *The Crisis, Adult Literacy Facts*. Retrieved from http://www.proliteracy.org/the-crisis/adult-literacy-facts

Roberts-Grey, G. (2008). Got coverage? *Essence*, *39*(7), 160–164.

Rumsfeld, J. (2002). Health status and clinical practice: When will they meet? *Circulation*, *106*(1), 5–7.

Ryan, R. M., & Deci, E. L. (2000). Self-determination theory and the facilitation of intrinsic motivation, social development, and well-being. *American Psychologist*, *55*(1), 68–78.

Seifert, T. L. (2004). Understanding student motivation. *Educational Research*, *46*(2), 137–149.

Seligman, H. K., Wallace, A. S., DeWalt, D. A., Schillinger, D., Arnold, C. L., Shilliday, B. B., . . . Davis, T. C. (2007). Facilitating behavior change with low-literacy patient education materials. *American Journal of Health Behavior*, *31*(Suppl. 1), S69–S78.

Smilkstein, G. (1978). The family APGAR: A proposal for family function test and its use by physicians. *Journal of Family Practice*, *6*(6), 1231–1239.

Spade, C. M., Fitzsimmons, K., & Houser, J. (2015). Reliability Testing of the Psychosocial Vital Signs Tool. *Journal of Psychosocial Nursing and Mental Health Services*, *53*(11), 39–45.

Spade, C. M., & Mulhall, M. (2010). Teaching psychosocial vital signs across the undergraduate nursing curriculum. *Clinical Simulation in Nursing*, *6*(4), e143–e151. doi:10.1016/j.ecns.2009.10.002.

Stephenson, P. (2006). Managing patient anxiety prior to providing education. *Clinical Journal of Oncology Nursing*, *10*(2), 241–245.

Stuart, G. W. (2005). Therapeutic nurse–patient relationship. In G. W. Stuart & M. T. Laraia (Eds.), *Principles and practices of psychiatric nursing* (8th ed., pp. 15–49). St. Louis, MO: Mosby Elsevier.

Tobias, S. (1994). Interest, prior knowledge, and learning. *Review of Educational Research*, *64*(1), 37–54.

Tunzi, M. (2001). Can the patient decide? Evaluating patient capacity in practice. *American Family Physician*, *64*(2), 299–306.

U.S. Census Bureau. (2012). *U.S. Census Bureau projections show a slower growing, older, more diverse nation a half century from now*. Retrieved from http://www.census.gov/newsroom/releases/archives/population/cb12-243.html

Weiss, B. D., Mays, M. Z., Martz, W., Castro, K. M., DeWalt, D. A., Pignome, M. P. M. J., & Hale, F. A. (2005). Quick assessment of literacy in primary care: The newest vital sign. *Annals of Family Medicine*, *3*(6), 514–522.

CHAPTER 5

Child Learner

OBJECTIVES

Upon completion of this chapter, you will be able to do the following:

- Describe the biologic changes, psychosocial stages, and developmental tasks characteristic of newborns through adolescents.
- List health education topics for newborn through adolescent clients related to biologic changes, psychosocial stages, and developmental tasks.
- Define pedagogy and apply it to teaching newborns through adolescents.
- Describe five steps that nurses as educators take to streamline the process of providing efficient yet personalized health teaching to children in a variety of settings.
- Identify health education topics when working with clients who have disabilities.
- List ways that nurses as educators work with families, are involved in the community, and work with health team members.

CHAPTER OUTLINE

Introduction
Biologic Characteristics, Psychosocial Stages, and Developmental Tasks
- Infants (Birth to 1 Year)
  - Biologic Characteristics
  - Psychosocial Stages
  - Developmental Tasks
- Toddlers (1 to 3 Years)
  - Biologic Characteristics
  - Psychosocial Stages
  - Developmental Tasks
- Preschool (3 to 4 Years)
  - Biologic Characteristics
  - Psychosocial Stages
  - Developmental Tasks
- School Age (5 to 12 Years)
  - Biologic Characteristics
  - Psychosocial Stages
  - Developmental Tasks
- Adolescence (13 to 19 Years)

  - Biologic Characteristics
  - Psychosocial Stages
  - Developmental Tasks
Implications for Health Education
- Promote and Retain Health
- Restore Health
Orientation to Learning
- Learning in Children
- Learning Styles in Children
- The Role of Play in Learning
- Practices That Encourage Child Learning
Pedagogy
- Implications for Health Education
  - Step 1
  - Step 2
  - Step 3
  - Step 4
  - Step 5
  - Step 6

Introduction

Understanding the development of children, including biologic characteristics, psychosocial stages, and developmental tasks, is fundamental to effective client education. A developmental task is a set of skills and competencies that are peculiar to each developmental stage and that children must accomplish or master to deal effectively with their environment (Wong, Hockenberry-Eaton, Wilson, Winkelstein, & Schwartz, 2008). Young clients react differently depending on their developmental stage. Differences in development not only affect clients' reactions to their condition but also their responses to and motivation for carrying out treatment recommendations. As the educator, you need to take into account the client's developmental stage based on an understanding of the health issues faced at that stage. Another important aspect of effectively teaching children is to know how children learn at different stages. This chapter describes child development in five major stages: infants (0–1 years), toddlers (1–3 years), preschoolers (3–4 years), school-age children (5–12 years), and adolescents (13–19 years). It looks at the concept of pedagogy and children's styles of learning at various stages. Your role as the educator is examined in working with pediatric clients who have disabilities, within families, groups, communities, and health team members.

Biologic Characteristics, Psychosocial Stages, and Developmental Tasks

Children grow, develop, and learn throughout their lives, from birth through adulthood. Development of the child learner refers to change or growth that occurs in a child during the life span from birth to adolescence. A developmental task represents our culture's definition of normal development at different points in the life span. A child's development is measured through biologic characteristics, psychosocial stages, and developmental milestones or tasks. Although there are universally accepted assumptions about human development, no two children are alike. Children differ in physical, cognitive, social, and emotional growth patterns. They also differ in their genetic background and the ways they interact with and respond to their environment. Psychosocial stages emphasize the development of healthy personality traits (Erikson, 1963). Developmental changes normally occur in an orderly sequence, in predictable patterns that are age related; however, there are differences in the rate or timing of the changes from one child to another. It is important to have an understanding of the sequence of development so you can respond to the learning needs of young clients and their parents. It is also important to be aware that regression in development may occur with stress and illness.

Infants (Birth to 1 Year)
Biologic Characteristics

Infants at birth have reflexes as their sole physical ability. A *reflex* is an automatic body response to a stimulus that is involuntary; that is, the infant has no control over the response. Many reflexes disappear within a few weeks or months after birth. The presence of reflexes at birth is an indication of normal brain and nerve development. If reflexes are not present or if the reflexes continue past the time they should disappear, this is considered an abnormal finding, and the infant should be seen by a healthcare provider for further evaluation (Wong et al., 2008). **Table 5-1** reviews the major infant reflexes and when they normally disappear.

There are a number of growth landmarks and physical changes that occur as infants grow in the first year. The weight gain of infants is particularly important. A newborn generally weighs between 6 and 9 pounds. A baby's size is influenced by a variety of factors, including the parents' size, gender, birth order, mother's health and nutrition, lifestyle choices during pregnancy, and medical problems. Babies often lose a few ounces in the first week after birth, but they regain the weight by the second week. By the end of the first month, newborns will generally have gained about 15 ounces. Between the ages of 1 and 3 months, a newborn generally gains about 6 ounces per week. Between the ages of 4 and 7 months, the weight gain is about 1.5 to 2 pounds per months. This rate typically slows a bit around 6 months of age to between 1.25 pounds per

Table 5-1 Common Infant Reflexes

Reflex	Response
Blinking	In response to a puff of air, the infant closes both eyes. The reflex disappears as the neurologic system matures within the first year.
Babinski	In response to stroking the side of the foot, the infant twists the foot inward and fans out the toes. The reflex disappears at about 1 year.
Grasping	In response to an object pressed against the palm, the infant attempts to grasp the object. The reflex disappears at 5 to 6 months.
Moro	In response to surprise movement or loud noise, the infant startles with the legs and head extending while the arms jerk up and out with the palms up and thumbs flexed. The reflex disappears at 3 to 6 months.
Rooting	In response to stroking the cheek, the infant turns the head toward the touch and attempts to suck. The reflex disappears at about 4 months.
Stepping	In response to holding the infant so that the feet barely touch a surface, the infant makes stepping movements. The reflex disappears at about 10 to 15 months.
Sucking	In response to inserting a finger or nipple into the mouth, the infant begins sucking. Voluntary movement occurs at around 2 months.
Glabellar	In response to tapping the forehead, the infant blinks. The reflex disappears as the neurologic system matures within the first year.
Plantar	In response to touching the ball of the foot, the infant curls the toes under. The reflex disappears at 9 to 12 months.
Tonic neck	In response to turning the head to one side, the reflex causes a relaxed baby to straighten the arm on that side and bend the other arm in the fencing position. The reflex disappears at 4 to 9 months.

Data from Wong, D. L., Hockenberry-Eaton, M., Wilson, D., Winkelstein, M. L., & Schwartz, P. (2008). *Wong's essentials of pediatric nursing* (6th ed.). St. Louis, MO: Mosby Elsevier.

month. By 8 months, the baby usually weighs around 2.5 times the birth weight. Between the ages of 8 and 12 months, weight gain is steady but at a slower pace. By the first birthday, an infant should weigh around three times the birth weight.

Psychosocial Stages

Erikson's theory of psychosocial development (1963) focuses on how children socialize and how this affects their sense of self. According to the theory, successful completion of each stage results in a healthy personality and successful interactions with others. Failure to successfully complete a stage can result in a reduced ability to progress; however, stages can be resolved successfully at a later time. Of the nine stages identified by Erikson, five relate to children (**Table 5-2**). The task in infancy is the development of *trust versus mistrust*. From the time of birth to 1 year, infants begin to learn to trust others based on the consistency of the responses of their caregivers. If trust

Table 5-2 Erikson's Stages of Psychosocial Development

Stage	Description
Trust versus mistrust Age birth to 1 year	■ Learns to trust others based on caregiver response. ■ If trust develops, gains confidence and trust; is able to feel secure when threatened. ■ Unsuccessful completion results in inability to trust and fear of the world.
Autonomy versus shame and doubt Age 1 to 3 years	■ Asserts independence, walks away from mother, and makes choices. ■ If encouraged, becomes confident and secure in own abilities. ■ If criticized, overly controlled, or not given the opportunity to assert self, may feel inadequate, become overly dependent, lack self-esteem, and feel shame or doubt.
Initiative versus guilt Age 3 to 6 years	■ Asserts self more frequently. ■ Plans activities, makes up games, and initiates activities with others. ■ Develops a sense of initiative, feels secure in ability to lead others and make decisions. ■ If discouraged through criticism or control, develops a sense of guilt; will remain a follower and lack self-initiative.
Industry versus inferiority Age 6 to puberty	■ Develops pride in accomplishments. ■ Initiates and completes projects, feels good about achievements. ■ Teachers play an increased role in development. ■ If encouraged and reinforced, feels industrious and confident about achieving goals. ■ If discouraged, feels inferior, doubts abilities, and may not reach potential.
Identity versus role confusion Puberty to adolescence	■ Transition from childhood to adulthood. ■ More independent, looks to the future: career, relationships, family, housing, and so forth. ■ Explores possibilities and forms own identity based on outcomes of explorations. ■ Can be hindered, resulting in a sense of confusion about self and role in the world ("I don't know what I want to be when I grow up").

Data from Erikson, E. (1963). *Childhood and society* (2nd ed.). New York, NY: W. W. Norton.

develops successfully, the child gains confidence and security in the surrounding world and is able to feel secure in future relationships. Unsuccessful completion of this stage can result in fear, anger, an inability to trust, and a sense of insecurity about the world. It may result in anxiety and a feeling of mistrust in the surrounding world.

The most important social task for the infant is the development of attachment to the primary caretaker, most often the child's mother. This forms the basis for attachment, which is the cornerstone of emotional development. *Separation anxiety* is another attachment behavior of infants characterized by the infant showing distress by crying when a familiar caregiver leaves (Wong et al., 2008). The first signs of separation anxiety appear at about 6 months of age and are clearly evident by 9 months of age. Separation anxiety is the strongest by 15 months of age and then begins to gradually weaken.

Developmental Tasks

Infant developmental tasks for this age group include the areas of motor development and cognitive development. Motor development follows cephalocaudal and proximodistal patterns, so that motor skills become refined first from the center and upper body and later from the extremities and lower body (Wong et al., 2008). Physical development is orderly and occurs in predictable sequence. The motor sequence of new movements for infants involves the following approximate sequence:

- Lack of head and trunk control: First few months after birth
- Lifts chin while lying flat: 1 month
- Raises chest while lying flat: 2 months
- Grasps rattle: 4th month
- Sits with support: 4th month
- Rolls over: 5th month
- Sits upright in a high chair: 4th to 6th month
- Sits without assistance: 8th month
- Crawling: 9th month
- Stands with help: 10th month
- Walks with help: 12th month
- Stands alone: 14th month
- Walks alone without support or help: 15th month
- Walks up stairs with help and runs clumsily: 18th month

The ages for each motor skill milestone are averages; the rates of physical and motor developments differ among infants depending on a variety of factors, including heredity, the amount of activity the infant participates in, and the amount of attention the infant receives (**Figure 5-1**).

Cognitive development refers to intellectual or mental development. It includes the activities of thinking, perception, memory, problem solving, language, and speech. Jean Piaget's theory of cognitive development in the 1920s challenged the then-prevalent thinking that children think like adults. Piaget's theory (1952) is based on the idea that a developing infant builds cognitive structures, or schemes, to understand and respond to physical experiences within the environment. Piaget posits that an infant's cognitive structure increases in complexity with development, moving from displaying reflexes, such as sucking and grasping, to highly complex mental activities, such as speech. Piaget's four stages of cognitive development are included in **Table 5-3**. The infant is in the *sensorimotor stage*, in which infants begin to understand the information entering

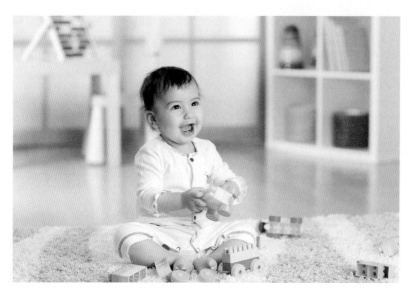

Figure 5-1 Infants Develop at Different Rates
© Oksana Kuzmina/Shutterstock

their senses and are able to interact with the world. During this stage, the infant learns to manipulate objects, although they will fail to understand the permanency of these objects if they are not within the infant's current sensory perception. Object permanence develops toward the end of the first year.

The most intensive period of speech and language development occurs during the first 3 years of life when the brain is developing and maturing. These skills appear to develop best when the infant is exposed to sounds, sights, and the speech and language of others. The beginning signs of communication occur during the first few days of life when an infant learns that crying will bring food, comfort, and companionship. The newborn also begins to recognize important environmental sounds, such as the mother's voice. As they grow, infants sort out the speech sounds or phonemes that compose the words of their language. Most infants recognize the basic sounds of their native language (National Institute on Deafness and Other Communication Disorders [NIDCD], 2014). **Table 5-4** reviews the developmental milestones of speech development of the infant.

Toddlers (1 to 3 Years)
Biologic Characteristics

During the toddler period, weight gain slows to about 4 to 6 pounds per year as the activity level increases. The physical appearance of the toddler includes a protuberant abdomen, accentuated lumbar lordosis (inward curvature of the spine), and a characteristic gait in which the feet are placed wide apart and the child appears to walk flat footed. The birth weight quadruples by the age of 2.5 years. A steady growth in height of 2 to 4 inches per year is expected. During this time, the child perfects the gross and fine motor skills that emerged during the first year by developing balance, coordination, stability, and an improved ability to manipulate objects. Emotional and physical readiness for toilet training begins at around 18 months.

Table 5-3 Piaget's Stages of Cognitive Development

Stage	Age	Characteristics of Stage
Sensorimotor	0–2	The child: ■ Learns by doing: looking, touching, and viewing ■ Learns through physical interaction with the environment ■ Builds a set of concepts about reality and how it works ■ Has a primitive understanding of cause-and-effect relationships ■ Develops object permanence at about 9 months
Preoperational	2–7	The child: ■ Is not able to conceptualize abstractly and needs concrete physical situations ■ Uses language and symbols, including letters and numbers ■ Is egocentric ■ Conservation marks the end of the preoperational stage and the beginning of concrete operations
Concrete operations	7–11	The child: ■ Starts to conceptualize, creating logical structures that explain physical experiences ■ Demonstrates conservation, reversibility, serial ordering, and a mature understanding of cause-and-effect relationships ■ Begins abstract problem solving and continues with concrete thinking
Formal operations	12+	The child: ■ Begins to develop an abstract view of the world ■ Is able to apply reversibility and conservation to both real and imagined situations ■ Demonstrates abstract thinking, including logic, deductive reasoning, comparison, and classification ■ Has an increased understanding of the world and the idea of cause and effect; can develop theories about the world

Data from Piaget, J. (1963). *The psychology of intelligence*. New York, NY: Routledge.

Table 5-4 Language Development: First Year

Age	Infant Response
Birth to 5 months	■ Reacts to sounds ■ Turns head toward sounds ■ Cries, coos, laughs ■ Makes noise when talked to ■ Looks at faces
6 to 11 months	■ Understands "no" ■ Says "da-da" and "ma-ma" ■ Tries to communicate by making gestures ■ Tries to imitate sounds

Data from National Institute on Deafness and Other Communication Disorders. (2014). *Speech and language developmental milestones*. Retrieved from https://www.nidcd.nih.gov/sites/default/files/Documents/health/voice/NIDCD-Speech-Language-Dev-Milestones.pdf

Psychosocial Stages

Toddlers are in Erikson's stage of *autonomy versus shame and doubt*. From the ages of birth to 1 year, children begin to learn how to trust others based on the consistency of the responses of their caregivers. Toddlers strive to develop a sense of autonomy within the boundaries of a trusting parental relationship. If trust develops successfully, the child gains confidence and security in the surrounding world. The child is then better able to develop affectionate and trusting relationships with family members and with adults outside the family. Unsuccessful completion of this stage can result in an inability to trust and therefore a sense of fear about the world.

Developmental Tasks

Toddlers are in Piaget's *preoperational stage* of cognitive development. A hallmark of this stage is egocentrism, or the tendency of children to recognize their environment only in terms of their own point of view. Toddlers think that parents and others share their thoughts. The toddler applies new knowledge of language and begins to use symbols to represent objects, such as pretending a broom is a horse. They may experiment with objects in their minds, first predicting what will happen if they do something to an object, then transforming their plans into action. To some degree, mental prediction and planning replace overt trial and error as growing toddlers experiment and attempt to solve problems. The toddler is now better able to think about things and events that are not present. Language development is proceeding rapidly in the toddler, but the ability to understand language is greater than the ability to express it, which creates frustration. **Table 5-5** reviews the milestones for language development at this stage.

Preschool (3 to 4 Years)

Biologic Characteristics

The preschooler has a steady growth rate of approximately 4 pounds of weight and 2 inches of height per year. The body lengthens, and the protuberant abdomen disappears. In terms of physical abilities, a 3-year-old can kick a ball, jump in place, build a tower of nine cubes, copy a circle, put on most clothing and shoes, and eat without assistance. By the age of 4 years, the child can climb a ladder, throw a ball overhand, hold a pencil, cut and paste, wash and dry hands, brush teeth, and ride a bike with training wheels. Most basic gross motor abilities have emerged. Existing skills are practiced and perfected, and the child develops mastery in applying motor skills to increasingly challenging and complex situations.

Psychosocial Stages

The preschooler moves through two of Erikson's stages of psychosocial development: the stage of autonomy versus shame and doubt, and the stage of *initiative versus guilt*. After developing basic trust, the child goes on to begin to plan activities, make up games, and initiate activities with others. If given this opportunity, the preschooler develops a sense of initiative and feels secure in the ability to lead others and make decisions. If this tendency is not encouraged, either through criticism or control, the child develops a sense of guilt. The child may feel like an annoyance to others and therefore remain a follower, lacking in self-initiative.

At 2 years and older, the preschooler develops rudimentary relationships with other children, which are usually characterized by *parallel play*; that is, play in the presence of, rather than in interaction with, other children. As the child progresses, social relationships increase outside the family,

Table 5-5 Language Development: Toddler Years

Age	Toddler Response
12 to 17 months	■ Attends to a book or a toy for a few minutes ■ Follows simple directions ■ Answers simple questions nonverbally ■ Points to objects, pictures, or family members ■ Says two to three words to label a person or object (pronunciation may not be clear) ■ Tries to imitate simple words
18 to 23 months	■ Enjoys being read to ■ Follows simple commands without gestures ■ Points to simple body parts ■ Understands simple verbs ■ Makes animal sounds ■ Starts to combine words such as "more milk"
2 to 3 years	■ Knows about 50 words at 24 months ■ Knows some spatial concepts such as in and on ■ Knows pronouns such as you, me, and her ■ Knows descriptive words such as big and happy ■ Says about 40 words at 24 months ■ Speech is becoming more accurate but may still leave off ending sounds; strangers may not be able to understand much of what is said ■ Answers simple questions ■ Begins to use more pronouns such as you and I ■ Speaks in two- to three-word phrases ■ Uses question inflection to ask for something (e.g., My ball?) ■ Begins to use plurals such as shoes or socks and regular past-tense verbs such as jumped

Data from National Institute on Deafness and Other Communication Disorders. (2014). *Speech and language developmental milestones*. Retrieved from https://www.nidcd.nih.gov/sites/default/files/Documents/health/voice/NIDCD-Speech-Language-Dev-Milestones.pdf

and interactive and cooperative play skills with peers are expanded. The preschooler also begins to imitate and practice social roles. Concepts of right and wrong are learned as the child begins to understand the nature of rules, which causes the child to experience guilt when doing wrong.

Developmental Tasks

Preschoolers are in Piaget's preoperational cognitive stage. A concrete thought process is evident in this stage by what Piaget calls *transductive reasoning*, which describes how the preschooler cannot think from the general to the particular or from the particular to the general. Piaget also describes the concept of *centering* as lacking in the preschooler's thinking. The child cannot consider more than one factor at a time when solving a problem or connect a reversible operation to the original act. This is called *irreversibility*. Piaget describes preschool-age children as preoperational because they do not yet use logic. They understand the world through magical thinking and have difficulty distinguishing between wishes and what really happens. They believe that thoughts and strong feelings can make things happen.

A major accomplishment in the preschool stage is the perfection of language skills and the use of language to communicate with others. During the preschool years, language progression depends on aptitude, the opportunity for using language, the quality and quantity of language used at home, and the child's range of experiences using language to communicate. It is also at this stage that grammar and syntax are refined, and vocabulary increases rapidly (**Table 5-6**).

School Age (5 to 12 Years)
Biologic Characteristics

The school-age child gains an average of 6 pounds and grows approximately 2 inches per year. Growth is marked by spurts and times of little growth as dictated by genetics. During these years, boys and girls are of similar size, but school-age children tend to be concerned about their rate of growth and what their height and weight will be. The child practices, refines, and masters complex gross and fine motor skills. Examples of gross motor skills for school-age children include balancing on one foot, tandem walking, hopping on one foot, pedaling a bicycle, and bathing self. Fine motor skills for this age group include drawing a person with three to six parts, cutting with a knife, tying a bow, drawing a diamond, and having good eye–hand coordination. This is also a time when the school-age child begins to lose baby teeth, and the permanent teeth emerge.

Psychosocial Stages

School-age children are in Erikson's stage of *industry versus inferiority*. In this stage, children begin to develop a sense of pride in their accomplishments. They initiate projects, see them through to completion, and feel good about what they have achieved. During this time, teachers play an increased role in the child's development. If children are encouraged and reinforced for their initiative, they begin to feel industrious and confident in their ability to achieve goals. If this initiative

---

Table 5-6 Language Development: Preschool Years

Age	Preschooler Response
3 to 4 years	■ Groups objects, such as food and clothes, together ■ Identifies colors ■ Uses most speech sounds but may distort some of the more difficult sounds, such as l, r, s, sh, ch, y, v, z, and th; these sounds may not be fully mastered until age 7 or 8 years ■ Uses consonants in the beginning, middle, and end of words; some of the more difficult consonants may be distorted, but attempts to say them ■ Strangers are able to understand much of what is said ■ Able to describe the use of objects such as fork, car, and so forth ■ Has fun with language; enjoys poems and recognizes language absurdities such as "Is that an elephant on your head?" ■ Expresses ideas and feelings, rather than just talking about the surrounding world ■ Uses verbs that end in -ing such as walking, talking ■ Answers simple questions such as "What do you do when you are hungry?" ■ Repeats sentences

Data from National Institute on Deafness and Other Communication Disorders. (2014). *Speech and language developmental milestones*. Retrieved from https://www.nidcd.nih.gov/sites/default/files/Documents/health/voice/NIDCD-Speech-Language-Dev-Milestones.pdf is not encouraged, if it is restricted by parents or teachers, the child will begin to feel inferior, doubting their abilities, and may not reach full potential. Relationships with people outside the family become more important to the school-age child. They develop friendships and participate in peer group activities. The child imitates, learns, and adopts age-appropriate social roles, including those that are gender specific. The child develops an understanding of rules that can be relied on to dictate proper social behavior and govern social relationships and activities. The child develops a sense of self as an individual with awareness of likes and dislikes and with special areas of skill. Introspection is possible at this age.

Developmental Tasks

School-age children are in Piaget's stage of *concrete operations*. During this stage, accommodation (the ability to modify schema to fit the world) increases. The child develops an ability to think abstractly and make rational judgments about concrete or observable phenomena that in the past the child needed to physically manipulate in order to understand. Some specific skills that develop at this time are the ability to classify items and put them in a series, recognize logical relationships among elements in a serial order, and understand that the quantity, length, or number of items is unrelated to the arrangement or appearance of the object or items (conservation). The school-age child can take into account multiple aspects of a problem to solve it. They understand that numbers or objects can be changed and then returned to their original state (reversibility). The child moves toward more cooperative interactions and develops the ability to understand other people's perspectives (**Figure 5-2**).

School-age children generally enter this developmental stage with the ability to understand and speak a language. School focuses on learning to read and write. Success in school depends on three things: the child having the visual ability to read, the auditory ability to perceive language spoken to them, and the fine motor skills for handwriting.

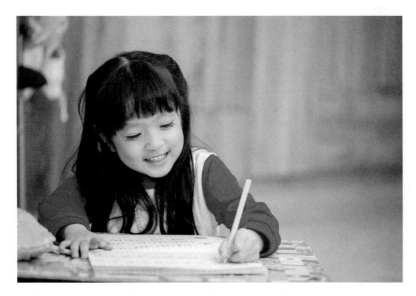

Figure 5-2 The School-Age Child Learns to Solve Problems
© Warongdech Digital/Shutterstock

Adolescent (13 to 19 Years)

Biologic Characteristics

Adolescence is a time of accelerated physical growth in weight and height; 15–20% of adult height and 50% of adult weight is achieved. This is also the time of onset of puberty, or sexual maturity, which signals the ability to reproduce. Females usually begin puberty 2 years earlier than males and experience their growth spurt earlier. Physiologic changes in puberty include the development of secondary sex characteristics. In females, the first sign of puberty is often breast development. Other signs are the growth of hair in the pubic area and armpits. Menarche, the onset of menses in girls, usually happens later in puberty, at around 13 years of age. In males, puberty usually begins with the testicles and penis getting larger. Then hair grows in the pubic area and armpits. Muscles grow, the voice deepens, nocturnal emissions begin, and facial hair develops as puberty continues. Even though the physical changes are usually sequential in nature and are mediated through the hormonal regulatory system, there are individual variations for onset and duration of puberty. Some adolescents may begin puberty earlier than normal, a condition called precocious puberty. Others may have delayed puberty, meaning the process begins later than normal.

Psychosocial Stages

The adolescent is in Erikson's stage of *identity versus role confusion*. This is a period of transition from childhood to adulthood. Adolescents want more independence and begin to look to the future in terms of career and future relationships. Social relationships center on their peer group, with decreased time spent with family. Group values often guide their individual behavior, and acceptance by peers becomes a critical part of self-esteem. Adolescents explore possibilities and begin to form their own identities based on the outcome of their explorations. Identity is defined as a coherent conception of the self, made up of committed goals, values, and beliefs. This sense of who they are can be hindered, which can result in a sense of confusion about themselves and their role in the world. Toward the end of this stage, identity becomes more individualized, and the adolescent develops a more stable sense of self that is separate from either family or peer group.

Developmental Tasks

Piaget's stage of *formal operations* describes the adolescent's cognitive development. This stage brings cognition to its final form. Adolescents no longer require concrete objects to make rational judgments. Abstract, theoretical, philosophical, and scientific reasoning become possible. At this time, they also develop an understanding of long-term cause and effect. Adolescents question, reinterpret, and revise their previous knowledge base. At this point, they are capable of hypothetical and deductive reasoning. There are many possible options for teaching adolescents because they can consider options from different perspectives. It is common for them to challenge current thinking and have a sense of idealism about the world as they move toward a formal thinking process.

Language development is largely complete by adolescence. Language at this stage exhibits evidence of reflective and abstract thought, with increasingly complex grammatical construction of speech and writing. Adolescents have the ability to define and discuss abstractions such as health, love, and peace. They are also aware that words can have multiple meanings. The use of slang is common. This is considered to be an opportune time developmentally to learn other languages.

Implications for Health Education

It is critical to understand child development to provide effective health education to children, their parents, and their caregivers. Knowledge of child development enables you to prepare client education plans based on realistic child expectations, and it increases the chances of adherence and success in promoting, retaining, and restoring health. As an educator, your knowledge and understanding of cognitive and perceptual behavior serves as a guide in counseling. Use this knowledge to influence behavior by listening to parental concerns, respecting values, and modeling behaviors that support the overall health of the child. As the child grows and is able to independently communicate, use understanding of growth and development to interact with the child in ways that acknowledge their verbal and physical abilities and encourage self-reliance.

Use age-specific strategies to prepare client education plans. Infants expand their gross and fine motor skills by being encouraged to reach and grasp and move toward objects. An example of this is placing toys safely in the crib that are black and white or brightly colored to attract attention and stimulate movement. Younger children, toddlers through preschool, have language skills that require concrete examples to help them understand information. A younger child will respond well to being told, "We always wash our hands before meals." An older child will want more explanation, to which the nurse can respond by discussing that this prevents germs that can make you sick.

As the child's gross and fine motor skills develop, it is helpful to supplement explanation with objects that the child can manipulate. When teaching about how to take blood pressure, having the child hold and examine the blood pressure cuff lets them gain familiarity with the equipment and gives a sense of mastery and trust. The preschool child enjoys pretend play, which is when the child remembers past experiences and replays them (Graca, Fowler, & Rosenstock, 2009). By pretending, the child is able to share fears and concerns and can gain a sense of mastery over the environment. Use this time to clear up misconceptions that are common in this age group because of magical thinking. Older children enjoy activities that involve peers and that are repetitive and entertaining. Games, including those on the computer, are fun and create a sense of mastery. **Table 5-7** summarizes psychosocial, cognitive, language, and teaching implications.

Promote and Retain Health

The focus of promoting health is on prevention of illness, whereas the focus of retaining health is on maintaining the present health status, assuming it is satisfactory. **Table 5-8** lists suggested topics to promote and retain health that are appropriate for children at various stages of development. These suggestions are not all-inclusive and need to be adapted to the circumstances of the individual client.

Restore Health

Restoration of health for children refers to working with children who have an acute or chronic illness or disability. The purpose of health education at this time is to help clients understand the nature of their health problem, the treatment regimen, and the limitations imposed by the health problem, disability, or injury. This may involve not only working with the client, but also with family members. **Table 5-9** explains the approach used by nurses as educators when teaching different age groups. The developmental stage is taken into account, and both the parent and the child are viewed as clients.

Table 5-7 Teaching Implications for Various Developmental Stages

Age	Psychosocial (Erikson)	Cognitive (Piaget)	Language	Teaching Implications
Infancy	■ Trust versus mistrust ■ 5–6 weeks: Responsive smile to families' faces and voices ■ Emotionally symbiotic with main caretaker ■ Individual temperament emerges in earliest weeks of life ■ Needs balance of rest, exercise, nutrition, love, strokes ■ Cuddliness varies	■ Sensorimotor: Basic reflex habits (e.g., sucking nipple within 2 weeks) ■ Higher levels later: 2–3 months ■ Looks for sounds ■ At 8–9 months develops object permanence ■ Thinks in pictures	■ Prelanguage sounds ■ Inner language: Recognizes objects ■ Audioreceptive: Recognizes spoken words	■ Teach parents and caregivers ■ Calibrate for their anxiety when child is very ill ■ Anticipatory guidance about growth and development, safety, and stimulation (talk and touch)
Early childhood 2 to 3 years	■ Autonomy versus shame and doubt ■ No! ■ Frustrated by personal and external limits ■ Egocentric ■ Needs to explore safely and to succeed	■ Sensorimotor: Still thinks in pictures ■ Starts development of object formation, representation, extension	■ Single three-word sentences: Nouns, verbs, and adjectives (ball, carry, soft) ■ At age 3, understands time (yesterday)	■ Needs safe play space, love, security ■ Find out routines, special words, comfort toy ■ Give positive, simple command ■ Read or make up relevant picture books ■ Most teaching through parent
3 to 6 years	■ Initiative versus guilt ■ Fears: Unknown, separation, strangers, disapproval, pain, punishment, own aggression ■ Roles: Male, female	■ Sensorimotor: Expanding imagination and concepts	■ Rapid growth ■ By 5 years has usual speech patterns	■ Encourage play to assess child and to teach ■ Give simple explanations (You will smell icky perfume) ■ See, hear, feel: Make tape and picture books, objects ■ Use timing: Tell child soon enough to allow processing but not to get panicky; allow only one stall ■ Positive commands (You hold the Band-Aid)

Stage	Psychosocial Development	Cognitive Development	Language	Implications for Health Education
Late childhood 6 to 12 years	▪ Industry versus inferiority ▪ Makes things ▪ Peer influence is important ▪ Developing parents and ego states	▪ Concrete operations ▪ Inductive reasoning ▪ Memory ▪ Conscience teachable in many cultures	▪ Good command of language; can use it to tell stories, ask questions, argue, tease	▪ Assess child's reading ability ▪ Likes mechanical explanations ▪ Help child gain content by participating in self-care and procedures ▪ Can pay attention to teaching ▪ Can do own hygiene, choose good food, recognize signs of illness
Adolescence	▪ Identity versus role confusion ▪ New and more mature relationships ▪ Sexual identity ▪ Changing body ▪ Becoming emotionally independent from parents ▪ Preparing for adult responsibilities, career, love ▪ Workable value system ▪ Social responsibilities ▪ Mood swings and ambivalence ▪ Fears loss of face	▪ Formal operations ▪ "One's thinking takes wings" (Piaget)	▪ Depends on IQ, culture, socioeconomic group ▪ Slang	▪ Ask for meaning of slang ▪ Use peers to teach and persuade ▪ Protect privacy ▪ Expect mood swings ▪ Be honest and straightforward ▪ Try to read between the lines of what a teenager is trying to say or does not say

Data from Babcock, D. E., & Miller, M. A. (1994). *Client education: Theory and practice.* St. Louis: Mosby.

Table 5-8 Suggested Topics to Promote and Retain Health

Nursing Assessment	Health Education Topics
Infant	<ul><li>Promotion of infant–parent bonding</li><li>Infant nutrition: Breastfeeding, formula feeding, introduction of solid food and weaning</li><li>Developmental milestones</li><li>Elimination patterns</li><li>Activity and exercise through stimulation and play</li><li>Sleep needs</li><li>Injury prevention</li><li>Sensory stimulation to promote cognitive and social development</li><li>Vaccinations</li></ul>
Toddler	<ul><li>Nutritional needs and preferences</li><li>Toilet training</li><li>Appropriate toys and activities</li><li>Rituals and security objects</li><li>Need for autonomy, temper tantrums</li><li>Parental frustration</li><li>Safety issues, injury prevention</li><li>Vaccinations</li></ul>
Preschooler	<ul><li>Nutritional needs and preferences</li><li>Dental care</li><li>Appropriate play activities and exercise</li><li>Choosing TV shows</li><li>Managing bedtime concerns</li><li>Imaginary friends and magical thinking</li><li>Vision and hearing screenings</li><li>Gender identification</li><li>Injury prevention</li><li>Health screenings</li></ul>
School age	<ul><li>Understanding of health</li><li>Balanced nutrition, prevention of obesity</li><li>Nocturnal enuresis, encopresis, and shy bladder</li><li>Sports activities, TV, video, and computer games</li><li>Developing socialization skills</li><li>Sleep walking, sleep talking, night fears</li><li>Health screenings</li><li>Attention-deficit hyperactivity disorder (ADHD)</li><li>Questions about sex</li><li>Coping strategies</li><li>Accident prevention</li></ul>

Nursing Assessment	Health Education Topics
Adolescent	<ul><li>Physical changes: Puberty</li><li>Common health issues: Acne, scoliosis</li><li>Diet and exercise: Prevention of obesity and eating disorders</li><li>Sexual behavior, contraception</li><li>Sexually transmitted diseases</li><li>Body image issues</li><li>Substance abuse: Alcohol and drugs</li><li>Injury and violence prevention</li><li>Health screening</li><li>Vaccinations</li></ul>

Table 5-9 Teaching Approach with Different Age Groups

Age Group	Clients/Parents	Nursing Approach
Infant (0–1)	Child	<ul><li>Observe the infant's physical condition: Weight and appearance</li><li>Observe child–caregiver interaction: Look for bonding behaviors</li></ul>
	Parent	<ul><li>Establish rapport</li><li>Use good listening skills to identify parent's concerns</li><li>Address parental anxiety and stress with calm demeanor</li><li>Assess parental educational level, literacy level, cultural influences</li><li>Encourage enjoyment of infants</li><li>Discuss balance of work and home life</li><li>Share knowledge of:<ul><li>Community resources</li><li>Developmental milestone</li><li>Importance of play for development</li><li>Preventive teaching</li><li>Infant safety</li><li>Nutrition</li><li>Health screenings and vaccinations schedule</li></ul></li></ul>
Toddler (1–2)	Child	<ul><li>Assess the quality of the parent–child relationship</li><li>Observe the physical status and growth of the child</li><li>Talk to and interact with the child on their level to initiate a relationship</li></ul>
	Parent	<ul><li>Establish rapport</li><li>Listen to parental concerns and encourage questions</li><li>Determine parental knowledge, literacy level, cultural influences</li><li>Be sensitive to signs of frustration with child's behavior</li><li>Provide appropriate teaching tools and resources</li><li>Share knowledge of:<ul><li>Community resources</li><li>Developmental milestones</li><li>Importance of play for development</li><li>Safety</li><li>Techniques of discipline and limit setting</li><li>Toilet training</li></ul></li></ul>

(continues)

Table 5-9 Teaching Approach with Different Age Groups   *(continued)*

Age Group	Clients/Parents	Nursing Approach
Preschooler (3–4)	Child	■ Talk to and interact with the child on their level to establish a relationship ■ Observe the child at play; listen to vocalizations and observe imaginary play ■ Observe the physical status and growth of the child ■ Teach children about procedures to be performed ■ Keep explanations simple ■ Allow children to express their fears
	Parent	■ Establish rapport ■ Listen to parental concerns and encourage questions ■ Determine parental knowledge, literacy level, cultural influences ■ Teach parents ways to respond to their child's questions ■ Provide appropriate teaching tools and resources ■ Share knowledge of: • Normal developmental milestones • Child's sexual curiosity • Imaginary play and magical thinking • Safety
School age (5–12)	Child	■ Observe the physical status and growth of the child ■ Develop rapport with the child by introducing yourself and asking about their interests and friends ■ Ask the child about their health and encourage questions ■ Explain procedures or teaching in clear, logical ways ■ Include child in the patient education process ■ Use appropriate tools and resources
	Parent	■ Establish rapport ■ Listen to parental concerns and encourage questions ■ Determine parental knowledge and literacy level ■ Help parents to foster child independence and praise accomplishments ■ Give parents tools for teaching ■ Share knowledge of: • Normal developmental milestones • School adjustment • Enuresis, encopresis • Sleepwalking, sleep talking • Learning disabilities • Obesity, nutritional teaching • Dental health • Safety, accidents, drowning, bicycles • Drugs, alcohol, smoking, sexual activity • Health screening: Vision, hearing • Use of TV, computer, cell phones, and video games

Age Group	Clients/Parents	Nursing Approach
Adolescent (13–19)	Child	■ Focus on establishing rapport based on openness and trust ■ Ask about bodily changes and sexual adjustment ■ Ask about family support and facilitate the family relationship ■ Ask about peer group and social, cultural influences ■ Ask about health concerns and answer questions ■ Advocate for the adolescent client ■ Be mindful of modesty and privacy issues ■ Use empathetic understanding; no lecturing ■ Provide appropriate teaching tools and resources ■ Share knowledge about: 　• Physical change in puberty 　• Sexual issues and contraception 　• Body image and eating disorders 　• Health issues and safety 　• Body piercing and tattooing 　• Scoliosis, acne
	Parent	■ Establish rapport ■ Listen to parental concerns and encourage questions ■ Determine parental knowledge, literacy level, cultural influences ■ Assist parents in understanding adolescent behavior ■ Encourage limit setting and fostering of adolescent independence ■ Help parents redefine their role in this transition phase

Data from Falvo, D. R. (2011). *Effective patient education: A guide to increased adherence.* Sudbury, MA: Jones & Bartlett Learning.

Orientation to Learning

Learning in Children

Most theorists believe that learning is something that occurs as the result of certain experiences that precede changes in behavior (Olsen & Hergenhahn, 2013). The experiences that precede learning are interactions with the environment. Athey (2007) and Piaget (1963) agree that children's interactions with their environment lead to mental actions through which they construct ideas or *schema* about what they are encountering. As they come across objects, situations, people, and ideas, they adjust and structure their knowledge to try to make sense of their experiences. Using this cognitive learning process, they build a framework for thinking and learning. Children's direct experiences and interactions with things and people around them are central to their learning (David, Goouch, Powell, & Abbott, 2003).

B. F. Skinner posits that learning is a change in overt behavior that occurs in response to events or stimuli that occur in the environment (1968). Reinforcement is the key element in Skinner's theory of classical conditioning. A reinforcer is anything that strengthens the desired response. It could be a smile, verbal praise, a good grade, or a feeling of increased accomplishment. Skinner also identifies negative reinforcers, which result in the increased frequency of a response when it is withdrawn (different from adverse stimuli or punishment, which results in

Table 5-10 Application of Cognitive and Behavior Learning Theories for Children

Learning Theory	Principles	Teaching Application
Cognitive theories of learning	Jean Piaget's cognitive development theory	■ Children will provide different explanations of reality at different stages of cognitive development. ■ Cognitive development is facilitated by providing activities or situations that engage learners and require adaptation. ■ Learning materials and activities should involve the appropriate level of motor or mental operations for a child of a given age; avoid asking children to perform tasks that are beyond their current cognitive capabilities. ■ Use teaching methods that actively involve children and present challenges.
Behavioral theory of learning	B. F. Skinner's operant conditioning theory	■ Behavior that is positively reinforced will reoccur; intermittent reinforcement is particularly effective. ■ Information should be presented in small amounts so that responses can be reinforced (shaping). ■ Reinforcements will generalize across similar stimuli (stimulus generalization), producing secondary conditioning.

Data from Kearsley, G. (2004). *Explorations in learning and instruction: The theory into practice database.* Retrieved from https://orion2020.org/archivo/cen/educational_theories_summary.pdf

reduced responses). Babies generally respond well to operant conditioning, which is a process of gradually shaping the infant's behavior. An example of this is an infant who learns that smiling elicits positive parental attention, which in turn causes the infant to smile at their parents more (Skinner, 1968). Babies generally respond well to operant conditioning. Cognitive and behavioral theories are applied to teaching in **Table 5-10**.

Learning Styles in Children

Learning occurs as children respond to environmental, social, emotional, and physical stimuli when trying to understand new information. Learning styles are the ways individuals process information. Sensory-based learning styles refer to three perceptual pathways or modalities of learning: visual (sight), kinesthetic (body, sensation, motion), and auditory (sound). The visual modality occurs when information is received best through visual stimulation (reading, pictures, movies, etc.). Approximately 40% of secondary students are visual learners. The kinesthetic modality occurs when information is received best via touch and hands-on activities (computer-assisted instruction, models, field trips, etc.). Approximately 50% of secondary students are kinesthetic learners. The auditory modality occurs when information is best obtained by hearing (being read to aloud, listening to songs, puppet shows, reciting songs or poems, etc.). Approximately 10% of secondary students are auditory learners (Carbo, Dunn, & Dunn, 1986). There is no right or wrong learning style. Most children show a preference for one style, as do nurses and parents. It is not unusual for the nurse and parents to prefer learning styles different from that of the child. To work effectively with children, it is important for you to understand your own, the child's, and possibly the parents' preferred learning styles. This understanding helps to produce more efficient, productive learning opportunities for children. Including activities that use other styles can be helpful in expanding children's areas of interest and ability to learn.

The Role of Play in Learning

Jones and Reynolds state that "young children learn the most important things, not by being told but by constructing knowledge for themselves in interaction with the physical world and with other children—and the way they do this is by playing" (1992, p. 1). In *play*, children expand their understanding of themselves and others, their knowledge of the physical world, and their ability to communicate with peers and adults. Children experience play through all the developmental stages. Infants and toddlers engage in activities that stimulate their senses and develop motor skills. Preschoolers play with other children, develop and refine motor skills, and use basic academic skills such as counting, reading, and writing. School-age children play formal and informal games with their peers, such as hopscotch, jump rope, and board, card, and computer games. Through these activities they enhance their coordination and physical abilities, refine their social skills, and build concepts such as cooperation and competition. In adolescence, play is more organized and structured as the need for orderly thinking is expressed through games with rules and in organized sports.

Play is so important that its significance in children's lives is recognized by the United Nations as a specific right (United Nations, 1989). The Association for Childhood Education International (ACEI) issued a position paper outlining the following beliefs about the importance of play in children's development (Isenberg & Quisenberry, 2002):

- Play is a dynamic, active, and constructive behavior and is an essential and integral part of all children's healthy growth, development, and learning across all ages, domains, and cultures.
- Play enhances learning and development for children of all ages, cultures, and domains.
- The forms and functions of children's play must be considered in the context of our knowledge about age-related play behaviors. Knowledge about how children play at different ages should guide the practice of all adults who work with children.
- Play is a powerful, natural behavior contributing to children's learning and development, and no program of adult instruction can substitute for children's own observations, activities, and direct knowledge.

The nurse as educator uses this knowledge of the importance of play to support child learning. Graca and colleagues (2009) describe *medical play* as developmentally appropriate activities that provide insight into how the child is coping with health events and can be used as a tool in successful teaching. Medical play allows opportunities to deal with both the physical and emotional stressors of health care and act as a mechanism to increase understanding. An example of using medical play is rehearsing activities before surgery. The child can manipulate equipment, such as an oxygen mask, and rehearse what it is like to have the mask in place. The nurse as educator uses knowledge of developmental milestones to choose play strategies that fit the child's need (**Figure 5-3**).

Practices That Encourage Child Learning

As an educator, you assume a big part in creating the climate and conditions that best promote children's learning. Involvement in learning is built on the confidence and trust that come from good relationships. First, build rapport with the child. It is important to promote self-esteem, confidence, and trust to create an environment conducive to learning. It is also important to involve children both physically and mentally in the learning process (David et al., 2003). Children should be encouraged to explore their world through movement, using all their senses to find out what they can do, what things are like, and what things mean. It is through this exploration that

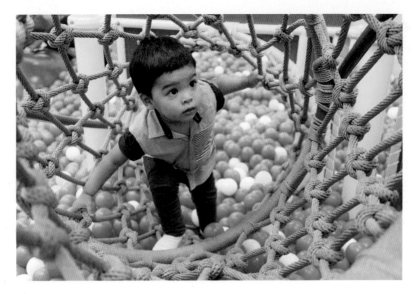

Figure 5-3 Children Explore the World Through Play
© Double_H/Shutterstock

they achieve understanding and form ideas from sensory experiences. Learning strategies should include these types of activities.

Provide support to cultivate, sustain, and extend children's explorations and recognize their accomplishments. You should also be aware that part of the active learning process is to allow children to make decisions and have control and independence as part of the learning process. Allowing children to decide what and how they do things increases their engagement in the learning process (David et al., 2003). This does not mean that children are left on their own to decide what and how they will learn, but it does mean the nurse can create situations for them to make decisions and then support them as they engage in learning activities. Making decisions helps children become managers of their own learning.

Another important aspect of active learning is to personalize the learning process. This means to build on what the child is familiar with, knows, and can do. Getting to know the child and their parents helps you understand how to stimulate and sustain the child's involvement and effort in learning (David et al., 2003). The pace and character of children's learning differ from one child to another because they have different interests, skills, and knowledge built on their experiences. This means that children learn the same thing in different ways, or learn the same thing at different times in their development. The range and character of learning activities should be planned to address these kinds of differences in a way that enables all children to find something that is relevant and that will engage and sustain their interest. Some children need additional support to become fully involved in learning activities.

It is important for you to consider how learning activities are presented. The context in which children experience things has a considerable effect on their willingness to become involved and their ability to connect with the ideas presented (David et al., 2003). Children want to understand the situation or circumstances in which they learn, so explanations should be simple and clear. When they find things they already know about and can latch on to, they have a base from which to explore new things. A final important factor you should consider is the importance of maintaining good working relationships with parents. Strong parental relationships provide essential information about the child's learning at home and help to provide insight into the things with which each child is familiar.

Pedagogy

Pedagogy is derived from the Greek word *paid*, meaning "child," plus *agogos*, meaning "leading," and is defined as the art and science of teaching children (Hiemstra & Sisco, 1990). In the pedagogic model, the teacher has full responsibility for facilitating learning, including what will be learned, when it will be learned, and whether the material has been learned. Pedagogy is also sometimes referred to as the correct use of teaching strategies and is described as being a didactic and traditional approach to teaching children. As the educator, you will use pedagogic principles when teaching young clients. One-to-one teaching with the child facilitates individual learning needs, provides for child and family interaction with the nurse, and protects confidentiality. Group teaching may be appropriate when the child can benefit from learning with others. Discussions and demonstrations often work well in groups.

Implications for Health Education

Health education occurs in a variety of situations, including clinics, hospitals, schools, colleges or universities, and community settings. Some situations offer the opportunity for advance planning, developing learning objectives, and arranging multiple teaching sessions. More often, there is no time for a formal teaching approach in the practice area. Woodring emphasizes that "economic realities require nurses to use both their time with patients and their teaching opportunities more efficiently" (2000, p. 505). Nurses are often placed in the position of needing to maximize time to teach the child and family. There is also an expectation that the child and family have learned the information presented and that the learning will be evidenced by positive health outcomes (Woodring, 2000). There are six steps that nurses as educators can take to streamline the process of providing efficient yet personalized health teaching in a variety of settings.

Step 1

The first step in building a trusting nurse–client relationship is to clarify the perceptions of the client and family about the health issue by asking questions. At the core of the teaching process remains the nurse–client relationship as described in the Miller-Stoeckel Client Education Model. Questions regarding client perceptions are drawn from the health belief model (see Table 1-3). For example: What is the need for care? What do you know about the problem? What is the seriousness of the condition? What impact is it having on your life? What are your goals for effective treatment? What are potential barriers to treatment? Careful attention to the answers and observations of the client as they respond helps establish the need for health education and begins the process of building trust. It is important to be attentive to the client's cultural background as the nurse analyzes client responses.

Step 2

A second step is consideration of the assessment factors that influence learning. It is important to assess the child's physical, psychosocial, and language development. It is also helpful to determine family support for treatment. Tools are available to assess the learning styles and literacy levels of both the child and parent (Davis, Nur, & Ruru, 1994; James & Galbraith, 1984). Assessment factors will weigh heavily when planning learning activities later. It is possible that how the child and family members learn may be discerned simply by observing their responses to activities that occur within the usual care situation, but assessment tools provide an efficient and quick way to gather this information.

Step 3

As an educator, you will draw on assessment data to establish mutual learning objectives that form the basis of the client education plan as part of step 3. The learning objectives should be reviewed briefly with the child and family to answer questions and determine if all learning needs are identified. You select teaching content appropriate to achieving the learning objectives and highlight the must-know information by separating information into small sections as part of the client education plan. It is important to consider current evidence-based practices as part of the plan.

Step 4

Selection of teaching strategies and instructional materials to carry out the client education plan is an important fourth step. Use assessment data to choose strategies and materials that accommodate learners' needs and abilities. It is important to take into account clients' cognitive stage, physical abilities, and language skills when planning activities. Reading capability and comprehension of the child and parent will help determine what instructional materials are appropriate. Learning materials should be age specific, interesting, and reflect the needs of the child. Remember that the cultural context of materials should be carefully considered as well. Brochures, pocket-sized flip charts, pamphlets, videos, and comic books depicting children of the client's race and ethnicity are suggestions for educational materials (Ebbinghaus & Bahrainwala, 2003). Samples of educational materials from pharmaceutical companies can be useful when return demonstrations are used.

Step 5

The fifth step is the implementation of the client education plan. Select a conducive learning environment to meet the learning objectives of the client education plan. Explanations should be simple and concrete with instructional materials that enhance understanding of the content. Speak slowly and clearly without extraneous noise interference. It is particularly important that you create an atmosphere that captures the child's interest. This may entail being adaptable and willing to offer the child options during the course of the teaching session. Pay close attention to body language that indicates distraction or lack of interest. It is particularly concerning if the child or parent does not ask questions. This is a clue that changes are needed in the teaching approach (Woodring, 2000). It is important for you to focus on the ultimate goal of the teaching session, child learning, not on maintaining a stubborn insistence on following the client education plan. A good way to determine how the teaching session went is to ask the young client or parent to summarize what has been learned at the conclusion of the session so you can correct any misconceptions related to essential content. Questions such as "Tell me in your own words how you plan to . . ." are helpful to evaluate understanding.

Step 6

Summative evaluation is the final step of the process. It not only evaluates content knowledge, but also allows the client to give the nurse feedback about what they liked or disliked about the

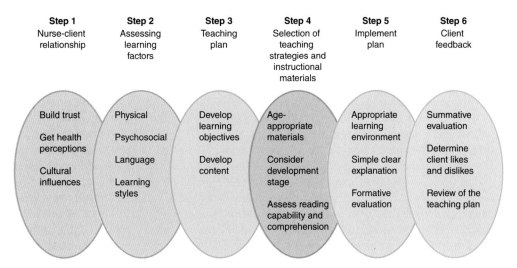

Figure 5-4 Stoeckel Health Education Process for Children

whole teaching and learning experience. Client evaluation may include return demonstration, short quizzes, or checklists. Evaluation of the learning experience includes asking the child and family about factors such as the setting, teaching strategies, instructional materials, pace of learning activities, and the nurse–client interactions. Ideally, you will see the child and family over time to assess long-term learning and provide reinforcement of essential content. This may involve scheduling follow-up teaching sessions, creating action plans for school use, and initiating a visiting nurse referral to provide ongoing education and support. **Figure 5-4** summarizes the steps of the health education process with children.

Educating Clients with Disabilities

The term *developmental disabilities* applies to children who are developmentally delayed, medically fragile, or who have intellectual or learning disabilities. Within each category of disability are extensive lists of syndromes, needed assessments, knowledge, therapies, and resources to care for this population. Societal changes have empowered persons with intellectual and developmental disabilities to more fully participate in community life (Cervasio, 2016).

Nurses play an important role in caring for children with developmental disabilities in a variety of healthcare and community settings. Roughly 5% of children ages 5 to 17 have disabilities (Disabled World, 2011), and it is estimated that approximately 13% of children in the United States have some type of special need (U.S. Census Bureau, 2000). The number of children with developmental disabilities continues to grow due to the use of scientific and technological advances that save the lives of premature infants and acutely ill children.

The most common disabilities seen in pediatric practice today are cerebral palsy, autism, and epilepsy (Centers for Disease Control and Prevention [CDC], 2016). Children with developmental disabilities require individualized and coordinated extended services, support, and assistance to function. The trend in healthcare has shifted needed disability services for these children away from institutions and toward inclusive community care settings (Nehring, 2004). Children with developmental disabilities require many advocates to seek out needed medical and nursing care, therapies, education, and equipment to integrate them into all aspects of community life.

Nurses in all practice settings must be prepared to provide nursing care, education support, training, advocacy, and leadership for children with disabilities. Nurses as educators may be asked to modify their approach to pediatric clients and their families to accommodate clients with disabilities. Disabled pediatric clients include those with autism; cognitive limitations; learning disabilities; visual, hearing, or physical limitations; and emotional disturbances or behavior disorders. Nurse educators and parents need to consider how children with disabilities respond to any form of stress brought on by illness or hospitalization. Children with disabilities generally have specific triggers, such as words, images, or sounds that signal danger or disruption to their feelings of safety or security. These are specific to each child but come from past experiences associated with traumas or seeing fear in adults. These cues can serve as warning signals that adults can read (National Association of School Psychologists, 2002). Examples of cues include certain facial expressions, changes in speech patterns, sweating, or becoming quiet and withdrawn. When adults observe these cues, they should provide assurance, support, and attention as quickly as possible. If cues are missed, children may escalate their behavior and lose control. If this happens, adults should remove the child to a safe place and allow them to calm down. Nurse educators and parents should work together to share information about triggers and cues.

Appropriate resources should be used that provide individual consideration for the child's developmental and emotional maturity. Activities that promote healing, such as making drawings or writing letters, may be important for children recovering from or facing illness. There are general guidelines that can be followed in preparation for teaching. They include preparing children for difficult vocabulary and concepts ahead of time. During the teaching session, the nurse may give explanations in small distinct steps, provide written and oral instructions that are age appropriate, and have the child repeat directions. The nurse will have greater results by being concise with verbal information. This approach is demonstrated by wording requests in a concise way, such as "Lisa, please sit" instead of "Lisa, would you please sit in the chair" (Bulloch, 2013). If a child has difficulty reading, the nurse can read or have a parent read. If a child has difficulty writing, oral responses can be accepted, or the child can dictate their thoughts to the nurse or parent.

All children benefit from concrete information presented at the proper level of understanding and maturity. The nurse educator and parents must consider how children with disabilities respond to teaching and anticipate their reactions. Strategies that have been effective for clients with disabilities in the past are the best strategies to implement, but understand that the steps might need to be more concrete and immediate. The nurse as educator should consider triggers and cues and anticipate rather than react to them. The nurse educator should expect some regression and deal with inappropriate behaviors calmly and consistently. Children need to know that despite changes and disruptions, they have a constant caring support system. Nurses must attain a core set of competencies to address the needs of children with disabilities. These competencies include:

- Communication skills including working with supportive communication devices, such as communication boards, basic sign language, and body movement.
- Critical thinking skills to promote comfort and safety.
- Working knowledge of wheelchair adaptations, walkers, seats, braces, and standing devices.
- Participating in activities of daily living require accessibility of adaptations for eating, grooming, and toileting.
- Education in schools necessitates individual accommodations for teaching and learning, as well as collaboration with school nurses.
- Ability to develop sensory integration plans.
- Behavior recognition and modifications skills and approaches to address behavioral problems.

- Professional interpersonal skills for the socialization of children.
- Safety and cultural awareness to enhance quality of life.
- Incorporation of family-centered collaboration with parents and primary caregivers. (Cervasio, 2016)

Educating Families

Families have considerable influence on children's health practices and the success of health education. As an educator you must consider the family as part of the unit of care when addressing the health education needs of children. Preparing client education plans for child clients without considering the family may result in less than adequate adherence to the treatment recommendations.

A *family* is a "group of individuals with a continuing legal, genetic, and/or emotional relationship. Society relies on the family group to provide for the economic and protective needs of individuals, especially children and the elderly" (American Academy of Family Physicians, 2003). Society's definition of family is rapidly expanding and has come to include single parents, biracial couples, blended families, unrelated individuals living cooperatively, and homosexual couples, among others.

It is important to determine who the immediate members of the family are, what roles they play within the structure of the family, their expectations about health care, and the nature of the relationships among family members. Not all families function the same way, so the nurse should assess this information by talking with clients and observing family interactions. A tool called the Family APGAR was adapted and introduced in the previous chapter to gain subjective information from clients to determine the level of support when learning new behaviors (Smilkstein, 1978). The tool addresses five aspects of family functioning; adaptive abilities, partnership, growth, affection, and resolve. This can give insight into family functioning when there is concern about family support. Child health issues disrupt family functioning. The extent of disruption is dependent on the seriousness of the illness, the family's level of functioning before the illness, socioeconomic considerations, and the extent to which the illness disrupts family functioning.

When you are aware of how the family operates, you can work to address their health education needs. The most effective client education is that which is compatible with the family's frame of reference and with which the client or family feels most comfortable. The nurse should assess the family's response to health teaching because the group's reaction can have a significant influence on the child's and parents' motivation to continue and cooperate with recommended treatment.

Kelo, Martikainen, and Eriksson (2013) describe patient education as a key intervention for promoting family health and empowerment of families. The concept of empowerment implies that client education provides knowledge and skills and increases self-awareness so that clients and family members can increase self-awareness and act in their own self-interest. Nurses facilitate empowerment of families by stating the objectives together with the child and the family, implementing child- and family-centered interactive methods, and using various evaluation methods.

Educating Groups and Communities

Nurses serve many different roles within the community. Public health nurses and school nurses assist children and families to take action to improve their health status. Often, this takes the form of teaching parents and children about healthy lifestyle choices. Public health nurses assist people in incorporating improved health behavior in their everyday lives. Ensuring children's health is critical not only for reducing child morbidity and mortality but also for increasing the likelihood of a healthier adult life. The primary goal of child health education in the community is to prevent major causes of disease, illness, and death during childhood. Health prevention teaching covers the topics of accidental injuries, infections, learning problems, and behavioral problems. The nurse may also work within school settings to develop action plans to support learning objectives.

Public health nurses educate clients concerning issues such as environmental risks, problems related to low family income, and psychological stress. Early detection and treatment of disease and disability require screening, counseling, and interventions for high-risk populations. For children from birth to age 10 years, screening includes measurement of height and weight, blood pressure, hearing, and vision. Counseling, or anticipatory guidance, relates to injury prevention, diet and exercise, substance use, and dental health. The nurse explains the importance of immunizations for children, which include diphtheria, tetanus, pertussis (DTaP); oral poliovirus; measles, mumps, rubella (MMR); *H. influenza* type B; hepatitis B; and varicella. For children older than age 10 years, additional screening recommendations include Pap smears and chlamydia screenings for sexually active females and assessments of problem drinking for adolescents. Counseling with this age group covers sexual behaviors, smoking, drinking, and other drug use. Immunizations for this age group include a tetanus–diphtheria booster for those aged 11 to 16 years. Hepatitis B and varicella vaccines should be given to those who did not receive them at earlier ages. High-risk populations include those who engage in high-risk sexual behavior or drug use and those with certain medical conditions.

Often, the nurse will inform families about services available to them. The nurse needs to be knowledgeable about community programs, which include programs such as health services for families with lower incomes, supplemental nutritional programs, child-care services, safe houses for people experiencing domestic violence, pediatric vaccine programs, and health education classes. One such nutrition program is the Women, Infants, and Children (WIC) program. WIC provides federal grants to states for supplemental foods, healthcare referrals, and nutrition education for people who have low incomes and/or are pregnant, breastfeeding, and nonbreastfeeding postpartum. It also provides help for infants and children up to 5 years of age who are found to be at nutritional risk. Another government service is Medicaid, which provides medical assistance for families with low incomes, mainly women and children. The Children's Health Insurance Program (CHIP) – formerly known as the State Children's Insurance Program (SCHIP) is a joint federal and state program that provides health coverage to low-income children and low-income pregnant women in families with incomes too high to qualify for Medicaid, but too low to afford private coverage. States have the flexibility to adopt their own eligibility standards so it is important for the nurse as educator to become familiar with the standards in the state in which you practice. (Chip Eligibility accessed on 5/15/2024 at https://www.medicaid.gov/chip/eligibility/index.html)

Educating Health Team Members

The nurse as educator works with multidisciplinary health team members in many settings. Each member of the team brings skills that contribute to the overall health of the child. Ideally, the team collaborates to develop individualized and comprehensive treatment plans that serve as the foundation for health education. Team members should include the child, family, primary care physician, specialty physicians if necessary, the nurse (nurse practitioner, home care nurse), and other healthcare professionals, depending on the need. Other team members could include a social worker, patient care coordinator, pharmacist, dietitian, respiratory therapist, occupational therapist, physical therapist, speech pathologist, radiologist, psychiatrist or psychologist, school teacher, and school nurse. It is important to view the child and family as an equal partner in the process of developing client education plans. This type of client education is a family-centered and community-based approach.

Summary

This chapter reviewed the biologic characteristics, psychosocial stages, and developmental tasks of infants, toddlers, preschool children, school-age children, and adolescents. Implications for health education were given for each age group. Orientation to learning in children involves how children learn, learning styles in children, and the role of play in learning. Specific teaching practices are used to promote child learning. Pedagogic concepts assist you as the educator in preparing client education plans. Working with clients with disabilities, families, groups, communities, and health team members brings together the importance of a multidisciplinary, holistic, community-based approach to health education for children.

Exercises

Exercise I: Deepen Sensitivity to Child Clients and Their Families

Purpose: Practice application of child learning theory.

Directions: Visit a preschool and gather a group of 6 to 10 preschoolers to complete the following tasks:

1. You are teaching a health education class to a group of preschoolers. Compose a health promotion song with gestures, using the tune of a popular nursery song or popular song—for example, "Safety the Snowman" (to the tune of "Frosty the Snowman").
2. Use props you have on hand to enhance the meaning of the song (e.g., bicycle helmets, street signs, etc.).
3. Share the songs with members of the class.
4. Discuss how you think the children learned the information.

Exercise II: Pretend Play

Purpose: Practice applying theory, discussed in this chapter, with children.

Directions: Role-play a baby doll clinic. Involve a nurse, children, and their dolls in a preschool setting to complete the following tasks:

1. Have the "mothers" come and see the nurse by walking into the pretend clinic or making an appointment on the pretend phone.
2. Have the nurse notice concern for the doll's health and ask what the mother wants (doll checkup or illness).
3. Have the nurse perform an examination, treatment, or give advice.

4. Ask a health or safety question about the doll.
5. Use real equipment or pretend you are using equipment.
6. With your peers, discuss what you learned by doing this exercise.

Exercise III: Helping Children with Chronic Illness

Purpose: Use your knowledge of child development and learning strategies.
Directions: Complete the following tasks in small groups:

1. Describe an adolescent with a long-term chronic illness. Include information such as age, developmental needs, amount of regression, and how the illness interferes with normal developmental tasks.
2. Design substitute experiences that would enhance the child's chances of meeting appropriate developmental needs.

Exercise IV: Group Teaching with Children

Purpose: Apply child learning theory to working in groups.
Directions: Role-play the following teaching and learning scenario with school-age children:

1. You are working with a group of fifth or sixth graders, discussing a topic of your choice.
2. Choose topics such as peer pressure, drugs, sex, abuse, eating disorders, or bullying.
3. Lead the children in role-playing and discussing a difficult situation.
4. Offer suggestions to address the problems that the children present—for example, how to develop drug-refusal skills or how to seek help for bullying.
5. With your peers, discuss what you have learned by doing this exercise.

Exercise V: Evidence-Based Nursing Practice

Purpose: Apply evidence-based nursing research to client education.
Directions:

1. Search the literature for nursing research applicable to health education for the child learner.
2. Describe how the findings could be applied to your practice in educating clients.

References

American Academy of Family Physicians. (2003). *Definition of family*. Retrieved from http://www.aafp.org/online/en/home/policy/policies/f/familydefinitionof.html

Athey, C. (2007). *Extending thought in young children: A parent teacher partnership* (2nd ed.). London, England: Paul Chapman Educational.

Babcock, D. E., & Miller, M. A. (1994). *Client education: Theory and practice*. St. Louis, MO: Mosby.

Bulloch, K. (2013). *How to adapt your teaching strategies to student needs*. Retrieved from http://www.Idonline.org/article/370

Carbo, M., Dunn, R., & Dunn, K. (1986). *Teaching students to read through their individual learning styles*. Englewood Cliffs, NJ: Prentice Hall.

Centers for Disease Control and Prevention. (2016). *Facts about developmental disabilities*. Retrieved at https://www.cdc.gov/ncbddd/developmentaldisabilities/facts.html

Cervasio, K. (2016). Inclusion of developmental disability nursing content into undergraduate nursing education: A renewed call for pediatric curricula reform. *International Journal of Nursing In Intellectual and Developmental Disabilities*, 6(1), Article 1.

David, T., Goouch, D., Powell, S., & Abbott, L. (2003). *Birth to three matters: A review of the literature compiled to inform the framework to support children in their earliest years*. (Research Report 444.) London, England: DfES.

Davis, E. C., Nur, H., & Ruru, S. A. (1994). Helping teachers and students understand learning styles. *English Teaching Forum, 32*(3), 12–15.

Disabled World. (2011). *Latest U.S. disability statistics and facts.* Retrieved from https://www.disabled-world.com /disability /statistics/census-figures.php

Ebbinghaus, S., & Bahrainwala, A. H. (2003). Asthma management by an inpatient asthma care team. *Pediatric Nursing, 29*(3), 177–183.

Erikson, E. (1963). *Childhood and society* (2nd ed.). New York, NY: W. W. Norton.

Falvo, D. R. (2004). *Effective patient education: A guide to increased adherence.* Sudbury, MA: Jones & Bartlett Learning.

Graca, S., Fowler, K., & Rosenstock A. (2009). Play—An educational tool in health care. In A. Lowenstein, L. Foord-May, & J. D. Romano (Eds.), *Teaching strategies for health education and health promotion: Working with patients, families and communities.* Sudbury, MA: Jones and Bartlett.

Hiemstra, R., & Sisco, B. (1990). *Individualizing instruction.* San Francisco, CA: Jossey-Bass.

Isenberg, J., & Quisenberry, N. (2002). Play: Essential for all children. (A position paper of the Association for Childhood Education.) *Association for Childhood Education International, 79*(1), 33–39.

James, W., & Galbraith, M. (1984). Perceptual learning styles: Implications and techniques for the practitioner. *Lifelong Learning, 8*(4), 23.

Jones, E., & Reynolds, G. (1992). *The play's the thing: Teachers' roles in children's play.* New York, NY: Teachers College Press.

Kearsley, G. (2004). *Explorations in learning and instruction: The theory into practice database.* Retrieved from https:// orion2020.org/archivo/cen/educational_theories_summary.pdf

Kelo, M., Martikainen, M., & Eriksson, E. (2013). Patient education of children and their families: Nurses' experiences. *The Pediatric Editorial Board, 39*(2), 1–9.

National Association of School Psychologists. (2002). *Coping with crisis-helping children with special needs: Tips for school personnel and parents.* Retrieved from http://www.nasponline.org/resources/crisis_safety /specpop_general.aspx

National Institute on Deafness and Other Communication Disorders. (2014). *Speech and language developmental milestones.* Retrieved from http://www.nidcd.nih.gov/staticresources/health/voice/NIDCD-Speech-Language-Dev-Milestones.pdf

Nehring, W. (2004). Directions for the future of intellectual and developmental disabilities as a nursing specialty. *International Journal of Nursing in Intellectual and Developmental Disabilities, 2*(1).

Olsen, M. H., & Hergenhahn, B. R. (2013). *An introduction to theories of learning* (9th ed.). Boston, MA: Pearson Prentice Hall.

Piaget, J. (1952). *The origins of intelligence in children.* New York, NY: International Universities Press.

Piaget, J. (1963). *The psychology of intelligence.* New York, NY: Routledge.

Skinner, B. F. (1968). *The technology of teaching.* New York, NY: Appleton-Century-Crofts.

Smilkstein, G. (1978). The family APGAR: A proposal for family function test and its use by physicians. *Journal of Family Practice, 6*(6), 1231–1239.

United Nations. (1989). *Convention on the rights of the child, G.A. res. 44/25, annex, 44 U.N. GAOR Supp. (No. 49) at 167, U.N. Doc. A/44/49 (1989). Entered into force Sept. 2, 1990.* Retrieved from http://www1.umn.edu/humanrts/instree/k2crc.htm

U.S. Census Bureau. (2000). *Census 2000 summary.* Retrieved from www.census.gov/hhes/www/disable/disabstat2k /table1.html.

Wong, D. L., Hockenberry-Eaton, M., Wilson, D., Winkelstein, M. L., & Schwartz, P. (2008). *Wong's essentials of pediatric nursing* (6th ed.). St. Louis, MO: Mosby Elsevier.

Woodring, B. C. (2000). If you have taught—have the child and family learned? *Pediatric Nursing, 26*(5), 505–509.

CHAPTER 6

Adult Learner

OBJECTIVES

Upon completion of this chapter, you will be able to do the following:

- Describe the biologic changes, psychosocial stages, and developmental tasks characteristic of early and middle adulthood.
- List health education topics for clients in early and middle adulthood related to biologic changes, psychosocial stages, and developmental tasks.
- Distinguish among goal-, activity-, and learning-oriented learners, and state which category best fits your motivation.
- Distinguish between pedagogy and andragogy.
- Describe how adult and child learners are alike and different in two of the assumptions of andragogy.
- Apply andragogic theory to teaching adult learners.
- Identify teaching and learning implications of educating individuals, families, groups and communities, and health team members.

CHAPTER OUTLINE

Introduction

This chapter discusses learning in adulthood and divides this period into early and middle adulthood. Learning and development are lifelong processes with identifiable features, including biologic characteristics, psychosocial stages, and developmental tasks. Learning and development are multidimensional and unique for each client, with implications for those who are seeking to promote, retain, and restore health.

Nurses work with clients of all ages who have different learning needs at different stages of development. This information is important because it affects what you teach and how you teach it. The first section of this chapter examines biologic characteristics, psychosocial stages, and developmental tasks, and their implications for nurses as educators. Andragogy, a theory of adult learning, and its underlying assumptions are examined. We describe how andragogy differs from pedagogy, the theory of how children learn.

Biologic Characteristics, Psychosocial Stages, and Developmental Tasks

Adulthood is divided into two periods: early and middle. This division is made because the biologic characteristics, psychosocial stages, and developmental tasks that accompany these periods are distinct. **Figure 6-1** illustrates the overlapping influence of these factors.

Early Adulthood (Early 20s Through 30s)

Biologic Characteristics

Clients complete their physical growth and experience peak functioning of the musculoskeletal system in their 20s. Laboratory findings are generally within normal limits. The health status of people at this age is generally uneventful unless severe illness or injury occurs. People who are pregnant have additional health concerns during pregnancy and lactation. The occurrence of chronic disease is unusual but can occur in this period (Ruchala, 2013; Santrock, 2023).

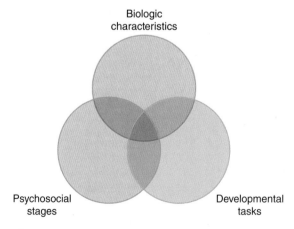

Figure 6-1 Factors Influencing Development Across the Life Span

Psychosocial Stages

Erikson's psychosocial stages for previous life stages are applicable to early and middle adulthood (1963). During puberty, the psychosocial stage is identity versus role confusion, from which a sense of identity develops. As young adults continue to mature, they move into Erikson's next stage, *intimacy versus isolation*, which is characterized by an increasing ability to love and care about others. They seek meaningful friendships and intimacy with others (Balakas, 2013). It is also during this stage that young adults clarify their values, understand themselves and others better, and develop a philosophy of life (Knowles, 1990).

Developmental Tasks

Becoming economically independent, establishing a career, and developing job-related skills are important tasks during this time. Making new friends and selecting a mate or significant other, starting a family, and rearing children are common tasks. Learning to get along with others at work, one's mate, and friends are other tasks. Dealing with ethnic and gender factors, changing role expectations in the United States, and the need for two-career families are stressors that influence these tasks (Santrock, 2023).

Middle Adulthood (40s Through Late 60s)

Biologic Characteristics

Clients in this stage begin to experience gradual physical changes, the rate of which can vary widely among individuals. Changes are influenced by genetic and lifestyle factors. Clients tend to gain weight, the skin begins to wrinkle and loosen, the hair turns gray, muscle mass and strength decline, and blood pressure and cholesterol levels may increase. Vision and hearing acuity decreases, biological females experience menopause, and biological men experience climacteric, which is similar to menopause. Cognitive functioning remains intact unless it is affected by illness or injury (Ruchala, 2013; Santrock, 2023).

Psychosocial Stages

Erikson's (1963) stage for this period is *generativity versus self-absorption and stagnation*, with a focus on helping the younger generation develop and lead useful lives. Generativity refers to the concern mature adults have for guiding the next generation. It includes being productive and creative. If they have children, parents may help them choose a suitable career. Cultural interests increase, as do social involvement and leadership responsibilities in organizations and the community (Knowles, 1990; Santrock, 2023). This is the longest of Erikson's psychosocial stages, covering the ages of 40 to 65 years.

Developmental Tasks

Clients are learning advanced job skills, often supervising others. Some are dealing with unemployment. If so, clients may be looking for new careers or educational opportunities to acquire new skills. Cultural interests increase, as does social involvement with others. As children leave home, spouses must readjust their marital relationship. If divorce occurs, further lifestyle adjustments are needed. Stay-at-home parents may return to the job market. These clients may have living parents who require time and financial attention. Because adults in this stage are still involved with raising their children and caring for parents who are aging, they are called the sandwich generation (Knowles, 1990; Santrock, 2014).

Implications for Health Education

How does this information help you become more sensitive and effective in your role as an educator? We now look at how this information helps you promote, retain, and restore the health of your clients.

Promote and Retain Health

The focus of promoting health is on prevention, whereas the focus of retaining health is on maintaining one's present health status, assuming it is satisfactory. With this in mind, **Table 6-1** lists suggested topics to promote and retain health that are appropriate for adult learners (Ruchala, 2013). These suggestions are not all-inclusive and will need to be adapted to the circumstances of the individual client.

Restore Health

Restoration of health for individuals in adulthood refers to addressing the needs of those who are experiencing an acute or chronic illness or disability. The purpose of health education at this time is designed to help clients understand the nature of their health problem, the treatment regimen, and the limitations imposed by the health problem, disability, or injury. This may involve working not only with clients but also with family members. **Table 6-2** suggests suitable topics related to the restoration of health (Ruchala, 2013). These suggestions are not all-inclusive and need to be adapted to the circumstances of the individual client.

Orientation to Learning

Houle (1961, 1980) found that adults continue learning for a variety of reasons. He identified three categories that describe adults' general orientation to learning: goal-oriented learners, activity-oriented learners, and learning-oriented learners.

Goal-Oriented Learners

Goal-oriented learners use their educational endeavors to accomplish clear and identifiable objectives. They often wait until their middle 20s to make a start on their education, and sometimes they wait much longer. Their educational activities tend to occur in episodes, each beginning with the realization of a need for an interest in expanding their skills and knowledge. Houle (1961, 1980) found that learning was a recurring pattern in their lives. These learners were not restricted to an academic setting or to any one institution or topic. They sought courses of instruction or other forms of learning when they became aware of a need. Exploration on the Internet, attending night courses, and enrolling in workshops were ways to add to their level of expertise.

Activity-Oriented Learners

Activity-oriented learners select activities that are likely to meet their need for human contact. They are course takers and group joiners. The course content or purpose of the organization is secondary to their social needs. These learners often begin their educational activities when their

Table 6-1 Suggested Topics to Promote and Retain Health

Nursing Assessment	Health Education Topics
General health habits	■ Eating a nutritious diet with dietary changes to control weight ■ Practicing regular oral hygiene and dental care ■ Obtaining adequate sleep ■ Knowing benefits of an exercise program ■ Managing physical stress ■ Coping with mental stress, such as depression ■ Minimizing risks of disease for which there is a family history, such as diabetes mellitus and cardiovascular disease
General living conditions	■ Avoiding exposure to hazardous cleaning supplies ■ Maintaining home safety for children and older adults (slip-resistant rugs, night-lights, nonskid adhesive textured strips in tub and shower, handrails on steps, grab bars in bathrooms, electrical outlets, etc.) ■ Maintaining cleanliness in the home ■ Managing family stress or abuse
Medications	■ Using prescription medications properly ■ Minimizing use of caffeine, tobacco, alcohol ■ Knowing the dangers of illicit drugs and avoiding them ■ Promoting medication safety with children in the home
Sexual habits	■ Preventing sexually transmitted diseases (STDs) ■ Knowing mode of STD transmission ■ Knowing partner's sexual history and practices ■ Practicing safe sexual practices ■ Recognizing STD symptoms
Pregnancy and children	■ Knowing about family planning ■ Addressing pregnancy and lactation issues ■ Knowing child growth and developmental stages ■ Obtaining immunizations ■ Parenting skills
Work site and employment	■ Maintaining a safe occupational environment ■ Avoiding exposure to hazardous substances ■ Minimizing economic stress ■ Minimizing job stress
Disease prevention	■ Getting routine health screenings, blood pressure checks ■ Knowing serum cholesterol levels ■ Performing monthly skin checks ■ Obtaining monthly breast exams and annual mammograms ■ Performing monthly male genitalia exams ■ Obtaining annual flu shots ■ Getting regular physical and screening exams

Table 6-2 Suggested Topics to Restore Health

Nursing Assessment	Health Education Topics
Acute illness	▪ Knowing the nature and cause of the health problem or disability ▪ Common conditions: Upper respiratory infections, urinary tract infections, minor surgery, substance abuse ▪ Understanding diagnostic tests ▪ Supporting and explaining treatment regimens ▪ Knowing hospital and clinic environment and routines ▪ Preventing spread of communicable illnesses ▪ Dealing with lifestyle changes ▪ Supporting continued physician supervision
Chronic illness	▪ Knowing the nature and cause of the health problem or disability ▪ Possible conditions: Multiple sclerosis, rheumatoid arthritis, hypertension, diabetes mellitus, AIDS, cancer, substance abuse ▪ Understanding diagnostic tests ▪ Using physical, occupational, and speech therapies ▪ Managing exacerbations and remissions ▪ Preventing complications ▪ Adapting to lifestyle changes ▪ Making environmental adaptations ▪ Using self-help devices ▪ Supporting and explaining treatment regimens ▪ Supporting continued provider supervision
Disability	▪ Knowing strengths and limitations due to disability ▪ Managing activities of daily living ▪ Building on abilities
Accidents	▪ Adapting to the nature of an injury and its impact on function ▪ Managing activities of daily living ▪ Building on abilities ▪ Addressing rehabilitation issues ▪ Preventing accidents and injuries ▪ Providing a safe home environment (slip-resistant rugs, night-lights, nonskid adhesive textured strips in tub and shower, handrails on steps, grab bars in bathrooms, etc.)

need to reach out to others becomes pressing. For example, divorce adjustment groups attract people who are attempting to fill specific needs. A young mother joins a La Leche group to fulfill her need for socialization and for support and information to breastfeed successfully. A divorced man takes a class in astronomy to talk to other people and ease his loneliness.

When setting up health education programs for adult learners, it is helpful to assess their interests via a survey. Although many adults indicate specific interests, a substantial number just want something to do and seek out classes for social reasons. You should become aware of community support groups and consider this category of learning activities whenever social isolation and loneliness are encountered. Newspapers periodically print lists of self-help and special interest groups. You should include such lists in your resource files and maintain connections in the community.

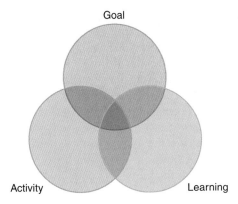

Goal

Activity   Learning

Figure 6-2 Primary Orientations to
Learning. Individuals Learn for Different
Reasons; Three Primary Orientations Are
Goal, Activity, and Learning

Learning-Oriented Learners

Learning-oriented individuals seek knowledge for its own sake. Often, they have been engrossed in learning all their lives and are avid readers. These individuals see themselves as lifelong learners and investigate everything of interest. They join groups, classes, and organizations they anticipate will be educational. An example of this is a learner who joins a book discussion group at the local library. When these learners travel, they prepare for trips by engaging in activities that make the trips more informative. They read about their destination in books, in periodicals, or on the Internet, or they might take a language course.

Figure 6-2 summarizes Houle's (1961, 1980) three orientations to learning. Most people fit into each of the categories at different times in their lives. People find that they emphasize one category more often than others. Houle concluded that most adults engage in continuing education every year, which they plan themselves. He also noted that people do not have to fit into only one category. His generalizations were meant to clarify motivations rather than to confine people to categories.

Andragogy

Malcolm Knowles, known as the Father of Andragogy in the United States, posited that adults learn differently than children. To explain this process, he developed a theory of adult learning, comprised of core adult learning principles that apply to all adult learning situations, called andragogy. His theory is about the art and science of how adults learn. Knowles's theory has its roots in the work of Abraham Maslow and Carl Rogers, who were concerned with self-actualization of the individual and a pragmatic philosophy that values knowledge gained from experience rather than formal authority (Knowles, Holton, & Swanson, 2011).

Knowles contrasted how children learn (pedagogy) in the formal education system with how adults learn (andragogy). The forces that impinge on educating young children have more to do with achieving than with learning. He cited passing tests, scoring high on the Scholastic Aptitude Test, and getting into college or graduate school as the goals of much formal education (Knowles, 1990). He noted that many assumptions that underlie the teaching methods used for adults were derived from pedagogy and are inappropriate for adults. He observed that adults learn best in informal, comfortable, flexible, and nonthreatening settings, and he consequently popularized a different set of assumptions, also called core principles, that apply to all adult learning situations (Knowles, Holton, & Swanson, 2005; Knowles et al., 2011). In these later publications, he wrote that the assumptions and core principles were the same. The six core principles of andragogy are (1) the learner's need to know, (2) the learner's self-concept, (3) the role of the learner's prior experiences, (4) readiness to learn, (5) orientation to learning, and (6) motivation to learn.

These principles should be viewed in a general sense and applied only as they fit the learners with whom you are working. They are also applied along with consideration of several variables, such as the context of the learning situation. For example, are you working with an individual or a group? Are you face to face with the learner or communicating online? A second variable to take into consideration is the differences in the nature of the subject matter. For example, are you teaching knowledge content, performance skills, or attitudes and values? For each type of subject matter, you will select appropriate teaching strategies. A third variable to take into consideration is individual learner differences. For example, what are the abilities, learning styles, and preferences among your learners? How does each prefer to learn? These variables and core principles or assumptions (Knowles et al., 2005, 2011) are discussed in the following sections, and healthcare examples are provided.

The Need to Know

Adults want to understand why they should learn something new before they are willing to learn it. In this case, you will need to be persuasive in explaining why your teaching is important. Others may recognize a gap in their current knowledge and realize they need more education in specific areas. Adult learners may also want to participate in setting the goals for learning. Adults who initiate new learning projects on their own spend considerable time and effort weighing the cost–benefit ratio before they expend large amounts of time and energy on new projects.

Application to Health Education

In your introductory remarks with adult clients in any individual or group teaching and learning situation, explain the importance of the instructional content and identify the benefits of learning it. Persuade them about the importance of learning the material by making it attractive and interesting. If you are working with a group, each individual has joined it for a different reason, so another approach would be to ask the clients what motivates them to be present and have them share their thoughts with the group. Some clients may want help developing learning objectives to address their self-identified knowledge gaps. As an educator, this gives you some sense of what motivates each individual and why they are present. Do this by asking questions such as the following:

- What do you hope to get from this lesson?
- What do you expect from our time together?
- What is the best outcome you hope for?
- Why have you come out on this beautiful (or awful) day?

Another approach is to set up situations in which clients discover for themselves the likely benefits of their efforts. For example, a first-time parent may have a multitude of questions about the care of their baby. As you work with the parent, ask her questions such as the following:

- What are your plans for caring for your baby at home?
- Have you thought about the equipment you will need at home to care for your baby?

- Will you have any help at home in caring for your baby?
- What are your concerns about the care of your baby?
- Is there anything that worries you about the care of your baby?

The Learners' Self-Concept

As individuals grow into adulthood, they increasingly see themselves as responsible beings in charge of their own lives and capable of making their own decisions. Having achieved maturity, adults wish to be respected and treated as being capable of self-direction. Any attempt to treat them as uninformed children in need of direction in the teaching and learning situation is considered demeaning. It is important to avoid talking down to clients.

Application to Health Education

This need for self-direction often presents a problem for you and clients because the situation may necessitate some client dependency. In the hospital, you have information about the acutely ill client's physiologic status, and you will be in a better position to decide what information is helpful for them to know. During certain stages of illness, the client may relinquish some control and trust your judgment and expert care. You can gently guide them in appropriate learning at this time.

Some clients who become dependent may respond with fear, bitterness, and sarcasm to relinquishing their independence. For example, an older man was rude to the nurses who cared for him while he was experiencing incontinence. He was accustomed to being the boss, and his strong self-concept was being challenged by the reality of his new dependency. The nurses were matter-of-fact and unperturbed while changing his soiled linen. As the nurses worked, they taught him that his incontinence was temporary and control would return with time and healing. They understood this response and treated him with respect and courtesy even though he was angry and rude.

Health problems may evoke feelings of unmet dependency needs in the client and complementary issues in you, such as the need to control. An example is a nurse who experiences a dependency problem when dealing with burn clients. The nurse thinks, "If only they would do what I say, they will learn that they will feel and look better in the long run. They do not understand that not moving will affect burn healing. It is up to me to teach them about the consequences of immobility before it is too late. They need to listen to me." This nurse wanted the clients to trust her advice and depend on her. In addition, the nurse is adamant about the nurse's role and her expected behavior of clients. In this case, the nurse as educator needs to reflect on her need to control and take a more empathetic approach to the clients.

The Role of the Learners' Prior Experiences

As people mature, they accumulate an expanding reservoir of experiences, both in quantity and quality. Based on these experiences, adults are able to handle more complex issues and make more thoughtful decisions that take into consideration a number of variables. Experience is something that happens to children, but for adults, experience is what defines them. A way to check out this assumption is to ask people of various ages, "Tell me about yourself." You will hear differences in the way children and adults answer. **Figure 6-3** shows adults in an active learning role.

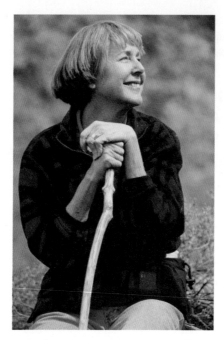

Figure 6-3 Experience Defines Older Adults
© Steve Mason/Photodisc

Application to Health Education

Adults bring a wide range of health experiences that nurses as educators can draw on as a group discusses common issues. Nurses guide the discussion by being a facilitator of learning and provide new information as appropriate. This is in contrast to lecturing to the group with little or no time for discussion. Some members of a group may have more experience with a particular issue than the nurse, and that person can become a resource for the group. For example, a small group of clients with diabetes met weekly to discuss their experiences in dealing with this disease. The nurse shared information about the physicians' medical regimen. Several clients in the group who had grappled with diabetes for more than 10 years explained the difficulties of balancing insulin intake, exercise, and nutritional requirements. By encouraging clients to share their experiences, the nurse tapped into a rich reservoir of experience to take advantage of the expertise of group members.

Adult clients learn better when strategies are employed that respect a broad base of knowledge and experience and that make use of it in the teaching and learning situation. Strategies such as discussion, laboratory, simulation, field experience, team projects, and other action-learning approaches are more conducive to the way adults learn and have strong experiential and integrating components. A good place to start is to ask adults what experiences they have had on the topic and then listen to how they interpret that experience and what it meant to them. For example, in teaching team members about a new urinary catheterization procedure, the nurse asked what their past experience has been. Have they done a similar procedure before? Were they familiar with the new equipment? What was their reaction to the new procedure? The nurse listened carefully to what was said and prepared the client education plan accordingly.

Sometimes having extensive experience is a hindrance to learning, according to Knowles (1990). Habits, biases, and presuppositions become a hindrance when the person is not open to looking at health issues in new and different ways. The nurse's role in these situations is to help clients examine troublesome and unresolved health issues and guide them in looking for alternative ways of doing things. Nurses can encourage clients to examine health habits that are not working for them and find creative ways to make changes.

In summary, it is important to recognize adult learners' experiences and contributions. If their experiences are ignored or devalued, they will likely reject efforts to learn in new ways. We believe this phenomenon is behind the resentment that some adults express when they return to school after years of earning a living and are not respected for what they have accomplished.

Readiness to Learn

It is assumed that children are ready to learn according to their biologic development and academic progress. Developmental readiness is also necessary for adult learning. The needs of adults, however, are related less to their biologic maturation and more to the developing roles in life that they have chosen or have had thrust upon them. A nurse's first pregnancy is an example. "I was a good student and did well in my OB/GYN experiences and state board examinations. Some years later, when I was pregnant, I went to childbirth education classes and was amazed at what I did not know. I listened with keen attention and made many associations that had not occurred to me when I was learning how to attend to women in labor and delivery. My increased interest was caused by a change in role. Now I was the one who was entering the role of pregnant woman and expectant parent."

Readiness to learn in the adult is associated with the ability to meet the developmental tasks associated with each stage in life. Adults face real-life situations and want to learn whatever will help them cope with their present circumstances and evolving social roles. Developing job skills and a professional identity, earning a living, meeting community responsibilities, establishing successful relationships, raising a family, and aging gracefully are some examples of these tasks.

Application to Health Education

Adults often seek out knowledge and skills based on a current health need at a particular time in their lives. Perhaps clients encounter a problem or situation and recognize that they do not have the knowledge or experience to handle it. Many adults are self-directed and find the information they need in the local library or in a class offering at a local college or community learning center. For example, a class titled "How to Remember" was offered in a setting that attracted retired citizens who had the time, energy, and resources to attend. The enrollment was high because the topic was on memory. Older people experience difficulty in remembering and find it a blow to their self-concept when they are forgetful. This workshop offered attendees an opportunity to address an important need.

Knowles (1990) noted that it is not always necessary to wait for readiness to learn to develop. You can foster readiness through experiences you create when you expose clients to successful role models. For example, encourage clients to participate in community-sponsored health fairs designed to prevent illness and detect early evidence of disease. When clients attend health education classes, they learn how to live more healthfully and how to prevent illness. By anticipating the future, clients can prepare themselves emotionally and intellectually if problems develop.

Orientation to Learning

Adults want to learn when it helps them perform a task or deal more effectively with current problems. This approach to learning is in contrast with learning that occurs in the formal educational system, in which the teacher decides what is to be learned and how the subject matter is to be organized. Adults want learning that helps them in the here and now, not learning that will be useful sometime in the future.

Andragogy assumes that adults learn better when life- or task-centered problems are the organizing factor. Adults are reluctant to expend their resources (time, money, and energy) to learn information, skills, and attitudes that they do not see as directly relevant to their current lives or problems they anticipate having. When you take a continuing education program or enroll in a degree-advancing program, you want to know how you can use it when you go to work tomorrow.

Application to Health Education

Adult clients expect nurses as educators to be knowledgeable and experientially familiar with the health issues they face. Clients expect health professionals to be in touch with real-life challenges in current society. They look for nurses who show empathy for their situation and respond to them in a professional manner. For example, one popular diabetic nurse was introduced to a group as "one of those nurses who works with diabetic clients in the clinic and has diabetes herself." Adults find information easier to grasp when it is presented in a practical life context. When clients ask for an example, they want you to present a real-life example to which they can relate. Another valuable approach is to set up a simulation or interactive exercise and offer clients the opportunity to role-play appropriate behavior in a safe setting.

Organization of content is important to learning and good teaching. Your challenge is to develop an effective client education plan. A good place to begin is the development of learning objectives to meet the client's needs. This should be a collaborative effort between you and the client. After the objectives are developed, the client education plan is organized. A good principle is to teach from the simple to the complex. Clients appreciate content that is presented from the simple to the complex and within a context to which they can relate. Other principles are to use a logical train of thought and to promote association. There are times when presenting the concept and then following it with more specific applications is the most effective way of teaching. There are other times when experiencing a number of events and then looking for their relationship to one another is more meaningful. The point is worth repeating. After the learning objectives are in place, organization of content is important. The most effective type of organization will vary with the objectives, the client, you, and the situation.

Motivation to Learn

According to Knowles (1990), the most effective motivators for adults are internal pressures and personal reasons; some examples are the desire for increased job satisfaction, self-esteem, quality of life, and so forth. Adults also respond to external motivators; for example, they may strive for a better job, a promotion, or a higher salary. Santrock (2023) calls these intrinsic and extrinsic motivators. Intrinsic motivators are like Knowles's internal pressures and are characteristic of an individual who does something for its own sake; for example, an adult may study literature because it is enjoyable. Extrinsic motivators are like Knowles's external motivators, which occur when an individual does something to obtain a reward or avoid a punishment, as noted.

Figure 6-4 Adult Learners Are Motivated for Intrinsic and Extrinsic Reasons
© Lisa F. Young/Shutterstock

Adults seek out learning experiences for a variety of reasons. Merriam, Caffarella, and Baumgartner (2007), quoting Boshier (1991), identify seven factors that motivate adults to continue learning: (1) improvement of verbal and written skills, (2) social interaction with others, (3) remediation of past deficiencies, (4) improvement of career or job status, (5) improvement of family relationships, (6) social stimulation, and (7) following interests and seeking new knowledge. These are broad-based and powerful motivators for adults seeking continued learning.

Carl Rogers (1961) and Abraham Maslow (1987) demonstrated that adults are motivated toward self-improvement and continued growth. In Maslow's terminology, adults strive for self-actualization. However, barriers such as negative self-concept, inability to access resources, time constraints, and programs that violate adult learning principles all interfere with the growth process. Our own experiences as clinicians and teachers working with clients of different ages and abilities lead us to believe that these principles have broad application. See **Figure 6-4**.

Application to Health Education

During times of illness and stress, clients are more motivated to make changes and modifications to improve their health status. Often, health-altering events cause clients to seek help for themselves or their family members. The nurse as educator asks, What is the nature of the client's problem, and what kind of adaptations will they have to make? How life-altering are these adaptations? Are they lifestyle changes, or do they involve a lengthy rehabilitation regimen? Is the client temporarily or permanently disabled? Depending on the seriousness of the health problem, clients undergo several stages of adjustment, and most become motivated to improve their health status.

Table 6-3 A Comparison of Assumptions of Pedagogic and Andragogic Approaches to Learning

Assumptions About Learning	Pedagogy	Andragogy
Need to know	Teacher driven; accepted by learner	Learner driven
Self-concept	Accepts direction from teacher	Self-directed
Role of experience	Happens to the learner	Integrally involved with self-concept; must be acknowledged
Readiness to learn	Biologic and academic development	Evolving social and life roles
Orientation to learning	Subject centered; selected by the teacher	Life centered; task and problem centered
Motivation	External approval from the teacher	Internal drives and life goals

Data from Knowles, M. S. (1990). The adult learner: A neglected species (4th ed.). Houston, TX: Gulf; Knowles, M. S., Holton, E. F., III, & Swanson, R. A. (2005). The adult learner (6th ed.). Burlington, MA: Elsevier.

Nurses also see clients who are undergoing stressful life situations that compound health problems they are experiencing. For example, consider clients who are going through role changes and life transitions, such as changing careers and requiring new skills, transitioning from childless couple to parents, and moving from being employed to unemployed. A life transition is the process that individuals undergo when their roles change dramatically, as in the death of a significant other, birth, marriage, divorce, moving from a stable environment, and making a radical work change. A life transition may force clients to make a paradigm shift in their thinking. As an educator, you can capture these moments when clients are amenable and motivated to hear your suggestions and encouragement. These times are what educators call teachable moments. It is a time when you have clients' full attention.

Table 6-3 compares the different assumptions of pedagogy and andragogy as they affect the approach to learning. This information is important because it influences how you approach clients of different ages. It is the theoretical knowledge that undergirds your client education plan and your approach to health education. Although the table makes a distinction between pedagogy and andragogy, the principles of andragogy have been reported to be effective in teaching younger clients (Knowles et al., 2005; O'Shea, 2003).

Experiential Learning

Learning in adulthood is also viewed from experiential learning theory, an approach that combines experience, perception, cognition, and behavioral learning theories. Personal experiences serve as sources of learning and contribute to adult development. Although experiential learning theory is applicable to individuals in all life stages from childhood to old age, we believe it is especially suitable for working with adult clients who have accumulated a wealth of life experiences.

Kolb developed a model for experiential learning (1984). From adults' concrete experiences, they formulate observations and reflect on those experiences. This leads to the formation of abstract concepts and generalizations, theories about effectiveness and ineffectiveness. Following this, adults test the implications of new concepts in new situations. Through personal experiences they continuously modify their thoughts, concepts, and ideas of the world and their environment. In this model, it is not necessarily the outcome that is important; the focus is on the process of learning.

Implications for Health Education

Teaching strategies that combine theory and practice with practical application are most effective for adults. Because learning is grounded in experience, not all experiences have resulted in accurate knowledge. Nurses as educators can implant new ideas and information to revise inaccurate perceptions. It is often helpful to begin teaching by asking learners what they know about the topic. If they express inaccurate beliefs and information, discuss them with the client. Nurses are responsible for modifying these beliefs by presenting accurate information, but they may encounter client resistance to new information. Clients must then decide if they will integrate, substitute, or reject this new information.

Educating Clients with Disabilities

Disabilities cover a wide range of conditions of the body and mind. The U.S. Census (2023) reported that one in four adults in the United States (27%), have some type of disability. The CDC categorizes disabilities into six dimensions: mobility, cognition, independent living, hearing, vision, and selfcare. Of those with disabilities, 41.6 have obesity, 21.9% smoke, 9.6% have heart disease, and 15.9% have diabetes. The World Health Organization categorizes disabilities in three dimensions: impairment (as in body structure or function), activity limitations (as in vision, hearing, walking, problem solving), and participation restrictions (as in activities of daily living and social activities). They further noted that at some point, almost everyone will be temporarily or permanently impaired, particularly those who live to old age (WHO, 2011).

This text limits the discussion of specific disabilities; rather, our focus is health education. Learning and developmental disabilities were covered in Chapter 5. Physical and brain disabilities are addressed in this chapter. Sensory disabilities, chronic illness, and cognitive issues are covered in Chapter 7.

Looking at the adult population addressed in this chapter, 10% of people aged 18 to 64 have disabilities (Disabled World, 2011). In this age group, you may see clients with a physical disability and brain disability. Physical disability refers to issues of mobility due to injury or disease. Brain disabilities are of two types, acquired brain injury and traumatic brain injury, and can be mild, moderate, or severe. The causes of brain disabilities are many but primarily the result of external forces (Disabled World, 2016).

Begin by assessing the client's functional ability and the nature, extent, and severity of the disability. Determine if the disability is new, long-standing, or requires adaptation to changing conditions. Is the health education setting a rehabilitation facility, a long-term care facility, or at home? Identify the client's learning needs and whether caretakers or family members should also be involved.

Determine which learning domain is the focus for your teaching. Is it in the cognitive, psychomotor, or affective domain or a combination of these? Consider that the client may have one of many learning disabilities. For example, learning disabilities affect information processing such as how people learn, understand, communicate, and remember information (Learning Disabilities Association of America [LDA], 2015). Clients with traumatic brain injury may be in an inpatient rehabilitation unit, at home, or in a long-term care facility. You need specific information about the rehabilitation program and how health education can facilitate it (Salazar et al., 2000). Clients with physical disabilities may need instruction in using crutches or other mobility aids. Next, establish objectives to address learning needs in collaboration with the client and the interprofessional team.

Remember that clients with disabilities are encouraged to be as self-sufficient as possible. If the disability is long-standing, the client knows their strengths and limitations and will guide you in determining the type and level of health education they desire. Your health education goal is to promote, retain, and restore health.

Educating Families

Illness affects not only the client but also the client's family and significant others. When clients need assistance from others, nurses must be sensitive to their wishes about the degree to which they want family and significant others participating in their health education. Some clients value their privacy, whereas other clients want family and significant others involved. If clients require procedures and follow-up care that they are unable to do themselves, they may request that others be involved. In all cases, it is important to avoid embarrassing clients by sharing unnecessary information with family or significant others. If clients want family and significant others involved, then reveal only information that is essential for communicating the health message.

Educating Groups and Communities

Many social groups, civic organizations, educational institutions, and industries are interested in health education and are looking for guest speakers. If you have a specialty area, consider making yourself available to these groups. It will build your confidence, and you will realize ways to contribute to your community. For example, nursing students were invited to present a program on healthful living to members of a local church. They each took a topic and kept their remarks pertinent and brief, and they supplemented the information with colorful audiovisual aids. They talked about the benefits of good nutrition, adequate sleep, daily exercise, and mental stimulation through a variety of activities. The audience listened and had questions following the students' presentation. Other nursing students met with female members of another church and taught them about early detection of breast cancer. They taught breast self-examination through a video presentation followed by demonstration of the technique on breast models. Both were successful events—many of the attendees scheduled mammograms at a nearby hospital.

When presenting health education to a group in the community, make it lively and interesting by using a variety of teaching strategies and instructional materials. Announce your presentation in advance by publishing it in a local newsletter or community newspaper to attract an audience. Doing so provides time for the audience to work it into their daily schedule. Also, give your presentation an interesting and catchy title, something that creates interest. Perhaps the place where you will make your presentation will help to advertise it. When making the presentation, use teaching strategies that encourage active participation, such as providing time for discussion. Also plan time for questions and clarification to ensure your message is understood. Active participation stimulates interest. Your presentation will be remembered longer if those attending actively participate.

Educating Health Team Members

Some of today's care providers have little formal healthcare training, such as nursing assistants, who usually receive about 6 weeks of training. Consequently, some health education may be directed to team members with whom you work. In planning health education for team members, you must know the provisions of the nurse practice act in your state to know the scope of practice for each team member, such as the nursing assistant, licensed practical nurse, and registered nurse. You must also know the general policies and practice guidelines of your employer. Acute care institutions have in-service education departments that handle continuing education for employees, but long-term care facilities may or may not.

If it is your responsibility to provide health education to team members, you should first assess their learning needs through either a formal or informal survey. You can also determine learning needs by observing team members as you work with them. While developing learning objectives, keep in mind the three learning domains—cognitive, affective, and psychomotor— and consider in which domain team members need health education. For example, does a team member lack knowledge about the client's health problem and rationale for treatment (cognitive domain)? Is a team member biased in their attitude toward caring for certain patients (affective domain)? Does a team member need to refresh their skills in performing nursing care procedures (psychomotor domain)? After you have determined the learning domain in which health education is needed, write the learning objectives. Your next step is to determine how the content should be taught and whether or not it can be done informally on the job or formally away from the patient care unit. After this decision is made, select teaching strategies and instructional materials to meet the team members' needs. Following your teaching, you need to assess the effectiveness of your teaching.

Summary

As adults deal with changes in their business, personal, and professional lives, they realize that learning is, indeed, a lifelong process. Learning in adulthood is influenced by needs related to biologic characteristics, psychosocial stages, and developmental tasks. Adults continue their learning for a variety of reasons, some to meet goals, others for social reasons, and still others for the love of learning. Health-related topics to promote, retain, and restore health are numerous and should be individualized for specific client situations.

The assumptions of andragogy were explored and contrasted to pedagogy. Adults engage in learning activities because they have a need to know, perhaps knowledge related to employment or personal issues. Adults want to be respected as competent and capable of self-direction, and they want to be valued for their life experiences. Other assumptions of andragogy include readiness to learn, orientation to learning, and motivation to learn. Health education opportunities occur with individuals, families, and groups or communities, as well as with health team members.

Exercises

Exercise I: Contrasting Pedagogy and Andragogy

Purpose: Test Knowles's ideas about adult learning.
Directions:

1. Identify children at different ages and say, "Tell me about yourself." Note the answer. If a child asks you, "What do you mean?" answer, "Oh, anything you want to tell me."
2. Repeat the preceding assignment with adults.
3. Note the differences and similarities between the responses of the children and the adults.
4. Discuss your findings with your colleagues.

Exercise II: Orientation to Learning

Purpose: Develop awareness of your own orientation to learning according to Houle.
Directions: Work in small groups to complete the following tasks:

1. Categorize your orientation to learning according to Houle's findings.
2. Discuss the implications this has for you as a learner and in your role as an educator.
3. Distinguish between andragogy and pedagogy.
4. Discuss how this information can be useful with clients.
5. Discuss your reflections with your peers.

Exercise III: Reflection Questions

Purpose: Become aware of how your orientation to learning affects your motivation, learning strategies, and topics of interest.
Directions:

1. What is your motivation for studying health education in nursing?
2. What strategies help you learn?
3. What aspects of nursing interest you the most?
4. What do you hope to gain from your formal education?

Exercise IV: Teaching Team Members

Purpose: Apply adult learning theory to teaching team members.
Directions: Role-play the following teaching and learning situations:

1. A newly certified nurse assistant is assigned to care for a client with a hip replacement. On the first postoperative day, the client requests a bedpan, and the nurse assistant asks you what she should do. How would you respond?
2. You observe a dietary aide responding to a client's request for more salt on her dinner tray. The client has congestive heart failure, and salt is prohibited. You meet the dietary aide as she is about to enter the client's room to deliver the additional salt. How would you handle this situation?
3. You are supervising a new registered nurse graduate who is administering heparin for the first time to a client with a clotting disorder. He asks you to help him properly administer the subcutaneous injection.
4. Your colleague needs to change a complex dressing on a hospitalized client, which is a new procedure for her. You are familiar with the procedure, and she asks you for help.

Exercise V: Evidence-Based Nursing Practice

Purpose: Apply evidence-based nursing research to client education.
Directions:

1. Search the literature for nursing research applicable to health education of the adult learner.
2. Describe how the findings could be applied to educating clients in your practice.

References

Balakas, K. (2013). Developmental theories. In P. A. Potter, A. G. Perry, P. A. Stockert, & A. M. Hall (Eds.), *Fundamentals of nursing* (8th ed., pp. 130–138). St. Louis, MO: Mosby-Elsevier.

Boshier, R. (1991). Psychometric properties of the alternative form of the education participation scale. *Adult Education Quarterly, 41*(3), 150–167.

Centers for Disease Control and Prevention. (2023). *Disability impacts all of us.* Retrieved from cdc.gov/ncbddd/disability andhealth/infographic-disability-impacts-all.html

Disabled World. (2011). *Latest U.S. disability statistics and facts.* Retrieved from https://www.disabled-world.com/disability /statistics/census-figures.php

Disabled World. (2016). *Disability: Definition, types and models.* Retrieved from https://www.disabled-world.com/disability /types/

Erikson, E. (1963). *Childhood and society* (2nd ed.). New York, NY: W. W. Norton.

Houle, C. O. (1961). *The inquiring mind.* Madison: University of Wisconsin Press.

Houle, C. O. (1980). *Continuing learning in the professions.* San Francisco, CA: Jossey-Bass.

Knowles, M. S. (1990). *The adult learner: A neglected species* (4th ed.). Houston, TX: Gulf.

Knowles, M. S., Holton, E. F., III, & Swanson, R. A. (2005). *The adult learner* (6th ed.). Burlington, MA: Elsevier.

Knowles, M. S., Holton, E. F., III, & Swanson, R. A. (2011). *The adult learner* (7th ed.). Burlington, MA: Butterworth-Heinemann, Elsevier.

Kolb, D. A. (1984). *Experiential learning.* Englewood Cliffs, NJ: Prentice Hall.

Learning Disabilities Association of America. (2015). *Adults with learning disabilities—An overview.* Retrieved from https:// ldaamerica.org/adults-with-learning-disabilities-an-overview/

Maslow, A. H. (1987). *Motivation and personality* (3rd ed.). New York, NY: Harper & Row.

Merriam, S. B., Caffarella, R. S., & Baumgartner, L. M. (2007). *Learning in adulthood* (3rd ed.). San Francisco, CA: Jossey-Bass.

O'Shea, E. (2003). Self-directed learning in nurse education: A review of the literature. *Journal of Advanced Nursing, 43*(1), 62–70.

Rogers, C. R. (1961). *On becoming a person.* Boston, MA: Houghton-Mifflin.

Ruchala, P. (2013). Young and middle adults. In P. A. Potter, A. G. Perry, P. A. Stockert, & A. M. Hall (Eds.), *Fundamentals of nursing* (8th ed., pp. 157–170). St. Louis, MO: Mosby Elsevier.

Salazar, A. M., Warden, D. L., Schwab, K., Spector, J., Braverman, S., Walter, J., . . . Ellenbogen, R. G. (2000). Cognitive rehabilitation for traumatic brain injury. *Journal of the American Medical Association, 283*(23), 3075–3081.

Santrock, J. W. (2014). *A topical approach to life-span development* (7th ed.). Boston, MA: McGraw-Hill.

Santrock, J. W. (2023). *A topical approach to life-span development* (11th ed.). New York, NY: McGraw Hill LLC.

U.S. Census Bureau. (2012). *Nearly 1 in 5 people have a disability in the U.S.* Retrieved from https://www.census.gov /newsroom/releases/archives/miscellaneous/cb12-134.html

World Health Organization. (2011). *World report on disability.* Retrieved from http://www.who.int/disabilities/world _report/2011/report.pdf

CHAPTER 7

Older Learner

OBJECTIVES

Upon completion of this chapter, you will be able to do the following:

- Discuss ageism and the subjective experience of the older client.
- Describe the psychosocial stages, developmental tasks, and physiologic changes that are characteristic of late adulthood and affect teaching and learning.
- List health education topics for clients in late adulthood related to psychosocial stages, developmental tasks, and normal physiologic changes.
- Identify common chronic diseases of older adults and their implications for health education.
- Describe the importance of cultural assessment of older adults from different ethnic backgrounds.
- Identify the implications of nutritional status on teaching and learning.
- Identify the teaching and learning implications of educating clients with disabilities; individuals, families, groups, and communities; and health team members.

CHAPTER OUTLINE

Introduction

Because people are living longer and healthier, you will encounter older clients in virtually every healthcare and community setting. Older clients, like their younger counterparts, are lifelong learners and have many lived experiences and much wisdom to share. The focus of this chapter is on providing health education to older adult clients. We do this by first looking at the concept of ageism that permeates U.S. culture. We then address the psychosocial stages, developmental tasks, and normal physiologic changes that are characteristic of late adulthood and their implications for teaching and learning. Nutrition and older adults from underrepresented ethnic groups are discussed as important aspects for health teaching. Some older clients have disabilities that nurses will encounter in their role as educators. It is common, for example, for them to have one or more chronic diseases and cognitive functioning issues related to memory and medication. These are important considerations for all clients, not just those who are older. The chapter concludes with a discussion of educating families, groups, and communities and health team members.

We define older adult learners as those who are age 65 years and older. This group numbered 54.1 million in 2019; which meant that 1 in every 7 persons in the United States (16% of the population) was an older American. This age group is projected to increase to 21.6% of the population by 2040. The older population is beginning to burgeon again as more than two-fifths (41%) of the baby boomer generation (those born between 1946 and 1964) is now 65 and older according to the most recent year for which data are available (Administration on Aging [AOA], 2021).

In 2019, 24% of those aged 65 years and older were members of racial or ethnic minority populations: 9% were African Americans, 9% were of Hispanic origin, 5% were Asian American, 0.6% were American Indian and Alaska Native, 0.1% were Native Hawaiian/Pacific Islander, and 0.8% identified themselves as being of two or more races (AOA, 2021).

The gender differences are increasing among those 65 and older. In 2019, of people aged 65 years and older, 30 million are women and 24.2 million men—a ratio of 125 women for every 100 men. At age 85 years and older, this ratio increased to 178 women for every 100 men. In 2019, there were 100,322 persons age 100 and older (AOL, 2021). These data suggest that aging is increasingly a women's issue.

Ageism

Ageism refers to the stereotypes (how we think), prejudice (how we feel), and discrimination (how we act) toward others or oneself based on age (World Health Organization, 2021). Ageism increased with the COVID-19 pandemic. Older adults were increasingly viewed as helpless, frail, and unable to contribute to society (Ayalon et al., 2021). As a nurse, you will be working with older clients, so it is important you examine your attitudes about aging. How you see older clients wittingly or unwittingly influences how you react and treat them. This, in turn, influences how they see and value themselves. This means confronting the myths and stereotypes about older people that research and experience have demonstrated are not true. For example, some people believe that many older adults are confused, lonely, and generally in poor health, none of which is true. Many older people live alone or with family members, have sufficient financial resources, and are in generally good health (Korem, 2013).

Health promotion and disease prevention for older adults are just as important as they are for all other age groups, including children. Health promotion activities, such as regular exercise, proper nutrition, and cessation of smoking and other harmful health habits, are effective in improving the quality of health among older adults regardless of their age. A person is never too old to improve their health by changing poor habits to health-promoting ones. Health promotion topics are fruitful areas for health education, and they enrich the quality of life regardless of age (Blais, 2014).

Psychosocial Stages, Developmental Tasks, and Physiologic Changes of Late Adulthood

The older population is increasing rapidly and has the longest developmental time span of any age group (Santrock, 2023). How people age is an individual process and varies greatly as people grow older. In addition to normal physiological aging and genetics, other factors influence aging, including the environment, economic circumstances, culture, lifestyle, and psychosocial variables. Each client must be assessed in terms of their unique circumstances and functional abilities. For example, some older learners may be cognitively competent and active in their daily lives, while others may have cognitive challenges and need assistance with the activities of daily living. Some older adults participate in walking and hiking activities, while others are more sedentary and limited in their physical abilities.

Because of this rapidly increasing population of older adults, demographers divide this age group into two time periods: young old adults (aged 65 to 84 years) and old adults (aged 85 years and older). In this section, we address the psychosocial stages, developmental tasks, and physiological changes of the young old adult and the old adult. In practice, each client is unique and deserves individual assessment and evaluation.

Psychosocial Stages

We view the psychosocial stages through the work of Erik Erikson (1963, 1982). The eighth developmental stage that he identified is *ego integrity versus despair*. In this stage, individuals engage in a life review. They evaluate the meaning of their lives, their accomplishments and failures, and their satisfactions and disappointments. It is a time of reflection, evaluation, interpretation, and often a reinterpretation of their experiences. Many look back with satisfaction, knowing they have done their best in spite of failures (integrity), whereas others look back with regret and see themselves as failures (despair). This stage holds the potential for growth, understanding, and the development of wisdom (Balakas, 2013; Santrock, 2023). Wisdom is the positive growth that comes from life's experiences and results in deeper insights, perceptions, and judgments.

Because the life span for humans continues to lengthen, Erik and Joan Erikson (Erikson & Erikson, 1997) further explored the 80- to 90-year-old age group and added a ninth stage by enhancing their eight stages. They reversed the order of each of the previous eight stages and added to the positive aspect as follows:

1. Basic mistrust versus trust: Hope
2. Shame and doubt versus autonomy: Will
3. Guilt versus initiative: Purpose
4. Inferiority versus industry: Competence
5. Identity confusion versus identity: Fidelity
6. Isolation versus intimacy: Love
7. Stagnation versus generativity: Care
8. Despair and disgust versus integrity: Wisdom

Placing the negative before the positive emphasizes how the negative aspects of each stage may potentially affect individuals in this age group. Physiologic aging changes occurring during this time result in daily difficulties and reevaluations. It is the final life-cycle stage when individuals must come to terms with declining independence, loss of control, and weakening self-esteem and confidence. Individuals who successfully deal with the negative aspects of this stage move on to gerotranscendence—that is, rising above the negative and celebrating the life that remains (Erikson & Erikson, 1997).

Robert Peck (1968) expanded upon Erikson's final developmental stage of the older adult ego integrity versus despair. Peck divided the final stage into three additional tasks: ego differentiation, body transcendence, and ego transcendence. The first task, *ego differentiation*, is developing satisfaction from the self as a person, rather than from an occupation role or a parent. The second task, *body transcendence*, is adjusting to the physical declines of aging, rather than becoming absorbed in health problems or physical limitations imposed by aging. The third task, *ego transcendence*, is having satisfaction when reflecting on one's life and accomplishments rather than dwelling on the prospect of death.

Maslow's hierarchy provides another framework for viewing the importance of individual needs. It is a theory of motivation that applies to older adults. At certain times in the older person's life, basic needs, such as nutrition, may be the most important, whereas at other times, the same individual may be engaged in self-actualization. It is important to assess each individual to determine present needs.

This is also a time of adjusting to transitions and new social roles. With longer lives, adults experience more losses, transitions, and adjustments to new social roles. Major losses include retirement, financial status, and possibly health. Social roles, relationships, and networks also change. The most difficult losses are usually related to the death of loved ones and friends (Korem, 2013). Your role as an educator in working with older adults is to help them successfully accept, adapt, and adjust to these psychosocial stages.

Developmental Tasks

Developmental tasks refer to the issues and problems that older adults face in living, including their changing social roles. Knowing about these tasks helps you understand the life stage clients are in and the common issues they face.

In late adulthood, many clients are adjusting to retirement and may use this time to explore new interests and find new activities. Many clients want to continue employment because it gives meaning to their lives. Others continue employment because of difficult economic times. Financial stress is particularly difficult to deal with when resources are limited or insufficient to meet daily needs. Declining financial resources may require a change in the living situation to which the individual must adjust. If clients are receiving a pension, Social Security, or welfare, they have to learn about that system and how to navigate it. The same is true with navigating Medicare and Medicaid (Knowles, 1990; Santrock, 2023).

Many retired adults expand their interests and hobbies during this time and find satisfaction in volunteer work. Many want to be useful and associate with like-minded individuals. The death of a spouse or significant other will require an adjustment in living. Roles change in retirement, and new ones have to be negotiated with the spouse or significant other, children, and grandchildren (Knowles, 1990; Santrock, 2023).

As the educator, you need to be tuned in to clients' changing social roles. Retirement, for example, is a major lifestyle rearrangement. For those who have identified themselves by their work without developing strong interests in other areas, retirement may be particularly difficult. These individuals may experience feelings of dependency, powerlessness, and helplessness. For clients about to retire or who are having difficulty adjusting to retirement, encourage them to gradually disengage from the work role. Help them identify other areas of interest and activities to pursue. Do not overlook the effect on the spouse when one marriage partner retires. Many at-home partners comment about the adjustments they have to make when their spouse retires and begins following them around the house all day.

Physiologic Changes that Affect Teaching and Learning

Older adults experience an increasing number of physiologic changes during this time; however, there is considerable variability in the rate and nature of these changes. Adults aged 65 to 84 years are increasingly healthier when compared with previous generations, and they can lead active, productive lives (**Figure 7-1**). They have substantial potential for physical strength and fitness and retain much of their cognitive capacity. Adults aged 85 years and older are losing some of their physical strength and agility and show a greater loss in cognitive skills. They also experience a decline in general health and well-being (Santrock, 2023). In evaluating the physiologic changes that occur with aging, it is important to distinguish between normal aging and pathologic processes. This section covers those physiologic changes that most affect teaching and learning. More complete information is found in medical–surgical textbooks.

The impact of biologic aging is evident in every body system and in the person's general appearance. While genetics is something that cannot be controlled, health habits and choices can be. Good health habits, preventive measures, and lifestyle patterns such as rest, exercise, nutrition, and stressors greatly affect the health of every individual. In the older person, the long-term accumulated effects of these patterns become more obvious. In this section, we highlight some physiologic changes and pathophysiologic problems that occur with aging and how they affect teaching and learning.

Figure 7-1 Many Older Adults Lead Active, Productive Lives
© Andresr/Shutterstock

Appearance

The most obvious signs of aging are seen in the skin. Wrinkling and sagging skin, thinning and graying hair, dryness, and pigmentation changes are common. Many skin changes are caused by exposure to sunlight, a problem that is addressed in much of health education today. Clients with diabetes or cerebral vascular accidents have decreased sensation and must be taught to prevent burns from heating pads, bathing, and cooking (Eliopoulos, 2014). The appearance of the body changes and alters the contours of earlier years. Body mass diminishes from the face and extremities and increases in the trunk, abdomen, and hips.

Musculoskeletal System

In the musculoskeletal system, muscle mass and strength diminish, bone mass declines, and degenerative joint changes can occur. Almost 30% of muscle mass is lost by the 70s. Older adults who regularly exercise retain more bone, muscle mass, and muscle tone compared to inactive individuals, providing an excellent opportunity for health education. There is a progressive loss of height, especially among females because of osteoporosis, which is demineralization of the bones (Roberts, 2014). Expect clients to fatigue more easily than younger ones. Their movements may be slower and more rigid. Taking frequent breaks and allotting sufficient time help compensate for this. Older clients are more comfortable sitting in padded chairs with arms.

Cardiovascular System

Cardiovascular changes occur with aging, as evidenced by a decrease in cardiac output, abnormal increases in systolic or diastolic blood pressures, and weak peripheral pulses, particularly in the lower extremities. Hypertension, if present, can lead to serious health problems such as heart failure, stroke, renal failure, coronary heart disease, and peripheral vascular disease. Collagen in the heart muscle increases and elastin decreases, affecting myocardial contractility. The heart valves become thickened and fibrotic from lipid accumulation and degeneration of collagen; fibrosis of the aortic and mitral valves is most frequently affected. The coronary blood flow decreases significantly. The number of pacemaker cells in the sinoatrial node and conduction cells in the atrioventricular node, the bundle of His, and bundle branches also decreases, which may result in conduction problems. Atherosclerosis and arteriosclerosis are common in the arterial walls, diminishing elasticity and vasomotor tone. Total peripheral resistance is increased, which results in an increase in blood pressure. These changes result from disease, environmental factors, lifetime health behaviors, and aging; they are not caused by aging alone. As a result, the older adult is less able to respond to physical and emotional stress (Disabatino & Bucher, 2014). Factors such as obesity, diet, activity, and habits have been implicated as etiologic factors, all of which have implications for nurse educators, particularly among younger adults.

Respiratory System

Lung function decreases as respiratory muscle strength and mobility of the ribs decline. Osteoporosis is often present, leading to dorsal kyphosis, a curvature in the thoracic spine. The anteroposterior diameter of the thorax increases, giving the chest a barrel-shaped appearance. The number of functional alveoli decreases, resulting in an increase in residual volume (the amount of air remaining after maximum expiration). The alveoli are less elastic and relatively more fibrous, which decreases the older person's ability to engage in physically taxing activities. Dyspnea may be evident on little exertion or stress (Eisel, 2014). With these respiratory changes, clients may fatigue easily and need their learning activities adjusted to their abilities.

Changes in the musculoskeletal, cardiovascular, and respiratory systems affect the older client's energy level, strength, and speed. Endurance certainly may be affected, but another influential variable is the person's usual activity level. Older people who lead very active lives tend to have remarkable endurance. They may be able to do a sustained activity familiar to them better than a younger individual who has less practice. Maintaining the functional ability of older adults—that is, maintaining their ability to live independently and perform the activities of daily living—is enhanced with regular exercise. Exercises also can reverse or slow declines in age-related motor performance (Fahlman, Topp, McNevin, Morgan, & Boardley, 2007). Nurses can encourage older adults to participate in exercises by teaching the benefits of a regular program. Ask older clients if they have noticed a decline in their strength and motor functioning. This focuses their attention on the topic, after which you can explain how exercise limits or reverses a decline, retains their independence, and maximizes their ability to engage in the activities of daily living (Schneider, Eveker, Bronder, Meiner, & Binder, 2003).

Exercise improves strength and endurance of people at all ages, including those who reside in nursing homes. Fahlman and colleagues (2007) found that a structured exercise program for older adults with limited functional ability increased their strength and endurance. For example, nursing students led older clients at senior centers in an exercise program. It was a lively activity, enjoyed by students and participants. If you are working with clients living in an institution, take into consideration their current rest and exercise routine when deciding on the best time to initiate teaching. Clients learn better when they are well oxygenated by an invigorated circulatory system and when they are rested enough to have the extra energy needed to focus on learning. Weinrich, Boyd, and Nussbaum (1989) recommend low-impact exercises during which their feet do not leave the floor. They also recommend slowing the speed of exercise and increasing the warm-up and cool-down time. As educators, focus on helping older clients retain as much physical strength and agility as possible.

Gastrointestinal–Urinary Systems

Bowel and bladder problems increase with age. Bowel motility decreases, resulting in constipation. Bladder capacity decreases and can result in urinary incontinence. To address bowel changes, nurses should teach clients the benefits of drinking adequate fluids, eating sufficient roughage, and getting regular exercise. Some medications have an effect on intestinal motility and need further evaluation. To address bladder changes, nurses should identify the cause of the incontinence, work with clients to establish a regular voiding schedule, and teach pelvic floor or Kegel exercises (Blais, 2014). Bladder capacity and urinary incontinence are conditions to be aware of when planning learning activities. Providing frequent breaks may be necessary.

Neurologic System

Functional changes in the neurologic system occur with aging. Neuron loss occurs, affecting the function of chemical substances (epinephrine and acetylcholine) that enhance or inhibit nerve impulse transmission. Degenerative changes in myelin can interfere with nerve conduction. Voluntary reflexes are slower, and the older person's ability to react quickly to stimuli is slowed (Lueckenotte, 2009). In addition to vision and hearing changes, other aging-related neurologic changes include decrease in memory, taste, smell, vibration and position sense, and muscle strength (Olson, 2014).

Some clients have benign essential tremors that affect their upper extremities, head, and voice, a condition commonly seen in older adults. Tremors also may be associated with pathology such as Parkinson's disease or with side effects of drugs (Millsap, 2007). The presence of tremors affects the type of learning activities in which these clients can successfully engage. Fine hand movements in manipulating equipment or writing tasks are difficult for these clients, so other learning activities should be selected.

Sensory Changes

Sensory changes have an effect on the lifestyle of older clients. The most important sensory changes affecting teaching and learning are vision and hearing impairments. Diminished functional ability in either or both interferes with the older client's ability to communicate orally and in writing. This leads to social isolation as clients avoid the strain of hearing a muted or indistinguishable conversation, embarrassment associated with responding inappropriately to the comments of others, or diminished mobility associated with loss of vision. All senses may be affected by aging, but vision and hearing are the most important to consider as you plan health education. Because of this, we address the functional declines in vision and hearing in greater depth and discuss how to use this information to adapt health education to the abilities of older clients.

Sensory Changes: Vision

In 2011, the National Health Interview Survey found that 12.2% of seniors aged 65 to 74 had some vision loss, as did 15.2% of those aged 75 and older. The leading causes of vision loss were age-related macular degeneration, cataracts, retinopathy, and glaucoma (AFB, 2013). The lens loses its ability to accommodate as it becomes less elastic, larger, and denser, resulting in a condition called presbyopia (farsightedness). The increased density plus the accumulation of loosened degenerative cells on the iris, cornea, and lens capsule result in increased scattering of light and sensitivity to glare. The lens becomes progressively yellowed and opaque, resulting not only in visual acuity difficulties but also in the inability to discriminate blues and greens. This is attributed to the decreased ability of the aging, yellowed lens to filter the shorter wavelengths of light (violet, blue, and green). It is easier for older clients to distinguish among warm colors, such as yellow, orange, and red (Linton, 2007). The use of these colors in teaching materials makes it easier for clients to distinguish them.

When teaching older clients, sit or stand in front of them so they have a full view of you. Clients should be able to see your face and mouth as you talk (Lueckenotte, 2009). If you are using visual aids, consider the impact of colors. For example, a color with a longer wavelength, such as yellow, printed on a white background would not be easy for older eyes to see because there is insufficient contrast between the two colors. A thick black outline surrounding the yellow material would improve readability. Even more effective is a background color, such as light blue, that contrasts with deep yellow lettering outlined in black.

We now examine functional visual changes (visual acuity, glare, dark and light adaptation, and loss of peripheral vision) that affect the teaching and learning process.

Visual Acuity

Virtually everyone will have visual difficulties related to the aging process, regardless of sex, race, ethnicity, or socioeconomic status. Many older adults wear glasses for reading or distance vision because of decreased visual acuity. Watch older clients for signs of difficulty. Note how clients read. How close do they hold a book to read? How much reading do they do? If institutional clients wear glasses, be sure they have them on and the lenses are clean to view your instructional materials. Older clients with presbyopia hold their reading materials at arm's length to focus clearly on the print. Symbols, letters, and objects that are small are more difficult to distinguish from one another. Diminishing ability to discriminate between stimuli is evident among older clients in terms of the size of words and pictures and their intensity and color. Small images, which project shorter light waves into the eye, are harder to distinguish, as are crowded or softly colored images. Larger and more intensely colored print is easier to see. There is enough of the image getting through the nerve pathways for clients to fill in the missing parts. Allowing space between each of the letters also helps.

This is harder to read for a person with aging eyes because the print is fine and there is a lot of it.

This print is easier to read.

Glare

Glare is a serious problem for older clients. It affects their ability to drive at night by leaving them virtually blind in its presence. Glare may come from a variety of sources, such as reflections off windows and shiny floors. Linton (2007) recommends soft incandescent lighting rather than fluorescent lighting to minimize glare. Sheer curtains or rugs can also help reduce glare. If you become involved with the production of instructional materials, avoid using slick, shiny, white paper, which is more likely to produce glare. If you are arranging lighting for older clients, make the light brighter but not glaring.

Dark and Light Adaptation

It takes longer for the eyes of older clients to adapt to dark and light. It takes more time for their eyes to adjust if the room is darkened for a DVD, video, or slide show. Plan for this extra time as you prepare the client education plan. When you turn the lights back on, clients need extra time to readjust their vision. Because pupils become smaller when the lights are turned on, less light is reaching the retina; thus, extra lighting is required (Linton, 2007). If you are using a physical model or object in teaching, consider placing high-intensity lighting on it. This increases the visibility of the model or object, which is preferable to increasing the light in the entire room. The level of intensity, however, needs to be balanced to avoid glare, which older eyes are more sensitive to.

Loss of Peripheral Vision

With the loss of peripheral vision, older clients are unaware of people and learning activities outside of their line of central vision. This may interfere with how your clients relate to others if you are teaching a group. They may not be aware of others sitting next to them or objects located in their peripheral visual fields. As a result, they may appear to lack social interaction skills or appear clumsy if they spill something or knock something over. They may not be able to see an object you refer to that is outside their visual field. Do your best to stay in the clients' line of central vision when teaching to address this condition.

Sensory Changes: Hearing

Some degree of hearing loss caused by changes in the inner ear or tympanic membrane inevitably accompanies the aging process. Approximately 63% of adults over 70 years old have some level of hearing loss while 80% of those over 80 years old have some degree of hearing loss. The two general causes of hearing loss are sensorineural hearing loss and conductive hearing loss (Erwin & Chen, 2023). Presbycusis is associated with aging and is the most common type of hearing loss. It begins in young adulthood and becomes evident usually after age 50 years. Initially, high-pitched sounds beyond the range of human speech are lost. Because these sounds have little functional significance, the individual is unaware of the loss. As the client ages, the loss eventually involves the sounds in the middle and lower ranges. It becomes problematic for clients when higher sounds are missed and only lower sounds are heard. Words sound distorted, and conversations are difficult to understand, especially in the presence of background noise (Linton, 2007).

With high-tone hearing loss, it is more difficult for clients to discriminate among consonants, such as *s*, *t*, *f*, *g*, *ch*, *sh*, *z*, and *th*, which have high frequencies. Clients with presbycusis have difficulty distinguishing among phonetically similar words. Words are distorted, and sentences make little sense. A sentence such as "I think he should go to the store" might be interpreted as "I wish we could go to the show." As hearing loss progresses, explosive consonants, such as *b*, *d*, *k*, *p*, and *t*, also become distorted (Miller, 1990).

Clients with presbycusis need more time to process information. Rapid speech is difficult for older clients to understand. If you speak rapidly, remember to slow down when you teach older clients. Lower your pitch, and speak more slowly and loudly. Face clients when you speak so they can see you. They may lip read to fill in what they do not hear. Reduce any background noise, or move to a quiet room. If clients wear hearing aids, be sure they are operational, in place, and turned on with sufficient volume (Lueckenotte, 2009).

Older clients in a group setting may not want to participate or answer questions for fear of appearing foolish. Hearing loss affects self-confidence and may lead to social isolation. Uninformed healthcare providers may assume that a hard-of-hearing client has dementia. Consider the example of a woman who was attempting to communicate with her mother-in-law. "My mother-in-law does not pay attention to anything I say. Even if I practically shout at her, it does no good. But let my husband come in the room and talk to her in a normal voice, and she hears every word he says." The nursing student responded with sensitivity to what may be symptoms of a family conflict. She explained the facts about sound waves to the woman and explained that a woman's voice is likely to contain higher sound frequencies. If she raises her voice in an effort to be heard, it is likely that she also raises the pitch. Tension also results in a rise in voice pitch. If the relationship is already tense, it is likely that the voice with which the woman begins to speak is already higher than her relaxed voice. These factors make her speech less intelligible to an aging person whose hearing is diminishing. The man who casually comes into the room is likely to speak in a lower-pitched voice, which has a longer wavelength.

Suspect hearing loss if older clients give inappropriate responses to questions, are unable to follow oral directions without cues, or frequently ask you to repeat a message. If clients watch you closely, turn an ear toward you, get unusually close to you, do not respond to loud environmental noises, speak too loudly or inarticulately, speak in a monotone voice, or avoid group settings, you should suspect hearing impairment (Miller, 1990). Remember, however, that not all older clients are hard of hearing. It is distressing for older persons to be spoken to as if they are deaf when they are not.

Implications for Health Education

Older adults experience many biologic and psychosocial changes in their lives and need different levels of help adapting to these changes. They are dealing with faltering health, decreasing strength, and biologic changes that alter or limit their activities. They are adjusting to losses, adapting to changing living circumstances, and changing their self-image. They may be enriching their lives by expanding their knowledge, developing new interests, and learning new skills. This is a time rich with opportunities for nurses to recognize unspoken and unmet needs and to take opportunities to provide health education. We now look at how this information helps you to promote, retain, and restore the health of older clients (**Table 7-1**).

Promote and Retain Health

The focus of promoting health is on prevention, whereas the focus of retaining health is on maintaining one's present health status, assuming it is satisfactory. Clients are never too old to start an

Table 7-1 Selected Physiologic Aging Changes and Teaching–Learning Implications

Physiologic Changes	Teaching–Learning Implications
Musculoskeletal: ■ Muscle mass and strength diminish ■ Bone mass declines ■ Degenerative joint changes ■ Loss of height ■ Demineralization of bone	■ Expect slower movements when teaching exercises ■ Observe for fatigue with physical activities and adjust accordingly ■ Take frequent breaks ■ Allow sufficient time for activities that involve movement ■ Provide comfortable seating ■ Increase warm-up and cool-down times
Cardiovascular: ■ Decrease in cardiac output ■ Orthostatic hypotension ■ Abnormal increases in systolic or diastolic blood pressure ■ Decreased coronary blood flow ■ Artherosclerosis and arteriosclerosis common ■ Conduction problems (atrial fibrillation)	■ Select activities based on client energy level, endurance, and speed ■ Select teaching times in midmorning when energy levels are high ■ Spread teaching sessions over several days rather than one lengthy session ■ Move slowly when rising from a sitting position ■ Adjust pace of activities based on client feedback
Respiratory: ■ Lung function decreases ■ Mobility of ribs declines ■ Functional alveoli decrease in number	■ Base activities on the level of exertion tolerated by the client ■ Encourage clients to maintain the highest level of functional abilities ■ Use oxygen safely if prescribed
Gastrointestinal and urinary: ■ Bowel motility decreases (constipation) ■ Urinary bladder capacity decreases (incontinence)	■ Provide frequent breaks ■ Provide liquids ■ Avoid embarrassment

(continues)

Table 7-1 Selected Physiologic Aging Changes and Teaching–Learning
Implications   *(continued)*

Physiologic Changes	Teaching–Learning Implications
Neurological: ■ Benign essential tremor common ■ Cognitive slowing ■ Decreased sensitivity to stimuli ■ May have decreased blood flow to brain	■ Allow additional time for teaching and learning ■ Adapt pace of teaching ■ Focus on essential information based on client interest ■ Repeat and reinforce important concepts ■ Reduce background noise and environmental distractions ■ Relate new information to current knowledge ■ Emphasize concrete rather than abstract information ■ Attend to nonverbal cues regarding comfort and questions ■ To evaluate learning, ask clients to demonstrate skills
Sensory changes, vision: ■ Decreased visual acuity ■ Sensitivity to glare ■ Decreased depth perception ■ Presbyopia or cataracts ■ Decreased adaptation to dark and light ■ Loss of peripheral vision ■ Poor night vision ■ Decreased ability to discriminate colors	■ Evaluate client's reading ability ■ Select instructional materials with large print ■ Use warm colors such as orange or red in printed materials ■ Stand in client's line of central vision ■ Choose age-appropriate, positive images for instructional materials ■ Provide sufficient lighting and reduce glare ■ Allow time for vision adaptation from dark to light ■ Encourage the use of corrective lenses or magnifying glass
Sensory changes, hearing: ■ Hearing acuity decreases (presbycusis) ■ Loss of high-pitched sounds ■ Distracted by background noise ■ Difficulty discriminating consonant sounds such as s, t, f, g, ch, sh, th, and z	■ Speak slower and slightly louder ■ Use words that are familiar and avoid medical terms ■ Lower the pitch of your voice ■ Let clients see your face and mouth ■ Select a quiet place for teaching ■ Repeat frequently as necessary ■ Confirm that clients have heard you by having them teach back the information

exercise program, improve their diet, and change unhealthful habits. **Table 7-2** lists suggested topics that are appropriate for older learners to promote and retain health (Hall, 2009; Lueckenotte, 2009). These suggestions are not all-inclusive and must be adapted to the circumstances of the individual client.

Restore Health

Restoration of health for older adults refers to people who are experiencing an acute or chronic illness or disability. The purpose of health education is to help clients understand the nature of

Table 7-2 Suggested Topics to Promote and Retain Health

Nursing Assessment	Health Education Topics
Biologic aging	■ Knowing normal age-related body changes ■ Knowing age-related changes to body system of interest
General health habits	■ Eating well-balanced, nutritious diet ■ Maintaining adequate hydration ■ Practicing oral hygiene and dental care ■ Knowing benefits of exercise program ■ Coping effectively with physical and mental stress ■ Visiting regularly with healthcare providers ■ Participating in meaningful activities
General living conditions	■ Maintaining home cleanliness ■ Evaluating need for mechanical aids to assist in activities of daily living ■ Making lifestyle adjustments ■ Preventing accidents and falls ■ Creating safe home environment (slip-resistant rugs, night-lights, nonskid adhesive strips in tub and shower, handrails on steps, grab bars in bathrooms, smoke detectors, etc.)
Disease and illness prevention	■ Avoiding risk factors (smoking, alcohol, etc.) ■ Modifying behavior to avoid risk factors ■ Obtaining immunizations (flu, pneumonia) ■ Having regular physical examinations ■ Screening procedures (mammograms, cholesterol, vision, hearing, blood pressure, blood sugar) ■ Knowing medications ■ Maintaining medication regimen and medication safety ■ Recognizing symptoms of depression
Sexual habits	■ Preventing sexually transmitted diseases ■ Knowing mode of disease transmission ■ Knowing partner's sexual history and practices ■ Using safe sexual practices ■ Recognizing symptoms
Community services	■ Knowing about community luncheon sites ■ Knowing community senior center services ■ Knowing county and state government senior services

their health problem, the treatment regimen, and how to deal with the limitations imposed by health problems, disabilities, or injuries. This involves not only working with the client but also with family members and caretakers. **Table 7-3** suggests topics related to the restoration of health (Baker & Heitkemper, 2014; Hall, 2009; Lueckenotte, 2009).

Nutritional Needs

Sufficient food intake and adequate nutrition are important to maintain health and prevent disease in older adults. Nutritional status is enhanced if sufficient food and adequate nutrition have been a pattern throughout life. Many factors affect nutrition in older adults, including age-related

Table 7-3 Suggested Topics to Restore Health

Nursing Assessment	Health Education Topics
Acute illness	■ Knowing the nature and cause of the health problem or disability ■ Common conditions: Urinary tract infections, fluid and electrolyte imbalance (hyponatremia, dehydration), pneumonia, hip fracture, dysrhythmias ■ Understanding diagnostic tests ■ Supporting and explaining treatment regimen ■ Orienting to hospital and clinic environment and routines ■ Adapting to lifestyle changes
Chronic illness	■ Knowing the nature and cause of the health problem or disability ■ Common conditions: Hypertension, cardiovascular disease, stroke, diabetes mellitus, cancer, arthritis ■ Understanding diagnostic tests ■ Supporting and explaining treatment regimen ■ Using physical, occupational, and speech therapies ■ Managing exacerbations and remissions ■ Preventing complications ■ Adapting to lifestyle changes ■ Adapting the home environment ■ Identifying and using self-help devices ■ Supporting continued provider supervision
Disability	■ Assessing strengths and limitations of disability ■ Managing activities of daily living ■ Building on abilities ■ Identifying and using self-help devices
Accidents	■ Knowing the nature of the injury sustained and the impact on function ■ Managing activities of daily living ■ Building on abilities ■ Assessing rehabilitation issues ■ Preventing accidents and injuries ■ Maintaining a safe home environment (slip-resistant rugs, night-lights, nonskid adhesive strips in tub and shower, handrails on steps, grab bars in bathrooms, smoke detectors, etc.)
Community services	■ Knowing about community luncheon sites ■ Knowing community senior center services ■ Knowing county and state government senior services

biologic changes, food preferences, financial status, lifestyle, medications, and presence of chronic disease. For healthy eating guidelines, review the USDA MyPlate from the U.S. Department of Agriculture available at https://www.myplate.gov/life-stages/older-adults. It includes dietary guidelines for the five food groups (fruits, vegetables, grains, protein, and dairy) that older adults need. The images are colorful and self-explanatory. The guidelines recommend eating a variety of foods from each food group with a focus on foods with potassium, calcium, vitamin D, dietary fiber, and vitamin B-12. Limit foods with added sugars, saturated fats, and sodium. To meet these guidelines, older adults may need to make small changes in their food and beverage choices. Older adults are advised to continue engaging in regular physical activities to maintain a desirable body weight. Proper nutrition is a broad topic that provides many opportunities for nurses to educate clients and their families (USDA Food and Nutrition Service, 2022).

Nutrition affects memory. The body is dependent on many nutrients to manufacture the neurotransmitters essential to learning. The B vitamins are essential ingredients in this process. Iron is essential for the transmission of oxygen to the brain, and water is vital to every metabolic process in the body. Many older adults who live alone do not eat a balanced diet. They may lack the motivation to prepare nutritious meals and may benefit from community programs such as Meals on Wheels or those offered at community senior centers.

Many older adults are also dehydrated and do not consume enough liquids daily. This occurs because of physiologic changes and a decrease in thirst sensation. Some older people tend to drink less in an effort to avoid the inconvenience or embarrassment of needing to empty their bladders more often. This problem of self-imposed dehydration may be exacerbated by a subculture among the older generation that considers bodily functions or attention to them as taboo. If clients are not properly hydrated, their health is endangered, and their ability to learn will be impaired (Eliopoulos, 2014).

Although more Americans value fitness, many older adults do not see the connections among exercise, cardiorespiratory functioning, and an oxygenated, nourished brain. Give clients information and choose a time to teach when they are more invigorated, such as when they are sufficiently rested and have the energy to learn so they are sufficiently stimulated to pay attention.

Ethnic Elderly

Some ethnic groups may view aging differently than white culture. Of the five major cultural groups in the United States, all show greater respect and reverence for older adults when compared with white culture (Purnell, 2013). For example, older adults in white culture are expected to live apart from their adult children and maintain their independence as long and as much as possible. Older adults in the African American culture enjoy closer family ties with extended family. Older adults in the Hispanic culture are respected and often live with large, extended families. Older Asians enjoy a high level of respect in the family, which increases as they age. The adult children are expected to take care of their aging parents. Older people in Native American Indian cultures enjoy a very high level of honor and respect for their accumulated knowledge and wisdom (Schmall, as cited in Wallace, 2006).

As with any age group, there is a great diversity of beliefs and values among older adults, both across ethnic groups and within any one ethnic group. A variety of factors affect how older adults from various ethnic groups approach health care, including cultural beliefs, social supports, socioeconomic status, and cultural values. Nurses often are the first healthcare provider to have direct contact with older adults and need to expand their expertise in interacting and caring for older persons. This includes being educated on the progression of normal aging and staying abreast of research to provide culturally competent care. It is essential that you conduct a thorough cultural assessment to identify the health beliefs and values of the older client, family, or group you are teaching. To avoid stereotyping, ask if there is a cultural or ethnic group with which older adults identify and what their beliefs are about health and illness (Eliopoulos, 2014). Your cultural assessment will identify the health practices of the client and the degree to which the client believes in and adheres to folk practices and Western health practices.

Clients who are immigrants or first-generation residents in the United States may adhere more strongly to the health beliefs and practices of their primary cultural affiliation. These immigrants, who may have come to the United States to join their children, have the unique challenge of relocating to a new culture and language late in life. The nurse as educator should be aware that the inability of older adults to acculturate may play a part in the lack of adherence to recommended health measures. Other clients from diverse ethnic backgrounds who have lived a lifetime in the United States are more likely to have become assimilated into U.S. culture, to have had some experiences with the nation's healthcare system, and to have better knowledge of its health practices. By assessing health beliefs, values, and practices, you can tailor your health teaching to the individual client.

Language may be a barrier in communicating with older adults from other cultures. The client may speak little or no English. In that case, it is better to use a qualified interpreter rather than a family member, especially when the topic is sensitive.

In providing health education, be sure your message is realistic in terms of the client's diagnosis, living situation, support network, educational background, and financial resources. For example, teaching an older Hispanic woman with diabetes about the importance of a daily intake of fresh fruits and vegetables may be meaningless if she has limited financial resources. Her situation could be compounded if she cannot drive and her family lives far away. It is also important to know that diabetes affects an estimated one-third of older Hispanic people, and the risk of depression among those with diabetes is 30% higher when compared to older adults without diabetes (Strunk, Townsend-Rocchiccioli, & Sanford, 2013).

A holistic approach to assessment may alter your teaching approach. For example, an older African American woman who has been on medication for hypertension for several years is found to have elevated blood pressure. After a lengthy discussion with the client, the nurse learns that the client had not been taking her medication. Because of her limited financial resources and the fact that her symptoms were not bothering her, she felt it was not necessary to take her medications. The nurse educator needs to be aware that a misconception in the African American population about hypertension and its treatment is that hypertension is an episodic condition rather than a chronic illness (Middleton, 2009). Establishing a trusting, ongoing relationship influences adherence to a treatment plan. Taking time to develop trusting relationships with clients in a culturally competent manner can increase adherence (Thomas & Stoeckel, 2016). By correcting misconceptions, the nurse can establish a relationship centered around providing culturally sensitive care. In this case, the older adult could also be referred to a social worker to address financial issues.

If an older client is undergoing treatment for a current health problem, inquire about what they are doing to treat it. The client may be engaging in a folk practice designed to ameliorate the condition. Listen carefully to the client's self-care practices and determine if these practices are helpful, neutral, or harmful; that is, if they should be preserved, accommodated, or restructured (DeRosa & Kochurka, 2006). Unless the practice is harmful, be supportive of it and view it as an adjunct to your nursing and medical interventions. Remember that the mind has a profound influence on health and healing, and we do not fully understand the extent of its influence. If clients' practices provide them with meaning and give them a sense of participating in healing, then the practices deserve our respect, not disdain.

Educating Clients with Disabilities

AOA (2021) reported that 19% of adults aged 65 and older reported they could not function at all or had a lot of difficulty in six domains. Twenty-two percent reported trouble seeing (even if wearing glasses); 31% reported difficulty hearing (even if wearing hearing aids); 40% reported trouble with mobility (walking or climbing stairs); 8% reported difficulty with communication (understanding or being understood by others); 27% reported trouble with cognition (remembering or concentrating); and 9% reported difficulty with self-care (such as washing all over or dressing). In this chapter, visual and hearing disabilities were addressed under physiological changes. This section continues the discussion of clients with disabilities under the headings of chronic diseases and cognitive functioning to include memory and medications.

Chronic Diseases

Chronic diseases are not a part of normal aging; however, the prevalence of chronic disease is higher among older adults. The increasing number of older Americans means that more of them need services from the healthcare system. People aged 65 years and older are less likely to have as many acute conditions as younger people; however, they are more apt to have at least one chronic condition for which they likely require assistance. Many have multiple chronic conditions. In 2019, 22.3% of those aged 65 to 74 assessed their health as fair or poor as compared to 29.3% of those aged 75 and over. The leading chronic conditions among adults age 65 and older in 2019 include: arthritis (48%); coronary heart disease (14%); myocardial infarction (9%); angina (4%); any cancer (25%); COPD, emphysema, or chronic bronchitis (10%); stroke (9% in 2017–2018); and physician-diagnosed and undiagnosed diabetes (29% in 2015–2018) (AOA, 2021).

Race and ethnic differences play a role in these conditions. For example, African-American and Hispanic Americans have higher rates of hypertension and obesity when compared to non-Hispanic whites. Asian Americans have higher rates of diabetes and high blood pressure when compared to non-Hispanic whites All groups are less likely to have health insurance coverage and thus do not receive care for preventable chronic illnesses. People of diverse racial, ethnic, and cultural heritage are less likely to get regular medical checkups, receive immunizations, and be routinely tested for cancer when compared with non-Hispanic white Americans (Carratala & Maxwell 2020).

Teaching older clients how to adapt to chronic diseases is a major theme in working with them. The causes of chronic diseases are multiple and are frequently related to lifestyle. Chronic diseases develop slowly over time. Older clients may not understand their illness, especially if it is characterized by exacerbations and remissions. Clients with chronic diseases may experience depression, which further compounds their ability to function. The depression may be related to the disease and the disability it inflicts or the many losses that older adults experience at this time in their lives. Working with older clients who have chronic diseases challenges you as the educator. Determine how well they understand their disease and the degree to which they are willing to adhere to the prescribed treatment. Clients need to be educated about how to prevent and manage crises, manage the therapeutic regimen, and control symptoms. They also need to know how to organize their time, prevent social isolation, and have a normal lifestyle and interactions with others despite disease. Refresh your memory about specific chronic diseases so you can answer questions that older clients may have.

Teaching related to general health is a fruitful area for educating older clients. General health measures are instrumental in improving health status and helping clients feel better. Consider teaching the virtues of exercising regularly, improving nutritional intake, controlling weight loss or gain, getting adequate rest, managing stress, and cooperating with the medical regimen. We have enjoyed teaching these topics, especially classes about exercises, to older clients during their noon meal at community lunch sites for senior citizens. The exercises we taught were suitable for the age of the clients and involved simple range-of-motion exercises. The clients perked up and began to smile and interact with one another in a way they had not before. Many said they felt better as a result of the classes.

Alcohol continues to be an underestimated and hidden problem for older adults. A national survey reported that around 11% of adults over age 65 report current binge drinking. Alcohol detoxification and excretion from the older body is less efficient than in younger counterparts and can lead to accidents, nutritional deficiencies, and damage that affect all body systems. Heavy drinking can make health problems worse, including diabetes, high blood pressure, congestive heart failure, liver problems, osteoporosis, memory problems, and mood disorders. Alcohol use and some prescription, over-the-counter medications, and herbal remedies are synergistic or incompatible. Medications that can interact badly with alcohol include aspirin, acetaminophen, cold and allergy medicine, cough syrup, sleeping pills, pain medication, and anxiety or depression medicine (NIH, 2023). Older adults need to be aware of these facts and should be taught to carefully regulate and monitor their alcohol consumption.

Finally, never assume that older adults are not interested in sex. Many individuals continue to be sexually active beyond the expectations and imaginations of their younger counterparts. Health education about sexuality in later years generates more interest than you might anticipate, even though many older adults were raised to not talk about sex. Keep in mind that older people with chronic diseases may need additional health education about meeting their needs (Kautz & Barnett, 2014). Consider the example of a 70-year-old female client seen in an outpatient clinic. She came in for her routine checkup and renewal of her prescription for vaginal Premarin (estrogen). She exercised regularly, ate nutritious meals, and maintained a long-standing sexual relationship with a 50-year-old man.

Social support networks are important for older adults. People who maintain relationships with others and remain active and involved with group activities fare better in terms of health and happiness. Self-help and peer support groups are also beneficial when clients are dealing with specific health problems. Your role as an educator is to foster these support networks.

Cognitive Functioning

If learning is the process of acquiring new knowledge, then memory is the process of retaining that knowledge over time. When memory falters or is lost completely, it is frustrating, particularly to older people. Memory is the "ability to retain or store information and retrieve it when needed" (Bjorklund & Bee, 2008, p. 107). Short-term memory loss is more commonly seen with aging than long-term memory loss. Short-term memory refers to remembering events in the recent past, whereas long-term memory refers to distant events (Williams & Mees, 2014). There is great variation in cognitive functioning among individuals as they age because people do not follow a predictable pattern.

Current research from longitudinal studies shows that some cognitive (thinking) functions decline with age, but other cognitive processes function at very high levels well into the later years. The decline that does occur is not as drastic as often believed, and individuals can compensate for the decline in ways that may not be noticeable (Bjorklund & Bee, 2008). These age-related changes in brain composition, cells, and synapses, do not necessarily affect thinking and cognition. The cognitive abilities of most healthy older adults show no noticeable evidence of decline (Baker & Heitkemper, 2014; Blais, 2014). Some are "cognitive super agers" who have memory performance comparable to people 20 to 30 years younger who are being studied at National Institute on Aging (NIA) (https://www.nia.nih.gov/health/how-aging-brain-affects-thinking).

It is a common misperception that older people become cognitively impaired as they age—that is, that they become confused, forgetful, and unable to manage their affairs. This is a myth because cognitive impairments are not part of normal aging. Keep in mind that most healthy older adults live without cognitive difficulties. Common changes in thinking that occur with aging include being slower to find words and recall names. Other examples are having problems with multitasking and experiencing a mild decrease in the ability to pay attention. Older adults who maintain a healthy lifestyle fare better when it comes to cognitive functioning. Studies have also documented the benefits of the Mediterranean-style diet and physical activity on memory, as well as the importance of engaging in mentally stimulating activities, and not smoking or drinking heavily. Older adults who engaged in four or five of these behaviors had a 60% lower risk of developing Alzheimer's compared to those who only followed one or none. People who followed two or three of the activities had a 37% lower risk (NIA, 2023).

The causes of memory loss are many. They include physiological causes, such as cerebrovascular changes, and pathologic causes like disease or trauma which cause a loss of neural cells. Psychosocial issues can lead to stress, depression, and social isolation (Williams & Mees, 2014). When older clients become aware of memory slippages, they often incorrectly conclude that something is wrong with their brain or that they are losing their mind. Believing this, they become fearful and anxious, which can interfere with the learning process and create a self-fulfilling prophecy. Memory loss does not necessarily mean brain disease because there are many causes of memory loss. Older clients may need to be reminded about the many memory tasks they perform daily that are accurate and important (Bjorklund & Bee, 2008).

Mild Cognitive Impairment (MCI)

The Mayo Clinic defines mild cognitive impairment (MCI) as the "stage between the expected decline in memory and thinking that happens with age and the more serious decline of dementia." It is an early state of memory loss seen in individuals who otherwise are able to function independently. MCI is characterized by memory loss, language difficulties and impairments in judgment and reasoning due to pathologic processes (Blais, 2014). MCI does not seriously affect the individual's ability to carry out activities of daily living. It may increase the risk of later progressing to dementia but some people with MCI never get worse, and a few eventually get better (Mayo Clinic, 2012). Dementia and Alzheimer's disease are more serious conditions that require physician evaluation and treatment.

Those with MCI have more memory or other thinking problems than other people their age. They are able to take care of themselves and do their normal activities, but may lose things, forget events and appointments, or take longer to think of a word or recall a name. Other common symptoms include: losing one's train of thought, inability to follow a conversation, difficulty making decisions, inability to finish a task, and showing poor judgment. Family and friends may notice these symptoms but they do not impact the person's daily life or affect usual activities (NIA, 2020; Mayo Clinic, 2023; Alzheimer's Association, 2023).

Memory problems that are serious include: asking the same questions over and over again, getting lost in well-known places, inability to follow recipes or directions, and becoming more confused about time, people, and places. Not taking care of oneself, eating poorly, not bathing, and behaving unsafely are also serious indicators (NIA, 2020). There is no proven treatment for MCI, but living a healthful lifestyle (nutritious diet, regular exercise, avoiding alcohol) can mitigate cognitive changes. Older adults who are experiencing MCI should visit their doctor every 6–12 months to track changes in memory and other thinking skills over time (NIA, 2020; NIA, 2023).

Teaching Memory Compensation Strategies

Clients may be aware of short-term memory deficits and become discouraged. Perhaps they cannot learn as much or as fast as when they were younger, but they can adopt new ways to adjust and successfully compensate for their forgetfulness. The goal is to live a productive and functionally independent life as long as possible. An important variable in memory and learning is the attitude of both clients and nurses. Your message and the client's internal messages (self-talk) matter. See **Box 7-1** Teaching Memory Compensation Strategies.

When teaching these memory compensation strategies, the nurse educator can approach the client in ways that facilitate learning. **Box 7-2** identifies helpful nurse educator approaches for clients dealing with forgetfulness.

We recommend that you encourage older clients to make a record of important information and keep it in a brightly colored folder. This may include the following: name of doctor, name of insurance, important identification numbers, names of medications, and important people's phone numbers. Keeping a diary of health issues is helpful, for example, noting the frequency of a particular problem or regularly recording vital signs. Clients should also place questions that occur between visits to the doctor or you in this folder.

"Do you understand?" is a tricky question and reveals only if the client acts cooperatively. Not all clients are assertive; many older clients try not to bother busy nurses. When they are feeling overloaded, clients may hide their feelings of ignorance, smile politely, and agree when they are asked this question. This type of response (with a half-hearted yes or a smile and a nod) may feel satisfying to a nurse who is very busy, but it is deceptive. When asked for specific feedback, the nurse may discover that the client understood very little. Eliciting this information is done by asking the client, "Tell me what you understand by what I said." Deception is also common whenever there is a perceived difference in status, such as between nurses and clients. Clients may not want to acknowledge they do not understand what the nurse said to avoid disappointing the nurse. Sometimes it may be necessary to check with the client's spouse or partner to see if the client understands and to learn how the client is doing.

Medication and Cognitive Functioning

Medications can interfere with cognitive functioning. Antimisiaris and Cheek (2014) cited surveys of older adults that found many take an average of five to six medications per day and noted that the number of prescriptions per person increases with age (Korem, 2013). Taking multiple medications is known as polypharmacy, which increases the risk of undesirable side effects and interactions among the medications. When asked what medications they take, clients vary in their reliability as historians. Nurses also vary in their interviewing skills and the amount of thought they give to clients' answers. It was common for older clients seen in a well-person clinic to list only their prescribed medications. They routinely omit herbs and over-the-counter medications, such as vitamins, laxatives, and pills taken for headache or upset stomach. They also may not mention medications prescribed by other doctors because they did not want to seem dissatisfied with the present providers. When working with older clients, teach them how drugs affect them, how multiple drugs can have untoward interactions in the body, and how to take drugs safely.

Box 7-1 Teaching Memory Compensation Strategies

Functional Area	Compensation Strategies
Daily routine	■ Follow a daily routine ■ Maintain a daily calendar with important dates and events ■ Create a daily To-Do list ■ Put purse, keys, phone, and glasses in the same place every day ■ Create memory aids and tools
Cooking	■ Stay in the kitchen while cooking ■ Set out ingredients/supplies ahead of time ■ Limit distractions (such as radio, TV)
Shopping	■ Make a written list ■ Shop during the least busy hours ■ Park car in the same place each time ■ Focus on one task at a time
Appointments	■ Highlight dates and times on a daily calendar ■ Arrange transportation ahead of time ■ Set reminder alarm (smartphone, mobile wrist technology, kitchen/stove timer)
Medications	■ Keep medications in a clearly visible location ■ Set reminder alarms (smartphone, mobile wrist technology, kitchen/stove timer) ■ Create association prompts (lunch time = medication due)
Finances	■ Put bills in one location ■ Pay bills at the same time each month ■ Use online and/or automatic payment methods ■ Balance accounts regularly (at least monthly)
Life style	■ Exercise regularly ■ Eat a well-balanced, nutritious diet ■ Get sufficient sleep, 7–8 hours/night ■ Maintain social contacts with family and friends ■ Learn new skills ■ Read new books ■ Volunteer in your community ■ Stay involved in activities that help both body and mind ■ Set a lower learning pace ■ Ask for help when you need it ■ Be patient with yourself

Data from National Institute on Aging (NIA), 2020. Tips for dealing with forgetfulness. Retrieved August 25, 2023, from https://www.nia.nih.gov/health/memory-forgetfulness-and-aging-whats-normal-and-whats-not; Farias, S. T., Schmitter-Edgecombe, M., Weakley, A., et al. (2018). Compensation strategies in older adults. *American Journal of Alzheimer's Diseases & Other Dementias*, 3393, 184–191. https://journals.sagepub.com; https://doi.org/10.1177/1533317517753361

Box 7-2 Nurse Educator Approaches

Approach	Nurse Educator Behaviors
Nonverbal	■ Be aware of tone, loudness of voice ■ Be aware of body language ■ Make eye contact ■ Gentle touch as appropriate ■ Show interest in client's concerns ■ Observe for client's reactions and understanding ■ Let client make the decisions ■ Be patient
Verbal	■ Call client by name ■ Speak slowly ■ Ask how they best learn (visual, hearing, kinesthetic) ■ Give short specific instructions ■ Focus on one task at a time ■ Associate memory with something important to client ■ Give written directions ■ Focus on the positive ■ If conflict, agitation, or stress arise, try distracting or changing topic

Data from NIA. (2020). Understanding memory loss: What to do when you have trouble remembering. Retrieved August 25, 2023, https://order.nia.nih .gov/sites/default/files/2022-06/understanding-memory-loss-nia.pdf

Educating Families

Older clients, as with their younger counterparts, value their privacy and do not wish to be overly dependent on their adult children. Often, family members or friends will need to be involved with the older person's care, and it is to them that you direct your health teaching. When this is necessary, be sensitive to the privacy concerns clients may have. Be respectful and avoid embarrassing older clients by sharing unnecessary information about them with others. When you teach family members or friends, reveal only the information that is essential for understanding the health message. If clients live alone and need assistance from family members or friends, identify the care needs and arrange mutually agreeable times for them to visit. If clients live with family, meeting the clients' care needs requires working around the family's employment and other routines.

Families may be aware that an older family member, neighbor, or friend is becoming forgetful but continues to adequately care for themselves. The Memory Compensation Strategies presented earlier are effective in teaching family members. Also important to teach are safety measures in the home. Urge family members to examine the older person's living area and bathroom. Be sure the usual pathways the person uses are free of clutter and tripping hazards. Remove or tack down throw rugs that might result in tripping. Bathrooms should be equipped with grab bars and other safety devices for getting in and out of tubs and showers. These safety tips and many others can be found on health-related websites.

Educating Groups and Communities

Senior citizen sites, community gathering places such as senior lunch programs, and assisted living and long-term care facilities provide opportunities for health education. Everyone is invited to participate, and many will do so if for no other reason than to enjoy companionship with like-minded individuals. This is also an opportunity to encourage team members to attend so they can update their knowledge about your health topic.

When you are presenting health education information to groups of older adults, be sure to make it lively and interesting. Announce your presentation in advance, and give it an interesting and catchy title that will capture their attention. The institution where you teach can help advertise your presentation in advance. If possible, use teaching strategies that encourage active participation, such as asking questions and waiting for responses and engaging clients in small group or short dyad learning activities. Your presentation will be more interesting and remembered longer if the attendees are active participants. Clients like to be given written materials they can read in privacy on their own. Brochures and handouts also reinforce your teaching.

Educating Health Team Members

As the number of older adults increases, there is a corresponding need for caregivers to provide healthcare services, whether in long-term care facilities or assisted-living residences. Providing these services is a growth industry in the United States. Many of today's caregivers have little formal training for their roles and responsibilities, especially in long-term care facilities in which the primary caregiver is a certified nursing assistant. Certified nursing assistants are supervised by a registered nurse; however, the ratio is often unbalanced, and the supervisor may be overloaded. Medicare and many states require that nursing assistants and other care providers undergo training. Because of this, there are multiple opportunities for you to provide health education for these valuable team members.

As with teaching adult learners, you must begin by knowing the provisions of the nurse practice act in your state and know the scope of practice for each team member: nursing assistant, licensed practical nurse, and registered nurse. You must also know the general policies and practice guidelines of your employer. Long-term care institutions may or may not have in-service education departments to provide continuing education for employees. If such a department is available, you can work with the staff to identify the education needs of the team members and plan for appropriate health education.

If no such department is available, it becomes your responsibility to provide health education to your health team members. In this case, you should first assess their learning needs. You can identify these as you work with health team members and become familiar with their capabilities and deficiencies. While assessing team members, remember the three learning domains—cognitive, affective, and psychomotor—and consider in which domain the team member needs health education. For example, does the team member lack knowledge about the client's medical and nursing diagnoses and the rationale for treatment (cognitive domain)? Does the team member's attitude show a lack of understanding or compassion toward clients (affective domain)? Does the team member know how to safely and accurately perform a needed nursing care procedure (psychomotor domain)? After you have determined the learning domain in which health education is needed, you can plan appropriate teaching strategies to address those needs. Your next focus will be to determine whether the content to be taught can be done informally on the job or if the team member needs formal teaching away from the nursing unit. After teaching, you need to assess the effectiveness of your teaching.

Summary

Because of the growing number and ethnic diversity of aging Americans, teaching and learning among this population are increasingly important. Older clients are different from younger and middle-aged clients in ways that significantly affect the planning and implementing of health education. Significant variables include psychosocial stages, developmental tasks, and physiologic changes associated with aging. Clients must be assessed individually to identify their particular characteristics and to plan health education that meets those needs. Suitable health education topics for assisting clients to promote, retain, and restore health were identified to include nutritional aspects of health teaching. Some clients have nutritional deficiencies that affect learning and are addressed through health education. Chronic disease is present in many older clients and affects client education plans. Many clients simply need more information about the nature of their chronic disease and how they can lessen its effect and work cooperatively with the physician to implement the treatment plan. Although researchers are not in agreement about the causes and extent of memory changes, many older individuals and their associates are aware of problems with short-term memory and associated mild cognitive impairment. Memory compensation strategies are identified for the nurse educator. Fortunately, a number of promising and tested remedies are available to those interested. The nurse who is helping older clients learn information, attitude changes, or skills to promote health can make use of research. As the educator, you can adapt learning theories and principles to enhance older clients' chances of success.

Exercises

Exercise I: Ageism

Purpose: Develop awareness of your own attitudes toward older people.

Directions: Debate the proposition that ageism negatively affects healthcare services given to older adults.

1. Divide into two groups, with each group taking opposing sides of the issue. Take 15 minutes to prepare your comments.
2. Reconvene as one group and debate the proposition.

Exercise II: Teaching Older Adults

Purpose: Identify suitable health education topics for older adults.

Directions: Divide into three groups and discuss the following client situations, all seen in a well-oldster clinic. Identify what health education topics are important to discuss with each client. Reconvene as a class and share your findings.

1. A thin 80-year-old female presents with a chief complaint of multiple subjective symptoms. Her objective findings included low sodium and chloride, elevated calcium, dry eyes and mouth, and other evidence of dehydration. She has a history of chronic obstructive pulmonary disease, long-standing alcoholism, osteoarthritis, and kyphosis.
2. An obese 65-year-old male has a chief complaint of increased hunger, thirst, and fatigue. He was diagnosed with adult-onset diabetes mellitus and appears motivated to learn better

self-care and self-management. His blood glucose was 240 mg/dL (65 to 99 is normal). He is employed at a local cafeteria where he eats two meals per day.
3. A slightly obese 85-year-old female presents with a chief complaint of constipation that has been a problem off and on for the past year. Subjectively, she complains of periodic abdominal discomfort. Her objective symptom includes a slightly distended abdomen.

Exercise III: Impact of Aging Physiology on Teaching and Learning

Purpose: Analyze the implications of aging physiology on teaching and learning.
Directions: Divide into small groups and discuss how the age-related changes in the following body systems affect teaching and learning:

1. Musculoskeletal system
2. Cardiovascular system
3. Respiratory system
4. Neurologic system
5. Sensory changes in vision and hearing

List teaching and learning strategies for dealing with each change you identify:

- Describe how the physiologic changes that occur with aging affect teaching and learning with older adults.
- Give an example of an older client you have worked with and how you adapted teaching to the client's physiologic changes.
- Describe the accommodations you have made when teaching a client with the following needs:
  - Chronic disease
  - Cognitive functioning
  - Nutritional

Exercise IV: Evidence-Based Nursing Practice

Purpose: Apply evidence-based nursing research to client education.
Directions:

1. Search the literature for nursing research applicable to health education for the older learner.
2. Describe how the findings could be applied to educating clients in your practice.

References

Administration on Aging. (2021). *2020 Profile of older Americans*. Administration for Community Living. U.S. Department of Health and Human Services. Retrieved from https://acl.gov/sites/default/files/Profile%20of%20OA/2021%20Profile%20of%20OA/2021ProfileOlderAmericans_508.pdf

Alzheimer's Association. (2014). *Mild cognitive impairment*. Retrieved from http://www.alz.org/dementia/mild-cognitive-impairment-mci.asp

Alzheimer's Association. (2023). *Mild cognitive impairment (MCI)*. Retrieved from https://www.alz.org/alzheimers-dementia/what-is-dementia/related_conditions/mild-cognitive-impairment

American Foundation for the Blind. (2013). *Special report on aging and vision loss*. Retrieved from http://www.afb.org/info/blindness-statistics/adults/special-report-on-aging-and-vision-loss/235

Antimisiaris, D., & Cheek, D. J. (2014). Polypharmacy. In K. L. Mauk (Ed.), *Gerontological nursing* (3rd ed., pp. 417–454). Burlington, MA: Jones & Bartlett Learning.

Ayalon, L., Chasteen, A., Diehl, M., Levy, B. R., Neupert, S. D., Rothermund, K., Tesch-Romer, C., & Wahl, H-W. (2021). Ageing in times of the COVID-19 pandemic: Avoiding ageism and fostering intergenerational solidarity. *Journals of Gerontology. Series B, Psychological Sciences and Social Sciences, 76*(2), e49–e52. doi:10.1093/geronb/gbaa051

Baker, M. W., & Heitkemper, M. M. (2014). *Chronic illness and older adults*. In S. L. Lewis, S. R. Dirksen, M. M. Heitkemper, & L. Bucher (Eds.), *Medical–surgical nursing: Assessment and management of clinical problems* (9th ed., pp. 61–78). St. Louis, MO: Mosby Elsevier.

Balakas, K. (2013). Developmental theories. In P. A. Potter, A. G. Perry, P. A. Stockert, & A. M. Hall (Eds.), *Fundamentals of nursing* (8th ed., pp. 130–138). St. Louis, MO: Mosby Elsevier.

Bjorklund, B. R., & Bee, H. L. (2008). *The journey of adulthood* (6th ed.). Upper Saddle River, NJ: Pearson Education.

Blais, K. (2014). Older adult. In C. L. Edelman, E. C. Kudzma, & C. L. Mandel (Eds.), *Health promotion throughout the life span* (8th ed., pp. 591–620). St. Louis, MO: Elsevier Mosby.

Carratala, S., & Maxwell, C. (2020). *Health disparities by race and ethnicity*. Center for American Progress. Retrieved from https://www.americanprogress.org/article/health-disparities-race-ethnicity/

CDC National Center for Health Statistics. (2014). *NCHS data on racial and ethnic disparities*. Retrieved from https://www.cdc.gov/nchs/data/factsheets/factsheet_disparities.pdf

DeRosa, N., & Kochurka, K. (2006). Implement culturally competent healthcare in your workplace. *Nursing Management, 37*(10), 18–26.

Disabatino, A. J., & Bucher, L. (2014). Nursing assessment cardiovascular system. In S. L. Lewis, S. R. Dirksen, M. M. Heitkemper, & L. Bucher (Eds.), *Medical–surgical nursing: Assessment and management of clinical problems* (9th ed., pp. 686–708). St. Louis, MO: Elsevier Mosby.

Disabled World. (2011). *Latest U.S. disability statistics and facts*. Retrieved from https://www.disabled-world.com/disability/statistics/census-figures.php

Eisel, S. J. (2014). Nursing assessment respiratory system. In S. L. Lewis, S. R. Dirksen, M. M. Heitkemper, & L. Bucher (Eds.), *Medical–surgical nursing: Assessment and management of clinical problems* (9th ed., pp. 475–496). St. Louis, MO: Elsevier Mosby.

Eliopoulos, C. (2014). *Gerontological nursing* (8th ed.). Philadelphia, PA: Wolters Kluwer Health/Lippincott Williams & Wilkins.

Erikson, E. H. (1963). *Childhood and society* (2nd ed.). New York, NY: W. W. Norton.

Erikson, E. H. (1982). *Life cycle completed: A review*. New York, NY: W. W. Norton.

Erikson, E. H., & Erikson, J. M. (1997). *The life cycle completed*. New York, NY: W. W. Norton.

Fahlman, M. M., Topp, R., McNevin, N., Morgan, A. L., & Boardley, D. (2007). Structured exercise in older adults with limited functional ability. *Journal of Gerontological Nursing, 33*(6), 32–39.

Farias, S. T., Schmitter-Edgecombe, M, Weakley, A., Harvey, D., Denny, K.G., Barba, C., Gravano, J. T., Giovannetti, T., & Willis, S. (2018). Compensation strategies in older adults: Association with cognition and everyday function. *American Journal of Alzheimer's disease & Other Dementias, Vol. 33*(3), 184–191. https://doi.org/10.1177/1533317517753361

Hall, A. M. (2009). Client education. In P. A. Potter & A. G. Perry (Eds.), *Fundamentals of nursing* (7th ed., pp. 361–383). St. Louis, MO: Mosby Elsevier.

Kautz, D. D., & Barnett, L. (2014). Sexuality. In K. L. Mauk (Ed.), *Gerontological nursing* (3rd ed., pp. 793–808). Burlington, MA: Jones & Bartlett Learning.

Knowles, M. S. (1990). *The adult learner: A neglected species* (4th ed.). Houston, TX: Gulf.

Korem, K. (2013). Older adults. In P. A. Potter, A. G. Perry, P. A. Stockert, & A. M. Hall (Eds.), *Fundamentals of nursing* (8th ed., pp. 171–191). St. Louis, MO: Mosby Elsevier.

Linton, A. D. (2007). Age-related changes in the special senses. In A. D. Linton & H. W. Lach (Eds.), *Matteson and McConnell's gerontological nursing concepts and practice* (3rd ed., pp. 600–627). St. Louis, MO: Saunders Elsevier.

Lueckenotte, A. (2009). Older adult. In P. A. Potter & A. G. Perry (Eds.), *Fundamentals of nursing* (7th ed., pp. 191–214). St. Louis, MO: Mosby Elsevier.

Mayo Clinic. (2012). *Mild cognitive impairment (MCI)*. Retrieved from http://www.mayoclinic.com/health/mild-cognitive-impairment/DS00553

Mayo Clinic. (2023). *Mild cognitive impairment (MCI)*. Retrieved from https://www.mayoclinic.org/diseases-conditions/mild-cognitive-impairment/symptoms-causes/syc-20354578

Middleton, J. L. (2009). A proposed new model of hypertensive treatment behavior in African Americans. *Journal of the National Medical Association, 101*(1), 12–17.

Miller, C. A. (1990). *Nursing care of older adults*. Glenview, IL: Scott, Foresman/Little, Brown Higher Education.

Millsap, P. (2007). Neurological system. In A. D. Linton & H. W. Lach (Eds.), *Matteson and McConnell's gerontological nursing concepts and practice* (3rd ed., pp. 406–441). St. Louis, MO: Saunders Elsevier.

National Center for Cultural Competence. (2003). *Policy brief 1: Rationale for cultural competence in primary care*. Retrieved from http://nccc.georgetown.edu/documents/Policy_Brief_1_2003.pdf and http://www11.georgetown.edu/research/gucchd/nccc/resources/cultural6.html

NIH, National Institute on Aging. (2020). *Tips for dealing with forgetfulness*. Retrieved from https://www.nia.nih.gov/health/memory-forgetfulness-and-aging-whats-normal-and-whats-not

NIH, National Institute on Aging. (2022). *Understanding memory loss*. Retrieved from https://order.nia.nih.gov/sites/default/files/2022-06/understanding-memory-loss-nia.pdf

NIH, National Institute on Aging. (2023). *How the aging brain affects thinking*. Retrieved from https://www.nia.nih.gov/health/how-aging-brain-affects-thinking

NIH, National Institute on Aging. (2023). *Facts about aging and alcohol*. Retrieved from www.nia.nih.gov/health/facts-about-aging-and-alcohol#effects

NIH, National Institute on Alcohol Abuse and Alcoholism. (n.d.). *Older adults*. Retrieved from http://www.niaaa.nih.gov/alcohol-health/special-populations-co-occurring-disorders/older-adults

Erwin, D.Z. & Chen, P. (2023). *Hearing Loss in the Elderly*. Retrieved May 27, 2024, from https://www.ncbi.nlm.nih.gov/books/NBK580566/).

Olson, D. W. (2014). Nursing assessment nervous system. In S. L. Lewis, S. R. Dirksen, M. M. Heitkemper, & L. Bucher (Eds.), *Medical–surgical nursing: Assessment and management of clinical problems* (9th ed., pp. 1335–1355). St. Louis, MO: Elsevier Mosby.

Peck, R. C. (1968). Psychological developments in the second half of life. In B. Neugarten (Ed.), *Middle age and aging* (pp. 88–92). Chicago, IL: University of Chicago Press.

Purnell, L. D. (2013). *Transcultural health care: A culturally competent approach* (4th ed.). Philadelphia, PA: F. A. Davis.

Roberts, D. (2014). Nursing assessment musculoskeletal system. In S. L. Lewis, S. R. Dirksen, M. M. Heitkemper, & L. Bucher (Eds.), *Medical–surgical nursing: Assessment and management of clinical problems* (9th ed., pp. 1489–1504). St. Louis, MO: Elsevier Mosby.

Santrock, J. W. (2023). *A topical approach to life-span development* (11th ed.). New York: NY: McGraw-Hill LLC.

Schneider, J. K., Eveker, A., Bronder, D. R., Meiner, S. E., & Binder, E. F. (2003). Exercise training program for older adults. *Journal of Gerontological Nursing, 29*(9), 22–31.

Strunk, J. A., Townsend-Rocchiccioli, J. T., & Sanford, J. T. (2013). The aging Hispanic in America: Challenges for nurses in a stressed health care environment. *MEDSURG Nursing, 22*(1), 45–50.

Thomas, O., & Stoeckel, P. (2016). Hypertensive black men's perceptions of a nurse protocol for medication self-administration. *Care Management Journals, 17*(1), 37–46.

Wallace, M. (2006). Older adult. In C. L. Edelman & C. L. Mandle (Eds.), *Health promotion throughout the life span* (6th ed., pp. 571–598). St. Louis, MO: Mosby.

Weinrich, S. P., Boyd, M., & Nussbaum, J. (1989). Continuing education: Adapting strategies to teach the elderly. *Journal of Gerontological Nursing, 15*(11), 17–21.

Williams, K., & Mees, K. (2014). Therapeutic communication with older adults, families and caregivers. In K. L., Mauk (Ed.), *Gerontological nursing* (3rd ed., pp. 97–121). Burlington, MA: Jones & Bartlett Learning.

World Health Organization. (2021). *Ageing:Ageism*. Retrieved from who.int/news-room/questions-and-answers/item/ageing-ageism

USDA Food and Nutrition Service, U.S. Department of Agriculture. (2022). Retrieved from https://www.myplate.gov/life-stages/older-adults

CHAPTER 8

Culturally Diverse Learner

OBJECTIVES

Upon completion of this chapter, you will be able to do the following:

- Define the terms *culture*, *ethnicity*, *acculturation*, and *culturally competent care*.
- Describe the six culturally based health education outcomes.
- Select a cultural assessment tool to assess clients from different cultural groups.
- Describe culturally related norms, beliefs about health and illness, family influences, and implications for health education for African American, Asian, Hispanic, and Native American clients.
- Describe verbal and nonverbal communication relevant to African American, Asian, Hispanic, and Native American clients.
- Identify five culturally based actions you can take to provide culturally congruent client education.
- Describe the supporting rationale for culturally based actions in providing culturally congruent client education.

CHAPTER OUTLINE

Introduction

This chapter examines the role of culture in the process of client education. *Culture* is defined as "the totality of socially transmitted behavioral patterns, arts, beliefs, values, customs, lifeways, and all other products of human work and thought characteristic of a population of people that guide their world view and decision-making" (Purnell, 2013, p. 6). Cultural factors include beliefs, values, moral principles, habits, dress, language, rules for behavior, economics, politics, dietary practices, and health care (Burchum, 2002). Not only do cultural factors relate to race and ethnicity, but also to behaviors and beliefs characteristic of particular social, ethnic, disabled, age, and gender groups. Ethnicity is identity with or membership in a particular racial, national, or cultural group and observance of that group's customs, beliefs, and language.

Knowledge of culture is a critical element in the process of delivering health education. All cultural and ethnic groups hold concepts related to health and illness and associated practices for maintaining well-being or providing treatment when it is indicated. The perception of health and illness is enculturated into members of a cultural group. In addition, the individual's socioeconomic, educational, geographic, religious, and other factors shape their cultural and ethnic health beliefs. Over time, *acculturation* may occur, which means that members of a group modify or give up traits from the culture of origin as a result of contact with another culture. Demographic changes anticipated over the next decade magnify the importance of addressing racial and ethnic disparities in health care.

Characteristics of Learners from Different Cultures

Shifting Demographics

The U.S. Census Bureau reports that the population of the United States is more racially and ethnically diverse than ever before. The majority population of English-speaking whites is giving way to a new influx of immigrants with many different cultures and ethnic backgrounds. Minority ethnic groups made up 37% of the U.S. population in 2013 but will comprise 57% of the population in 2060. It is projected that the U.S. population will continue to be older and more racially and ethnically mixed (U.S. Census Bureau, 2012). By 2043, the population of people belonging to minority ethnic groups will become the majority in the United States; however, no single group will make up a majority. The non-Hispanic white population will remain the largest single group. Nonwhite underrepresented ethnic groups are projected to comprise 57% of the population (King, 2014). This change is not occurring only in the United States. Demographic changes are occurring in many countries worldwide…. As a result of this multicultural phenomenon, the cultural competence of nurses is becoming more critical to ensure positive outcomes for an increasingly diverse client population. Nurses must also realize that addressing cultural diversity goes beyond knowing the values, beliefs, practices, and customs of African Americans, Asians, Hispanics/Latinos, and Native Americans/Native Alaskans. In addition to racial classification and national origin, there are many other facets of cultural diversity. "Religious affiliation, language, physical size, gender, sexual orientation, age, disability (both physical and mental), political orientation, socioeconomic status, occupational status and geographical location are but a few of the faces of diversity" (Campinha-Bacote, 2003, p. 1).

It is important not to stereotype people of different cultures, but to cultivate an appreciation for individual cultural variations. Andrews notes that having an understanding of culture, either your own or others, does not necessarily bring about respect and understanding: "Nursing students, nurses, and other health care providers must have positive experiences with members of other cultures and learn to genuinely value the contributions all cultures make to our multicultural society" (2012, p. ix).

Healthcare Disparities

The health and life expectancy of Americans are improving, but racial and ethnic minority populations have not benefited equally from this progress. Complex sociologic, cultural, political, and economic factors account for this. A major concern is that even those non-white clients with equivalent access to the healthcare system receive lower-quality care than white patients for many medical conditions (Smith et al., 2007). These differences in *health disparities* were revealed in the 2002 Institute of Medicine report, *Unequal Treatment: Confronting Racial and Ethnic Disparities in Health Care*. Despite improvements in the overall health status of the U.S. population in the past few decades, disparities in health status among ethnic and racial minority groups continue to be a serious local and national health challenge. Populations with health disparities have increased incidence of diseases, as well as morbidity and mortality, when compared to the general population. Experts have also noted that without new and more effective interventions, health disparities will be difficult to eliminate and may become an even larger problem as racial and ethnic minority groups become a greater proportion of the U.S. population (Smith et al., 2007). Because of this, eliminating health disparities is one of the most important priorities of Healthy People 2020 (U.S. Department of Health and Human Services, 2010).

To meet the needs of different cultural groups, nurse educators must be aware of social determinants of health and how to assess them. Key factors that make up *social determinants of health* include economic stability, neighborhood and physical environment, education, accessibility of food, social and community context, and healthcare system. Outcomes of these social determinants of health affect mortality, morbidity, life expectancy, healthcare expenditures, health status, and functional limitations. Without understanding these important factors, the nurse educator cannot develop an effective and realistic educational plan. See **Table 8-1** to view social determinants of health and factors that should be considered when assessing clients of all cultures.

Cultural Competence and Cultural Humility

Definition of Cultural Competence

Campinha-Bacote defines *cultural competence* as "the process by which the health care professional continuously strives to achieve the ability and availability to effectively work within the cultural

Table 8-1 Social Determinants that Impact Disparities

Economic Stability	Neighborhood and Physical Environment	Education	Accessibility to Food	Community Context	Healthcare System
■ Employment status ■ Income ■ Excess expenses ■ Debt ■ Medical bills ■ Poverty	■ Housing instability ■ Transportation ■ Safety ■ Parks ■ Crime and violence	■ Literacy ■ Language ■ Childhood education ■ High School graduation ■ Vocational training ■ Higher education	■ Hunger ■ Access to healthy options ■ Affordability of food ■ Transportation to access food	■ Social integration ■ Number of support systems ■ Discrimination ■ Incarceration ■ Social cohesion	■ Health coverage ■ Provider availability ■ Provider linguistic and cultural competency

Data from Healthy People 2020. (2016). *Approach to social determinants of health.* Retrieved from https://www.healthypeople.gov/2020/topics-objectives/topic/social-determinants-of-health

context of a client (individual, family, community)" (1998, p. 6). This process requires nurses to see themselves as becoming culturally competent, rather than being culturally competent. Cross, Bazron, Dennis, and Isaacs (1989) further describe cultural competence as a developmental process that evolves over an extended period of time that includes both individuals and organizations at various levels of awareness, knowledge, and skills along the cultural competence continuum. Practicing cultural competence brings about the practice of *culturally competent care* that is considered to be "the knowledge, skills, and attitudes required to provide quality clinical care to patients from different cultural, ethnic, and racial backgrounds" (Harvard Medical School, 2009). The American Nurses Association recognizes the need to provide culturally competent care. It states in the association's code that nurses should "practice with compassion and respect for the inherent dignity, worth and uniqueness of every individual" (2001, p. 4).

Campinha-Bacote Cultural Competence Model

Campinha-Bacote's model, the process of cultural competence in the delivery of health services, includes the components of cultural desire, cultural awareness, cultural knowledge, cultural encounters, and cultural skill (conducting culturally sensitive assessments) (Campinha-Bacote, 2002). Because cultural competence is an important attribute of the nurse as educator, the five key concepts of the model are described further.

Cultural desire is the most critical concept of cultural competence because it is the nurse's desire that brings about the entire process of cultural competence. This desire must come from the nurse wanting to engage in becoming culturally competent, not from having to participate in the process. The nurse takes a humble approach to client differences and, as educator, examines their personal motivation to work with clients of different cultures. In this important first step, the nurse as educator asks, How will I develop the willingness and patience to work with clients who are different from me?

Cultural awareness is the self-examination and in-depth exploration of one's own cultural background. This process involves the recognition of the nurse's biases, prejudices, and assumptions about individuals who are different. This means examining past experiences and considering how to handle biases and assumptions. The nurse asks the question, How will I develop the skill to be objective and open to cultural differences?

Cultural knowledge is the process of seeking and obtaining a sound educational foundation about diverse cultural and ethnic groups. Obtaining cultural knowledge about the client's health-related beliefs and values involves understanding how clients interpret their illnesses and how their view of the world guides their thinking, doing, and being. It is in this part of the model that stereotyping is addressed. Campinha-Bacote states that "no individual is a stereotype of one's culture of origin, but rather a unique blend of the diversity found within each culture, a unique accumulation of life experiences, and the process of acculturation to other cultures" (2003, p. 7). The nurse as educator makes a commitment to learning about other cultures and to grow and evolve in that knowledge.

Cultural encounter is the process that encourages the nurse to directly engage in face-to-face interactions with clients from different cultural backgrounds. Interacting with clients from various cultural groups has the potential to refine or modify nurses' beliefs about cultural groups and aids in preventing stereotyping. It is important to note that interacting with only three or four members from a specific ethnic group does not make one an expert on the cultural group, but these encounters give the nurse as educator valuable experiences to draw from. As the nurse approaches the role of educator, it is advisable to look for opportunities to expand knowledge of other cultures either locally or even internationally.

A final component of Campinha-Bacote's model, *cultural skill*, is the ability to collect relevant cultural data regarding the client's presenting problem and accurately performing a culturally based physical assessment. Cultural assessment is defined as "a systematic, comprehensive examination of individuals, families, groups, and communities regarding their health-related cultural beliefs, values and practices" (Campinha-Bacote, 2002, p. 184). As part of achieving cultural skill, a variety of more in-depth cultural assessment tools are presented here. These tools should be selected and used to meet the specific needs of the learning situation. The nurse as educator should be aware that the way these tools are implemented through the nurse–client interaction is important. Cultural skill brings all the knowledge from the components of the model together to create a culturally competent client interaction.

Definition of Cultural Humility

Cultural humility is a concept that has been studied in the field of counseling and psychology but that has relevance to the role of nurse educator. It is defined by Hook, Davis, Owen, Worthington, and Utsey (2013) as "the ability to maintain an interpersonal stance that is other-oriented (or open to the other) in relation to aspects of cultural identity that are most important to the client" (p. 354). This approach views the act of gaining knowledge about culture as a process that is ongoing rather than as an end product of arriving at being culturally competent. It refers to having an ongoing attitude toward being open to learning about the culture of our clients and of ourselves.

Three factors address the journey of cultural humility. The first is a lifelong commitment to self-evaluation and self-critique (Tervalon & Murray-Garcia, 1998). This step highlights the fact that we are never done learning about our cultural roots or those of others. We must remain committed to continued learning. The second step is a desire to address the power imbalances that exist in society (Tervalon & Murray-Garcia, 1998). Nurse educators and clients should learn from each other, recognizing that the client brings expertise about their life that the nurse must consider and listen to. It is also about recognizing the concept of "white privilege." Finally, cultural humility means working as partners with people and groups who advocate for others (Tervalon & Murray-Garcia, 1998). Perspectives about culture are bigger than our individual selves. This confirms the major idea that cultural humility is about constantly expanding our attitudes and understanding of culture.

Cultural Assessment Models

Andrews/Boyle Transcultural Nursing Assessment Guide for Individuals and Families

Andrews and Boyle (2012) offer an extensive in-depth assessment tool titled the Andrews/Boyle Transcultural Nursing Assessment Guide for Individuals and Families. The major categories in this guide include cultural variations and cultural aspects of the incidence of disease, communication, cultural affiliations, cultural sanctions and restrictions, developmental considerations, economics, health-related beliefs and practices, kinship and social networks, nutrition, religion and spirituality, and values orientation. The guide focuses on a holistic cultural approach to the health history and the physical examination.

Leininger's Sunrise Model

The Sunrise Model is part of Leininger's Theory of Cultural Care Diversity and Universality and includes seven assessments of culturally congruent nursing care. They include a holistic approach that looks at cultural values and lifeways; religious, philosophical, and spiritual beliefs; economic factors; educational factors; technological factors; kinship and social ties; and political and legal factors (Leininger, 1991).

Purnell's Model for Cultural Assessment

Purnell's Model for Cultural Assessment includes domains of culture for assessing ethnocultural attributes of individuals, families, or groups (Purnell, 2013). The 12 domains are inhabited localities and topography, communication, family roles and organizations, workforce issues, bicultural ecology, high-risk behaviors, nutrition, pregnancy and childbearing practices, death rituals, spirituality, health practices, and healthcare practitioners. The strength of this model includes the domain of bicultural ecology that identifies specific physical, biologic, and physiologic variations in ethnic and racial origins. This is a source of information on cultural variations in physical assessment for nurses as educators.

Giger and Davidhizar's Transcultural Assessment Model

Giger and Davidhizar's Transcultural Assessment Model consists of six cultural phenomena that go across all cultures and that affect nursing care. They are communication, space, social organization,

Table 8-2 Culhane-Pera and Colleagues' Levels of Cultural Competence

Level 1: No insight about the influence of culture on health care
Level 2: Minimal emphasis on culture in healthcare settings
Level 3: Acceptance of the role of cultural beliefs, values, and behaviors on health, disease, and treatment
Level 4: Incorporation of cultural awareness into daily healthcare practice
Level 5: Integration of attention to culture into all areas of professional life

Data from Esposito C. L. (2013). Provision of culturally competent health care: an interim status review and report. *The Journal of the New York State Nurses' Association*, 43(2), 4–10. PMID: 25109038.

time, environmental control, and biological variations (Giger & Davidhizar, 2008). The model applies these concepts to 23 specific cultural groups that are found in the United States.

Assessing Cultural Competence

Nurses should take time to self-evaluate their progress in becoming culturally competent. The following two tools take slightly different approaches to examining cultural competence, but both help the nurse as educator reflect upon the role of culture in client care. Campinha-Bacote and Narayan state that cultural awareness is "a continual self-examination of one's own prejudices and biases toward other cultures" (2000, p. 213). Campinha-Bacote (2002) provides a mnemonic, *ASKED*, to help nurses assess their cultural awareness:

A is for awareness

S is for skill

K is for knowledge

E is for encounters

D is for desire

Nurses as educators ask themselves if they have *awareness* of biases and prejudices; if they have the *skill* to conduct a cultural assessment; if they have cultural *knowledge*; if they have experiences *encountering* people of different cultures; and if they have the *desire* to be culturally competent. This self-assessment assists the nurse when working with clients from various cultural and ethnic groups.

Culhane-Pera, Reif, Egli, Bake, and Kassekert (1997) describe five levels of cultural competence with respect to health care. With this tool, nurses can track their progress in becoming culturally competent as they advance through the levels (**Table 8-2**).

Culturally Congruent Client Education

The definition of *culturally congruent client education* is drawn from the concept of culturally congruent care, initially conceptualized by Leininger, who defines culturally congruent care as "those cognitively based assistive, supportive, facilitative, or enabling acts or decisions that are tailor made to fit with individual, group, or institutional cultural values, beliefs, and lifeways in order to provide or support meaningful, beneficial, and satisfying health care to well-being services" (1991, p. 49). Schim, Doorenbos, Benkert, and Miller further explain Leininger's definition by saying that "culturally congruent care is a holistic construct, heavily influenced by negotiated experiences, meanings, mutual understandings, and respect" (2007, p. 105). We use this as a foundation to define culturally congruent client education. Culturally congruent client education involves providing meaningful and useful education for clients by incorporating diverse ways of knowing from the viewpoint of various cultural groups. It is a harmonious approach to working with clients that shows sensitivity and respect for individual cultural differences and a willingness to collaborate with them to meet their health education needs. Culturally competent nurses who are educators welcome client collaboration and cooperation. They have a foundation of knowledge about client cultures and reflect on their own personal cultural values and beliefs. This self-examination helps them understand how their beliefs influence the way they teach.

The need for culturally congruent client education is based on the fact that clients respond culturally to health and illness. In the United States, healthcare disparities are a leading cause of morbidity and mortality among underrepresented groups and those of lower socioeconomic status. Because of this, it is important that nurses incorporate cultural perspectives into all facets of health education delivery (Anderson, Scrimshaw, Fullilove, Fielding, & Normand, 2003). This approach addresses the need to promote equal access to quality health care and equal treatment of clients.

Stoeckel Culturally Congruent Client Education Model

The increasingly multicultural profile of the U.S. population requires that nurses provide culturally congruent care. Providing culturally congruent client education has the potential to improve health outcomes, increase the efficiency of healthcare professionals, and result in greater client satisfaction with services (Brach & Fraser, 2000). The Stoeckel Culturally Congruent Client Education Model brings together the concepts presented in this chapter to summarize the essential framework of what it means to provide culturally congruent client education. The three major components of the model are culturally based actions, rationales, and culturally based client education outcomes (**Figure 8-1**).

Culturally Based Actions

The *culturally based actions* in this model begin with developing cultural competence. This chapter provides Campinha-Bacote's cultural competence model that identified the steps in the process of becoming culturally competent: cultural desire, cultural awareness, cultural knowledge, cultural skill, and cultural encounters.

The second culturally based action is using *culturally specific client assessment tools* to develop individualized client education plans. This chapter presented in-depth assessment tools by a variety of authors and a focused assessment option to gather client information. The nurse chooses the cultural assessment tool that is appropriate for the situation.

The third culturally based action is using *knowledge of cross-cultural communication techniques* to interact with clients in developing client education plans. A preserve–accommodate–restructure approach (DeRosa & Kochurka, 2006) is taken in working with clients so that cultural practices are preserved, except for those that hinder the client's health. The LEARN technique—L: listen, E: explain, A: acknowledge, R: recommend, N: negotiate—is an example of cross-cultural communication (Berlin & Fowkes, 1983). It is a negotiation framework that supports a cross-cultural approach to client communication.

Culturally based actions	Rationale	Culturally based client education outcomes
1. Develop cultural competence	Clients seek out nurse educators of their own race/ethnicity	Increase client understanding of and adherence to treatment recommendations
2. Use culturally specific client assessment tools	Use of interpreters and linguistically appropriate instructional materials results in better understanding and communication	Increase client willingness to access health information
3. Use cross-cultural communication techniques		Increase client integration of health information into activities of daily living
4. Use diverse interprofessional team members and interpreters	Cultural competence awareness results in greater knowledge and sensitivity to ethnic/racial variations in health beliefs/practices	Increase client satisfaction with and confidence in health education
5. Use linguistically and culturally appropriate teaching strategies and instructional materials	Cultural competence awareness gives nurses knowledge of their own beliefs/behaviors and how they impact diverse populations	Increase confidence in nurses as educators and the healthcare system

Figure 8-1 The Stoeckel Culturally Congruent Client Education Model

The fourth culturally based action is to use *diverse interprofessional team members and interpreters* that reflect the client's culture. Clients from underrepresented ethnic groups are more likely to access and use healthcare services when they encounter health professionals of their own race and ethnicity (Purnell, 2013). The correct use of interpreters or bilingual team members is an important culturally based action that allows for cultural congruency. A lack of interpreter services is a significant factor associated with client dissatisfaction and poor comprehension.

The fifth culturally based action is using *linguistically and culturally appropriate teaching strategies and instructional materials* to enhance and support learning. This action involves providing culturally appropriate oral and written language services to clients with limited proficiency. This action increases client adherence to treatment and improves the quality of health education.

Rationales

Nurses as educators gain knowledge through developing cultural competence, which includes becoming aware of their own beliefs and behaviors as well as those of clients. The use of assessment tools facilitates gathering clients' cultural data that can be used to build individualized client education plans. When possible, nurses of the clients' race or ethnicity should be involved in teaching clients. A goal for the future is to engage culturally diverse nurses to meet this need. The use of interprofessional team members, interpreters, and linguistically appropriate instructional materials results in better understanding, adherence to treatment plans, and improved cross-cultural communication.

Culturally Based Client Education Outcomes

Culturally based actions result in meeting the needs of underrepresented populations. The desired culturally based client education outcomes meet the needs of non-white populations by increasing client understanding of treatment and adherence to treatment recommendations. When nurses take the recommended culturally based actions, clients are more willing to access health information. This increases their satisfaction with health education and increases their confidence in nurses as educators. These outcomes result in clients who are better able to integrate health teaching into their activities of daily living.

Culturally Specific Client Assessments and Concerns

Cultural factors affect client education interactions. It is important for the nurse as educator to have an understanding of the cultural factors that shape learners from different cultural groups. Stressors and adaptive behaviors may present considerable barriers to effective client education unless nurses are sensitive to their origins and meanings and are willing to take them into account when working with clients (Falvo, 2011). By taking time to investigate a client's past experiences and cultural perceptions, the nurse takes steps to build rapport with clients, which is a basic component of effective nurse–client relationships.

Clients accept or reject the information provided by a nurse based on whether they perceive the information as truthful, in their best interest, and congruent with their beliefs. To gain a better understanding of factors related to teaching and learning with cultural groups, we have chosen to present information on four ethnic minority groups: African American, Asian American, Hispanic, and Native American. They are the major ethnic minority populations in the United States as traced by the U.S. Census Bureau. Four aspects of each group's culture that impact health education are examined: *cultural norms* (aspects of the culture that impact the teaching and learning process), *family influence* (impact and involvement of family in the teaching and learning process), *beliefs about health and illness* (including religious influences and folk medicine that influence clients' perception of health care), and *implications for health education*. Knowledge of these aspects provides insight for nurses as educators in planning and implementing client education plans, but caution is needed to avoid stereotyping. Never assume that all clients from one ethnic group hold the same beliefs.

African American

Cultural Norms

The U.S. Census Bureau reported that the Black population is expected to increase from 41.1 million to 61.8 million in 2060 (2012), which is about 14.7% of the total population.

In preparing to work with African American clients, the nurse should be aware that the initial client approach and the initial impression you give are very important. Because interpersonal relationships are highly valued among African Americans, it is important to focus on developing a sound, trusting, and respectful relationship. This begins with consideration of the way that clients are greeted and referred to. Be aware of intracultural variations within the cultural group; for example, different generational groups may have a particular way in which they wish to be identified. Younger clients may want to be called African American; older clients may prefer the terms Negro or colored, and middle-aged clients may refer to themselves as Black or Black American (Campinha-Bacote, 2008). Most African Americans prefer to be greeted formally, with Mr., Mrs., Ms., or Miss, along with their surname, because the family name is respected and indicates pride in family heritage. Unless invited, it is best to use the last name and appropriate title instead of first names. It may be necessary to clarify preferences with clients.

The attitude of healthcare professionals is one of the most significant barriers when working with African Americans. Research shows that African American clients feel they are often treated unfairly or disrespectfully because of their race (Kaiser Family Foundation, 2001). Because of this, African Americans may be suspicious of healthcare professionals and may seek out a physician or nurse only when absolutely necessary. Treating clients with respect is the foundation of the nurse–client relationship. *Respect for persons* has been broadly defined as the recognition that all persons have dignity and inherent worth. Expressions of respect include treatment with dignity and respect for autonomy and involvement in healthcare decisions. These expressions are associated with clients' satisfaction with care and increased adherence to treatment regimens. Beach and colleagues (2005b) suggest that clients can determine when clinicians demonstrate a valuing attitude. These perceptions correlate with whether the client was treated kindly or rudely. Respectful treatment of African American clients includes acknowledging clients appropriately as described previously, shaking hands, using eye contact, listening intently, and giving physical and mental comfort.

Family Influence

Understanding African American families is an important aspect of teaching clients. Traditional family structure of husband and wife is often found, but many African American families have a *matriarchal system* with a single mother, aunt, or grandmother heading the household. The role of the grandmother is one of the most central roles in the African American family and is afforded great respect (Campinha-Bacote, 2008). A growing number of grandparents are functioning in the primary parental role. African American women are expected to assist family members in maintaining good health and determining treatment if a family member is ill. It is important for the nurse to recognize the importance of African American women in disseminating information and in assisting family members in making decisions (Cherry & Giger, 2008). If present, an African American man should also be included in the decision-making process. Some African American families have large supportive extended family networks. It is important to include involved, extended family members in planning and implementing client education plans where appropriate because they could unknowingly sabotage the clients' progress if they are not informed.

Health Beliefs

Spiritual and religious orientation is important in some African American families, with the majority participating in Protestant denominations. Belief in God and the use of prayer and participation in formal religious service may be part of religious practices. The church community is viewed as a viable support system in developing health-promoting behaviors, and the nurse may consider a partnership with faith-based communities to support client learning.

Figure 8-2 The African American Family
© Patricia Marks/Shutterstock

There is evidence that African American folk medicine is practiced in all areas of the United States, but the extent of its use is not known. *African American folk medicine* is an offshoot of African cultural heritage in the rural South. It can involve treatment by folk practitioners who use witchcraft, voodoo, and magic. Folk medicine may be used for a variety of reasons: lack of access to traditional healthcare services, inability to afford the cost of health care, or humiliating experiences when encountering the mainstream healthcare system (Cherry & Giger, 2008).

Folk medicine perceives illness as either a natural or an unnatural occurrence. Natural illness occurs because a person is affected by natural forces without adequate protection. Unnatural illnesses are perceived as either a punishment from God or the work of the devil, which are more difficult for the nurse to address. Death is viewed as a natural part of living and is handled through strong religious beliefs (Campinha-Bacote, 2008). It is important for the nurse to assess if folk remedies are being used, and if so to assist the client in sorting out what is helpful, neutral, or harmful. This is part of the assessment information necessary to prepare the client education plan.

Implications for Health Education

When setting up teaching sessions with African American clients, keep in mind that they may prefer a closer personal space and that extended family may accompany them. When teaching how to perform psychomotor skills, structure the learning activities in ranked order to produce maximum learning results. If timing is involved with an activity, it is important to be clear about when timing is flexible and when it is not, such as with the giving of medication. Keep in mind that a client education plan that is congruent with the client's beliefs has a better chance of being successful. The most common health concerns for African Americans requiring health education are listed in **Table 8-3**.

Of particular concern at this time to nurse educators is that African American females are 2 to 6 times more likely to die from complications of pregnancy than white females, depending on

Table 8-3 Other Common Health Concerns Requiring Health Education: African Americans

Ethnic/Racial Group	Most Common Disorders Requiring Health Education
African American	■ Heart disease ■ Hypertension ■ Stroke ■ Cancer ■ Asthma ■ Influenza/pneumonia ■ HIV/AIDS ■ Homicide ■ Obesity ■ Sickle cell anemia

where they live (American Medical Association, 1999). Nurse educators including childbirth educators are in a unique position to instruct pregnant people about the risks of unhealthy lifestyle factors and delayed prenatal care. Contraception information can be added to the educational plan to help reduce the risk of unintended pregnancy during the postpartum period. In addition, childbirth efforts should be extended to more females living in poverty.

Additional teaching approaches by nurse educators include:

- Asking questions to better understand clients and factors affecting their lives.
- Helping clients, and those accompanying them, to understand the urgent maternal warning signs and when to seek medical attention right away.
- Helping clients manage chronic conditions or conditions that may arise during pregnancy like hypertension, diabetes, or depression.
- Recognizing and working to eliminate unconscious bias in themselves and in their practice on an ongoing basis.
- Responding to any concerns clients have.
- Recommending doulas for additional support in labor, delivery, and postpartum.
- Providing all clients with respectful quality care (CDC, 2023).

Asian American

Cultural Norms

The U.S. Census Bureau projects that the Asian American population will double from 15.5 million in 2012 to 34.4 million in 2060 (2012). Its share of the total population will rise from 5.1% to 8.2% in the same period. Asian Americans emigrate from more than 20 countries and speak more than 100 languages. The Asian American population is diverse and represents people from a variety of countries and cultures. The largest subpopulations are persons of Chinese, Filipino, Japanese, Asian Indian, Korean, and Southeast Asian ancestry. Recent Asian immigrants represent the highest foreign-born percentage among all racial and ethnic groups in the United States.

Establishing rapport with Asian American clients begins with establishing trust. It is important to remember as you approach Asian American clients to be aware that their values include hard work, acceptance of what life brings, respect for nature, self-control, respect for elders, and loyalty to family. Cultural values stress politeness in verbal discourse, and if mistrust develops, you may find the client reluctant to discuss lifestyle issues and behaviors. Many Asian Americans view relationships in health care as hierarchical and therefore expect the health professional to take charge (Beach et al., 2005a). Clients may not want to participate in making decisions about their treatment and may appear passive in the process. Nurses as educators should acknowledge their role and use it to their advantage when working with clients. This can be particularly effective in encouraging patients to adopt healthy behaviors and adhere to client education plans. It is important, however, that the client not feel intimidated by the nurse. Feelings of intimidation may prevent the client from telling the truth about customs, beliefs, or behaviors that may impact the success of the client education plan. You should also be aware that some clients may silently decide not to adhere to recommended treatments (Beach et al., 2005a).

Asian American clients view health from a variety of perspectives and often combine Eastern and Western perspectives of health. They use acupuncture, acupressure, and herbs in combination with dietary therapy, Western medicine, and supernatural healing to achieve maximum results. When beliefs contradict each other, however, some Asians will not adhere to Western medicine. It is also important to be aware that clients do not always disclose the use of *complementary and alternative medicine (CAM)*, which can increase the chances of adverse interaction with conventional Western treatments. Clients may be reluctant to share their use of these methods, fearing disapproval from the nurse and worrying that they might appear disrespectful of Western traditions. To determine the use of CAM, you should ask clients directly and clearly what remedies they use. Nurses need to educate themselves about traditional Asian approaches to healing and encourage their clients and their healers to collaborate for the client's good. A common belief of Asian clients is that Western medicine is very potent and that it can cure illness rapidly (Beach et al., 2005a). This belief may manifest itself by the client reducing dosages. Clients also may stop medications as soon as symptoms are relieved. These are all areas that require attention when preparing client education plans.

When meeting older Asian people, it is a sign of disrespect to look them straight in the eyes. A limp handshake from Asian clients is a way of showing humility and respect. For many, physical contact such as a handshake or a hug between a man and a woman is interpreted as a sexual advance. For some Asian subcultures, it may be appropriate for you to first address the oldest male in a group or family before greeting other members (Beach et al., 2005a). Be aware that a lack of facial expression or a low level of verbal communication may not indicate a lack of emotion or opinion. Neither does it indicate agreement with the diagnosis or recommended treatment. Try to determine your clients' true feelings or opinions before accepting their apparent acquiescence of the treatment plan. Asian clients tend to be more comfortable with a health professional who shares their language and culture, perhaps because they believe that a person of their own culture will not dismiss their traditional Asian practices and home remedies (Beach et al., 2005a).

Family Influence

Traditionally, the Asian family unit is strong, stable, and cohesive for all its members. The family plays a critical role in the ongoing development and support of children through adulthood. The importance of the extended family, emphasized in Asian culture, often results in the extended family being highly involved in the client's care and medical decision making (Beach et al., 2005a). Family members can provide valuable information regarding the client's diet, health behavior, daily activities, and types of alternative medications used. Their involvement in a treatment plan may be vital to the client's ability to adhere to the recommended client education plan. Families may decide what the client will eat, when to take medication, whether to exercise, and when to seek medical attention. The family also exerts influence on youth to prevent antisocial and self-defeating behaviors.

Many Asian immigrants experienced stressful and painful episodes in their native countries that affect their health and influence their perception of the U.S. healthcare system. The effects of war, migration, detention camps or torture, and experiences associated with adjustment to the U.S. culture are all major factors that might result in mistrust, fear, or helplessness and prevent the client from taking an active role in their health care.

Nurses as educators need to be sensitive to the diversity and generational differences within the Asian population and decide on an individual basis whether it is culturally appropriate to involve family members. The culturally competent educator will discuss with the client the patterns of decision making in the family. Understanding and respecting complex and often delicate interactions among family members enables nurses to use the client's family as a valuable resource rather than an intrusion into the nurse–client relationship (Beach et al., 2005a).

Health Beliefs

Asian medical tradition centers on a belief in the interconnectedness of the mind, body, and spirit and the need for balance and a holistic approach to the treatment of illness. Buddhism and other Eastern philosophies teach that art and science coexist and that healing is spiritual as well as scientific (Yee, Mokuau, & Kim, 1999). A common belief held by many Asians is that of *Taoism*, which originated in China. Tao, or the way, is based on the idea of balancing the natural processes and forces of yin and yang. *Yin* is negative female energy associated with cold and water, and *Yang* is positive male energy associated with heat and fire. These forces remain in balance through a combination of practices of holistic medicine, acupuncture, herbalism, and meditation. Beliefs

Figure 8-3 The Asian Family
© Monkey Business Images/Shutterstock

about health and illness strongly influence clients' behavior. They may avoid the wind, be reluctant to go out after surgery, or refuse to have blood drawn (Beach et al., 2005a). Many Asians perceive life in fatalistic terms and may feel less able to do something about their illness. Beliefs in supernatural spirits may result in reliance on religion or spiritual healing rituals in addition to Western medicine. All these factors influence your approach to teaching Asian clients.

Implications for Health Education

As an educator, you need to provide strong encouragement because Asian clients need assurance that the recommended treatment plan is the right thing to do. This may mean urging family members to encourage the client. Being an advocate also means helping to locate other supportive healthcare providers. In some communities, Asian American organizations (temples, churches, benevolent association, cultural associations, etc.) serve as focal points for social and other activities. Developing contacts with and working through these community-based organizations can be a useful way for you to develop an understanding of the health and social needs of clients (Beach et al., 2005a). Be aware that Asian clients usually expect something concrete, such as prescriptions for medications, at the conclusion of a teaching session for the meeting to live up to their expectations. Without this, they might be reluctant to return for routine teaching visits or preventive care. Also be aware that Asian females may prefer to work with a female educator.

In March 2020, there was an alarming increase in racial discrimination and racially motivated violence toward Asian Americans. This disturbing fact is attributed to the blame placed on China for causing the COVID-19 pandemic discovered in Wuhan (Lee, 2021; Kim & Tummala-Narra, 2022). Anti-Asian discrimination has been a part of the Asian American experience since the initial migration of Asians to the United States, but this rise in violence contributed to the isolation, illness, and economic difficulties of the pandemic (Kim & Tummala-Narra, 2022). Asian hate crimes have occurred in a wide variety of locations, potentially causing Asian American clients to feel unsafe in spaces they previously felt were safe, including hospitals and clinics.

The term "Asian American" encompasses more than 50 distinct ethnic groups, in which more than 30 different languages are spoken. Asian Americans are one of the fastest-growing ethnic groups, with a projected increase in population to 6.2% by 2025, and 8.9% by 2050 (Iwamasa, 2012). As the population of Asian Americans continues to grow and become more diverse, the demand for appropriate services will continue to grow as well. Asian American diversity is tremendous, but several cultural beliefs are held in common: strong family structures, respect, adaptability, and, for first-generation immigrants, widespread use of traditional therapies (Juckett et al., 2014).

Asian clients pose significant challenges for nurse educators due to having radically different ideas of disease causation, differing communication styles, and physical presentations of mental illness. Additional challenges include that while the incidence of mental illness among Asians is comparable to that of the general population, Asian Americans are less likely to report such problems or to use mental health services due to the stigmatization of mental illness in Asian culture (Juckett et al., 2014). Symptoms of mental illness may be subconsciously converted into the more socially acceptable medium of physical illness, which "saves face" and preserves family honor. These cultural values affect the willingness of Asian Americans to seek professional psychological treatment. Asian Americans have been found to underutilize traditional mental health services. In addition to cultural values such as stigma and loss of face, limited English proficiency, differing conceptualizations of distress, and limited access to culturally competent services also contribute to low treatment utilization rates (Juckett et al., 2014; Lee, 2021).

Suggested approaches for nurse educators working with Asian Americans follow:

- Create safe spaces in outpatient and inpatient settings for Asian American clients. This includes displaying welcoming images and literature and ensuring racial diversity of clients and clinicians in pamphlets, brochures, and posters around the office. The nurse educator should be willing to accommodate requests to move a roommate who has made discriminatory remarks (Lee, 2021).
- The nurse educator should understand that Asian Americans are immensely diverse in many ways and not make assumptions about a client's experiences and adherence to traditional cultural values and practices.
- When taking a history, the nurse educator should assess whether Asian American clients feel safe in their homes, in their neighborhoods, or on public transit. The nurse educator should assess for clients' personal experiences of racism and oppression and use relevant screening questions and instruments.
- When suspecting racism, use targeted screening for depression, anxiety, and substance use to reveal symptoms that patients may have previously dismissed. If a client reports having experienced a hate crime, it is appropriate to treat the incident as a traumatic experience. Taking a more thorough history of the incident and using a post-traumatic stress disorder (PTSD) screening instrument to assess the patient for psychological distress and loss in function.
- When developing a teaching plan, the nurse educator should use the results of the history, physical exam, and screening tools to guide teaching strategies. Keep in mind that mental issues may be expressed in physical findings.
- A part of the teaching plan can be referral of Asian clients to organizations such as STOP AAPI Hate and Asian Americans Advancing Justice. Referral to colleagues in social work and case management should also be a part of the teaching plan.
- Multilingual Asian Americans or language services should be used, when possible, to improve communication and understanding of the educational plan. Mental health treatment providers should be trained and educated in culturally competent treatment methods.
- The nurse educator should provide convenient times for teaching sessions and help with transportation, if possible, to assist Asian American clients in making appointments (Juckett et al., 2014; Lee, 2021; Iwamasa, 2012).

Other common health concerns for Asians requiring health education are listed in **Table 8-4**.

Table 8-4 Most Common Disorders Requiring Health Education: Asians

Ethnic/Racial Group	Most Common Disorders Requiring Health Education
Asian	■ Cancer ■ Heart disease ■ Stroke ■ Accidents ■ Diabetes ■ Tuberculosis ■ Liver disease

Hispanic

Cultural Norms

The U.S. Census Bureau projects that the Hispanic population will double from 53.3 million in 2012 to 128.8 million in 2060 (2012). At the end of this period, nearly one in three U.S. residents will be Hispanic, up from one in six in 2013. This will continue to make Hispanics the largest ethnic minority group in the United States. Hispanics are classified as one ethnic group, but they are actually multiple, culturally similar ethnic subgroups. The subgroups that make up the Hispanic population in the United States are Mexicans, Puerto Ricans, Cubans, Central Americans, South Americans, Dominicans, and other Hispanics and Latinos.

When working with Hispanic clients, it is important to be aware of the different terms used to refer to Hispanics. The U.S. Census Bureau (2012) uses the term *Hispanic* to describe any person, regardless of race, creed, or color, whose origins are in Mexico, Puerto Rico, Cuba, Central or South America, or some other Hispanic region. *Latino* or *Latina* refers to a person of Latin American or Spanish-speaking descent who is living in the United States. The terms *Hispanic* or *Latino* may be used interchangeably (Zoucha & Zamarripa, 2003). It is not recommended to use the terms *Chicano*, *Mexicano*, or *Xican* unless the client refers to themself in these ways because these terms may be considered derogatory. The term *Tejano* is used to describe a Texan of Hispanic descent. It is important to ask clients how they would like to be referred to.

Several cultural characteristics impact the way that Hispanic clients perceive interactions with healthcare professionals. The concepts of *respecto* (respect), *personalismo* (personal relationships), and *confianza* (trust) are important concepts for the nurse to be aware of when interacting with Hispanic clients (Gonzalez, Owen, & Esperat, 2008). Respecto is a behavior that shows differential attention toward others based on age, sex, social position, economic status, and authority. It is important for you to show respect by addressing Hispanic clients by their surname and title in English or Spanish, such as Mrs. Rodriquez or Señora Rodriquez, and by avoiding a condescending attitude. Hispanic clients may avoid eye contact with authority figures. To be respectful, personal or private questions should be approached in an indirect way to avoid client embarrassment. Personalismo is about the nurse conveying to the client that they want a personal relationship. This is demonstrated by being friendly and taking interest in the client's life. This is shown by engaging in a greeting that inquire about how they are doing and puts the client at ease. Personal contact and touch are acceptable parts of the relationship and are considered important aspects of the nurse–client relationship. Hispanic clients prefer to be close and are comfortable with the nurse giving a handshake, sitting closer, leaning forward, and giving a comforting pat on the shoulder or other gestures that indicate interest in the client. Hispanic clients demonstrate stronger attachment to the healthcare provider than to the healthcare institution and will follow the provider if they move (Beach et al., 2005a). This emphasizes how strongly they value personal relationships. Confianza, or trust, develops over time in relations with Hispanic clients. When trust is established between the nurse and the client, it becomes more likely that the client will value the time spent with the nurse and be more likely to adhere to client education plans.

It can be frightening for clients who cannot speak English to enter the U.S. healthcare system. Studies show that Hispanic clients view nurses who attempted to speak some Spanish as caring and respectful (Gonzalez et al., 2008). It is common for Hispanic clients to appear agreeable on the surface and to be courteous, but if they disagree they may not carry out the suggested treatment. It is uncommon for Hispanic clients to be aggressive when interacting with healthcare professionals, but their response may be silence or not adhering to the client education plan. Joking by the nurse is considered rude, insulting, and offensive, and it may cause stress and result in a negative response (Gonzalez et al., 2008). When under stress, Hispanic clients may revert back to using their native language. Hispanic clients also may prefer educators of the same gender.

Family Influence

Family is a highly valued part of Hispanic life, and family involvement is often critical in providing health care to the client. Family matters take precedence over work and all other aspects of life. Hispanic families are large, and respect for parental authority is emphasized. Typical Hispanic families are *patriarchal*, with the male family members having the dominant role as head of the household. They are the decision makers. Hispanic men typically have a strong sense of machismo. This is an attitude that the man is wiser, smarter, stronger, and more knowledgeable (Zoucha & Zamarripa, 2003). Hispanic women defer to men and have subdued qualities. Mothers may influence family decisions but do not play a dominant role. Any dishonor or shame that may occur for an individual family member is considered a reflection on the entire family. Older Hispanics are respected and may live with married children if they are not self-sufficient. Changes in these patterns are seen in more educated clients and families with higher socioeconomic status. Overall change to a more egalitarian family structure is slow to happen.

Many clients live in multifamily arrangements that include extended family who offer social and economic support. The term familismo describes the Hispanic belief in family interdependence that curtails exposure to outside influences, and that may be a major cause of resistance to change (Gonzalez et al., 2008). An important aspect of Hispanic families is that they are the main source of assistance before seeking out assistance from the community. By including family members, nurses as educators can build greater trust and confidence and in turn increase adherence to client education plans.

Figure 8-4 The Hispanic Family

© Feverpitch/Shutterstock

Health Beliefs

Hispanics believe in an external *locus of control*, which is the belief that outside forces control their lives. For some Hispanics, health is viewed as the result of good luck or a reward from God. Some also believe in the theory of hot and cold imbalances. The basis of this belief is that illness is caused by prolonged exposure to hot or cold. Many of the illnesses are digestive in nature. To ensure good health, both hot and cold foods must be taken into the body. It is important for the nurse to be aware that the use of self-medication with alternative therapies is prevalent in Hispanic culture, and this information is seldom reported to healthcare professionals. The nurse should understand that Hispanics will have more respect for the nurse who accepts the spiritual and folk basis of their health beliefs (Gonzalez et al., 2008). If the client education plan is incongruent with folk beliefs, the nurse as educator should attempt to find compromises or solutions to resolve the incongruence and allow clients to maintain their belief system while following the plan. Folk healers are part of *curanderismo*, which views illness from a religious and social perspective rather than the Western scientific perspective. *Curanderas*, *santera*, and *espiritistas* are folk healers who are sought out to treat illness and are preferred over the medical community because they are personal, less dehumanizing, know the family, and are an integral part of the Hispanic community (Gonzalez et al., 2008).

Implications for Health Education

Begin with an assessment of the Hispanic client's ability to communicate and understand English. Establishing rapport is an essential part of building a trusting relationship. There should be continuous evaluation of learning by questioning and return demonstration; problem solving should be encouraged. You need to understand the perceived causes for folk-related diseases and show respect for cultural differences, such as amulets that the client might wear to protect from the *evil eye* or evil spirits. Also be aware that some Hispanics feel that medication is always necessary, and many may not believe their illness is being treated adequately unless medication is ordered (Beach et al., 2005a). Your long-term goal working in the Hispanic community should be to gain an understanding of folk medicine beliefs and try to establish a relationship with the healers in the hope of eliciting acceptance and understanding of the rationale for the client education plan. You need to be aware of the client's cultural health beliefs to have an effect on the client's behavior and recovery.

Alarming statistics indicate that there is increased morbidity and mortality among Hispanic men who are less likely to seek medical care than Hispanic women (Agency for Health Care Research and Quality, 2019; Department of Health and Human Services, 2021). Hispanic males have a higher incidence of obesity and hypertension and an increased rates of diabetes, end stage renal disease, colorectal cancer, liver disease, and HIV (Daniel-Ulloa et al., 2023). Hispanic males' avoidance of seeking medical care is an urgent concern and requires attention by nurse educators.

The reason for not seeking care is related to Hispanic men striving to be recognized and respected as men and the expectation that they will follow certain culturally determined roles, attitudes, and norms to prove their manhood within the family unit and the broader community. Hispanic men may avoid routine medical screenings to appear "brave and self-sufficient." This strong sense of masculinity, or "machismo," is ingrained in Hispanic culture. It is anticipated that Hispanics' share of the population will grow to 28% of the U.S. population by 2060 (Anft, 2017). As that number grows, researchers worry that the nation could face costly consequences as long-ignored conditions lead to serious illness and disability. Additional reasons Hispanic men may not seek care include: lack of health insurance, low income, lack of adequate transportation, and lack of care providers who are bilingual and culturally competent (Ariel Gelrud Shiro et al., 2023)

Nurse educators face challenges helping Hispanic men manage health problems, practice preventative medicine, and live healthy lifestyles.

Teaching approaches that aid nurse educators working with Hispanic men include:

- The nurse educator should ensure interpersonal communication by providing Spanish language access. Properly communicating with patients in their native language improves comprehension of medical instructions and guidelines, reduces misunderstandings, and ensures accurate exchange of information. Explaining medical information in language and terms your patients understand increases medical compliance. Interpreters should be used and not family members.
- The nurse educator should partner with Hispanic caregivers when possible. When patients see healthcare professionals who share their background, it creates comfort and understanding within the nurse–client relationship. Working with caregivers of their own culture encourages male patients to better engage in their care and treatment plans. Hispanic men should be actively involved in their care rather than passively acquiescing to instructions. When clients are connected with their healthcare provider, healthcare outcomes are improved.
- The nurse educator should respect and incorporate Hispanic culture when working with Hispanic men. Several normative values must be recognized in clinical settings with male clients. These include simpatía (kindness), personalismo (friendliness), and respeto (respect). Simpatía emphasizes politeness and conflict avoidance. Personalismo, a personal connection, can be achieved by asking about the patient and their family (Juckett, 2013). Because people stand closer to each other in most Latino cultures, physical proximity is also perceived as being more personable. Respeto implies attentive concern for the patient and respect of their personhood and age, especially if the patient is older. Older patients should be addressed as señor rather than by their first names. Using don with the given or full name indicates even greater respect for older male patients (Juckett, 2013).
- The nurse educator should respect the cultural value of modestia (modesty). Hispanic men may be conservative about modesty, and physical exposure should be negotiated as the examination warrants. A chaperone is often appreciated if a same sex caregiver is not available.
- The nurse educator should advocate for Hispanic men by helping them access affordable care and insurance when possible.
- The nurse educator should offer flexible scheduling and convenient times for Hispanic men that work alternative hours so they can attend client care meetings.
- The nurse educator should provide Spanish-language medical handouts and client teaching forms.

The most common health concerns for Hispanics requiring health education are listed in **Table 8-5**.

Table 8-5 Most Common Disorders Requiring Health Education: Hispanics

Ethnic/Racial Group	Most Common Disorders Requiring Health Education
Hispanic	■ Heart disease ■ Cancer ■ Accidents ■ Stroke ■ Diabetes ■ Hypertension ■ Obesity ■ HIV/AIDS

Native Americans

Cultural Norms

The number of Native Americans and Native Alaskans in the United States is 3.9 million, and it is projected to increase by more than half to 6.3 million in 2060. This will increase their share of the population from 1.3% to 1.5%. The Bureau of Indian Affairs recognizes more than 500 different Indian tribes, with the largest number being Cherokee and Navajo (Hanley, 2008). Native Alaskans are divided into five cultural and linguistic groups: Interior Indians, Aleuts, Southeast Coastal Indians, Northern Eskimos, and Southern Eskimos (Davidhizar & DeLapp, 2008). For the purposes of this discussion, Native Americans and Native Alaskans are referred to as Native Americans.

The first meeting with Native American clients is considered a time for building rapport and not for carrying out essential work. Native Americans may introduce themselves by stating the clan and the location of their home. They often initially appear silent and reserved; quiet voice tones are usually used when speaking. On initial greeting, they may extend a hand and touch the hand of the other person lightly out of respect, but touch is generally reserved for those people the client knows well. Eye contact is to be avoided, and pointing at another person should not be done because it is considered rude.

Family Influence

Family is very important to Native American clients and includes all members of the extended family. The primary goal of the family is the development of children and adolescents. They follow the concept of *clanship*, in which the nuclear family and extended family are in close relationship (Hanley, 2008). Usually a male member of the family is looked upon as the leader; however, all members of the family may be involved in healthcare decisions. A family member may travel long distances to be with an ill family member. Although men are seen as important, grandmothers and mothers are often at the center of many Native American traditions (Zoucha & Zamarripa, 2003).

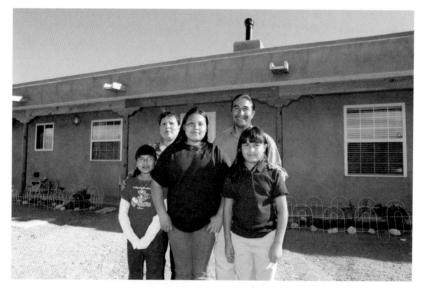

Figure 8-5 The Native American Family

Courtesy of U.S. National Archives and Records Administration.

Elders are a source of cultural information and can provide advice and support to the nurse. The time orientation for many Native Americans is focused on the present, which affects how they perceive future events. This may result in difficulties knowing when to take medications and the importance of being on time for appointments. Many Native Americans believe that the shared space of the *hogan*, or round open room, provides spiritual security and a sense of trust (Hanley, 2008). Some clients may not feel comfortable outside their normal surroundings.

Health Beliefs

Native Americans believe that wellness is a state of harmony with one's surroundings and with families. Illness results from something that the client has done to cause disharmony. When they are ill, they may seek out the services of a medicine man to find out what is causing disharmony. The different types of medicine men and women include diagnosticians, singers, and herbalists. The use of the healing ceremony is used to return to a harmonious state. The *Blessingway ceremony* attempts to remove ill health by means of stories, songs, rituals, prayers, symbols, and sand paintings (Hanley, 2008). They have *jish*, or medicine bundles, containing symbolic and sacred items, such as corn pollen, feathers, stones, arrowheads, and other instruments used for healing and blessing (Hanley, 2008). Pain is considered something that must be endured, and clients may not ask for pain medication. An important cultural belief is that Native Americans should not touch a dead or dying person because they believe that the spirit of the deceased may contaminate them. They also may avoid discussing the topics of death and dying. They blend traditional beliefs with Western health practices.

Implications for Health Education

It is important to remember that Native American beliefs depend on clients' personal experiences and the degree of acculturation into U.S. society. If the client uses folk medicine, it is important for you to determine which cultural health practices are beneficial, neutral, or harmful to provide culturally congruent care. When teaching Native Americans, you should be aware that they are comfortable with extended periods of silence, so allow them adequate time for information processing. You should use straightforward and easily understood language and clarify misconceptions in a direct manner.

Nurse educators should have awareness of serious issues that have affected Native Americans for decades. Native American and Alaska Native communities have struggled with high rates of assault, abduction, and murder of women. Community advocates describe the crisis as a legacy of generations of government policies of forced removal, land seizures, and violence inflicted on Native people (U.S. Department of the Interior Indian Affairs, 2023). The Bureau of Indian Affairs (BIA) estimates that there are 4,200 missing person and murder cases that have gone unsolved, and most are female. The Missing and Murdered Indigenous Women USA (MMIWUSA) organization's mission is to combat the widespread issue of violence against native people (Nelson et al., 2020). They aim to serve Indigenous families in the United States who are affected by violence and poverty.

The troubling trends in violence should be of concern to nurse educators because we know violence perpetuates negative health outcomes. Native Americans are disproportionately impacted by domestic violence, sexual assault, psychological aggression, child abuse, and other forms of neglect, which are all concerns that increase the risk of human trafficking (Nelson et al., 2021). Native American communities across the country are finally beginning to address this problem. Nurse educators can use their caring and expertise to address the needs of Native American communities to help end the epidemic of missing and murdered Indigenous women and girls.

Suggested approaches for nurse educators working with Native Americans follow:

- Nurse educators should receive up-to-date training on prevention, detection, and appropriate treatment for victims of domestic assault and violence.
- Nurse educators should advocate for violence prevention education for Native American families and communities.
- Nurse educators should support and advocate for basic social determinants of health such as safe housing, access to health care, education and job training, and social support within Native American communities.
- In the United States, 574 tribal nations exist, each with their own unique traditions, religious beliefs, languages, and cultures. If the nurse educator is uncertain of a client's cultural beliefs, it is acceptable to ask questions. Native families will not consider you rude if you ask questions. Instead, it demonstrates a healthy recognition of their expertise on their background, values, and experiences. When you are honest about the limits of your knowledge, Native clients are more likely to trust your sincerity in offering respectful and effective care.
- Nurse educators should build a caring nurse–client relationship to gain the client's trust and help them feel physically and emotionally safe. If a client refuses a procedure or treatment, respond with understanding rather than pressuring them into compliance. Treatment options should involve collaboration with the client and their family to develop a teaching plan that prioritizes their spiritual needs and well-being (AORN, 2021).
- Nurse educators should ask older Native clients and their families about their preferences and then build teaching plans around those wishes as much as possible. When their wishes cannot be accommodated, explain why. Do not try to rush patient interactions or interrupt family members. The nurse educator should slow down and listen. You'll create a friendlier rapport and learn more about the patient's cultural practices and expectations. Older Native Americans deserve recognition for their wisdom and experience; they deserve accessible resources and culturally sensitive care (AORN, 2021).
- Provide Native American families, who have missing family members, with information about where to go for help and what needs to be done. The link for the guide entitled *When Your Child Is Missing: A Family Survival Guide* is included here: https://ojjdp.ojp.gov/publications/family-survival-guide.pdf

Additional common health concerns for Native Americans requiring health education are listed in **Table 8-6**.

Table 8-6 Most Common Disorders Requiring Health Education: Native Americans

Ethnic/Racial Group	Most Common Disorders Requiring Health Education
Native American	<ul><li>Heart disease</li><li>Cancer</li><li>Accidents</li><li>Diabetes</li><li>Stroke</li><li>Alcohol abuse</li><li>Hepatitis</li><li>Obesity</li><li>Sudden infant death syndrome (SIDS)</li></ul>

Cross-Cultural Communication

Cross-cultural communication factors must be considered when nurses interact with clients and their family members from cultural backgrounds that differ from their own (Andrews, 2012). To be culturally competent, the nurse as educator needs to examine ways in which people from various cultural backgrounds communicate. Research has shown that communication between healthcare professionals and clients is linked to client satisfaction, adherence to medical instructions, and health outcomes (Stewart et al., 1999). This discussion on cross-cultural communication focuses on verbal and nonverbal communication, focused communication tools, and the use of interpreters. These factors are reviewed for the four major cultural groups: African American, Asian, Hispanic, and Native American.

Verbal Communication

Some African American clients speak in what is called African American English. This dialect, a mixture of English, Creole, and West African languages, is sometimes misinterpreted as uneducated but is actually a way to share unique cultural ideas and symbolize racial pride and identity (Campinha-Bacote, 2003). You may have to seek clarification if words are not understood. The volume of African American voices is sometimes louder than those of other cultures, but this should not be interpreted as anger or aggression.

A hallmark of Asian communication is to think before speaking and to be polite. When working with Asian clients, you may find that they respond with "yes" to a question as a way of being polite or avoiding conflict, even when they do not understand the question (Hoang & Erickson, 1985). Also, some Asian clients may feel uncomfortable about giving and receiving compliments or saying "thank you." Their communication style is based on a cultural tradition that emphasizes self-humility in social situations. An interpreter may be needed to communicate with Asian clients.

For Hispanics in the United States, an inability to speak and understand English can be a serious complication to receiving healthcare services. Most Hispanics speak some English, but many continue to speak Spanish at home with family. Communication may be complicated by the fact that Hispanics often learn a mixture of English and Spanish, which makes it difficult for you to understand. An interpreter may be required to facilitate communication. Hispanic clients expect that nurses will give direct eye contact when interacting with them, but they do not reciprocate with direct eye contact. When looking at or admiring a Hispanic child, it is important to touch the child to avoid giving the child the "evil eye" (Gonzalez et al., 2008).

Communication with Native American clients may require you to use interpreters because many still speak native tribal languages. Another complicating factor when developing client education plans is that many of the native languages do not have equivalent single words in the English language, which makes understanding difficult. Native Americans consider silence essential to understanding and may pause after questions to carefully consider the answer.

Nonverbal Communication

African American clients are generally more comfortable with touch and a close personal space. You will see more demonstrative facial expression and use of animated gestures when talking. Using humor is acceptable with African Americans and can be a way to release feelings and reduce stress. Asian clients often will be serene and stoic, suppressing negative emotion. Asians consider the head sacred, so it is not polite to pat the head (Giger & Davidhizar, 2008). Be aware that the lack of facial expression of Asian clients or a low level of verbal communication may not indicate a lack of emotion or opinion. It is important to determine Asian clients' true feelings or opinions before deciding what they think. Hispanic clients are often tactile in their relationships and show affection for each other. They may appear agreeable on the surface to avoid confrontation, especially during health education. Dramatic body language is used when Hispanic clients describe emotional problems (Gonzalez et al., 2008). If a disagreement develops, Hispanic clients may become silent and not adhere to the client education plan. Native American clients prefer listening to speaking and rarely practice small talk except among close acquaintances. In social situations when they are angry or uncomfortable, Native Americans may remain silent. Often, they will avoid eye contact and may look at the floor while you are talking as a way of showing they are listening intently.

Focused Cultural Assessment Tools

A thorough cultural assessment helps you as the educator to develop a client education plan that, if possible, should be done in advance of the teaching session. Specific assessment tools for an in-depth cultural assessment were described earlier in the chapter and can be selected based on client needs. Often, however, a client presents with a specific problem that needs immediate attention. In this situation, it is important to first assess how the client views current health problems and what care they believe is needed to resolve it. Kleinman (1980) developed the following list of questions that you can use to gain better insight into the client's perception of their illness:

1. What do you call your problem (sickness)? What name does it have?
2. What do you think caused your sickness?
3. Why do you think it started when it did?
4. What does your sickness do to you? How does it work?
5. How severe is it? Do you think it will last a short time or a long time?
6. What do you fear most about your sickness?
7. What are the chief problems that your sickness has caused for you?
8. What kind of treatment do you think you should receive? What are the most important results you hope to receive from the treatment?

When you have an understanding of the client's perception of the health problem, there may be a need to negotiate the plan of care. The *LEARN* model is a framework for creating new health patterns through effective listening, education, and negotiation (Berlin & Fowkes, 1983). When using this framework for health education, you should first attempt to understand, then to be understood, and finally to negotiate a client education plan that fits the client's cultural framework. Negotiation includes a preserve–accommodate–restructure approach (DeRosa & Kochurka, 2006). You should preserve cultural practices that help the client achieve their health goals and accommodate neutral cultural practices that neither help nor hinder the client. *Negotiation* is called for in restructuring harmful cultural practices that might risk or impair the client's health. This approach of honoring cultural values and practices helps the client feel respected and comfortable, and it is more likely that they will adhere to the treatment plan.

L: Listen with sympathy and understanding to the patient's perception of the problem.
E: Explain your perceptions of the problem.
A: Acknowledge and discuss the differences and similarities.
R: Recommend treatment.
N: Negotiate agreement.

Use of Interpreters

Interviewing non-English-speaking clients requires a bilingual interpreter for full communication. This requirement is in line with The Joint Commission standard RI.01.01.03 that states, "The hospital respects the patient's right to receive information in a manner in which he or she understands" (The Joint Commission, 2014). Even a person who has basic English skills may need the services of an interpreter when placed in teaching situations that require give and take. Whenever possible, use a bilingual team member or trained medical interpreter. The interpreter should possess a high level of fluency and a strong sense of ethics. Family members, children, or friends are not good choices for interpreting. Using them violates confidentiality, plus they are not trained to understand medical terminology. A professional interpreter has the special skills needed to fully understand what the nurse and client want to say and to make messages clear in two languages. In addition, a qualified interpreter knows the role, limitations, and responsibilities of an interpreter.

If possible, the interpreter should meet the client ahead of time to build rapport. Arrangements should be made in advance because the teaching session will take more time. Prepare ahead of time and focus on the major teaching points and prioritize information. During the session, the nurse, client, and interpreter should sit so they form the points of a triangle. The nurse should look at the client when speaking. Two different interpretive styles are possible in the teaching session: line by line and summarization. The line-by-line approach ensures accuracy but takes more time. Information needs to be presented on a concrete level because abstract conceptualizations do not readily translate and may confuse the client (Putch, 1985). The nurse must choose words carefully and use gestures sparingly. A normal tone of voice should be used, not too fast or too loud. The nurse and client should say only a sentence or two so the interpreter will have time to interpret. Simple language, without medical jargon, should be used. Summary translation is faster and works well when teaching simple procedures with which the translator is already familiar. The interpreter summarizes the points that the nurse wants to teach. The interpreter and the nurse observe the nonverbal messages throughout the teaching session. At the end, it is important to ask the client to confirm understanding of what was taught.

The use of on-site medical interpreters or translators is only one way that language access services may be available to nurses. There are also telephone interpreter services, video medical interpreting services, translation software for written materials, bilingual clinical staff, and language classes for staff.

Linguistically and Culturally Appropriate Teaching Strategies and Instructional Materials

Linguistic competence is the capacity of an organization and its personnel to communicate effectively and convey information in a manner that is easily understood by diverse audiences, including persons with limited English proficiency, those who are not literate or have low health literacy skills, and individuals with disabilities (Goode & Jones, 2006). To address cultural linguistic competence, the *National Standards on Culturally and Linguistically Appropriate Services Standards (CLAS)* were developed by the U.S. Department of Health and Human Services Office of Minority Health (2001) to ensure that all people entering the healthcare system receive equitable and effective treatment in a culturally and linguistically appropriate manner. Standard 6 mandates that healthcare organizations must provide competent language assistance from interpreters and bilingual staff to clients with limited English proficiency. The standards are intended to be inclusive of all cultures, not limited to any particular population group. They are designed to address the needs of racial, ethnic, and linguistic population groups that experience unequal access to health-care services. These standards serve as guidelines for nurses and can be accessed online through the Office of Minority Health.

The Patient Protection and Affordable Care Act (2010), Title V, defines health literacy as "the degree to which an individual has the capacity to obtain, communicate, process, and understand basic health information and services to make appropriate health decisions." This is similar to the definition provided by Healthy People 2010 (2009). Research shows that health literacy is the single best predictor of client health status (Campinha-Bacote, 2008). Low health literacy affects older people, immigrants, people experiencing poverty, and ethnic minority populations. It is often brought about by inadequate communication between clients and nurses. Clients frequently attempt to hide their inability to read, and the nurse cannot judge literacy level solely by a client's years of education. Clients with low reading ability and comprehension skills may not be able to express what is not understood and therefore may choose to conceal their low literacy skills (Maurer & Smith, 2004). Ways to assist clients with low health literacy include limiting the amount of medical jargon, using pictures or models to explain important health concepts, assuring understanding with demonstration techniques, and encouraging clients to ask questions. Goode, Brown, Mason, and Sockalingam (2006) identified six principles to create culturally competent health materials that should be considered when choosing, adapting, or creating health-promoting instructional aids:

1. Acknowledge the unique issues of biculturalism and bilingual status of both healthcare providers and service populations.
2. Incorporate client preferences in choosing instructional materials. Health messages should demonstrate respect for client uniqueness and cultural differences.
3. Involve members of the target population in the creation of instructional materials.
4. Use the family as the focal point of intervention when developing health messages.
5. Base health education and promotion on cultural aspects of epidemiology (concepts of causation and cure).
6. Education and promotion should exist in concert with natural and informal healthcare and support systems within the community.

Culturally appropriate teaching strategies and instructional materials are necessary when the client's culture dictates how a problem should be addressed. These teaching strategies and instructional materials include the following:

- Use a variety of teaching strategies and instructional materials that are specific to the culture and language. This includes written materials (posters, brochures, etc.), short films, computer-assisted instruction, group teaching, and websites.
- Consider clients' cultures and language skills when developing learning objectives, teaching strategies, and instructional materials.
- Facilitate comparable learning opportunities for clients with differing characteristics and learning styles. For example, consider learning opportunities for clients who differ in race, sex, disability, ethnicity, religion, socioeconomic status, and ability.
- Incorporate learning objectives for personal development based on cultural beliefs, and clearly communicate the learning objectives.
- Use concrete terms, choose words that do not have multiple meanings, and avoid medical jargon and slang.

- Give clients an overview of the client education plan and tell them about the learning objectives. Relate the plan to previous learning, and summarize the main points.
- Provide frequent review of the content learned.
- Facilitate independence in thinking and action by helping clients find answers themselves.
- Promote on-task behavior by keeping clients actively involved.
- Check with clients during the teaching session to see if they have any questions about what they are doing and if they understand the content.
- Provide frequent feedback and reinforcement.

DeRosa and Kochurka (2006) developed a six-step approach to providing culturally competent care, which we have adapted for nurses to provide culturally congruent health education.

Summary

This chapter looked at the importance of cultural competence for nurses who provide health education. Changing demographics and disparities in health care are powerful reasons that require nurses to become culturally competent. Becoming culturally competent is a developmental process and involves self-awareness and insight into the workings of other cultures. To provide meaningful health education, it is important for nurses to adapt the Stoeckel Culturally Congruent Client Education Model, which looks at culturally based actions, their rationales, and outcomes.

Exercises
Exercise I: Health Beliefs and Home Remedies

Purpose: Examine the health beliefs of various cultural, ethnic, and racial groups.
Directions:

1. Divide into small groups composed of individuals who are most culturally, ethnically, and racially alike.
2. Discuss how your parents and grandparents (a) defined good health and poor health, and (b) list the home remedies they used to treat individuals in poor health.
3. Share your findings with the entire class. How were your findings similar and dissimilar?
4. What did you learn about individuals who are supposedly alike?

Exercise II: Health Beliefs and Home Remedies

Purpose: Examine the health beliefs of various cultural, ethnic, and racial groups.
Directions:

1. Divide into small groups composed of individuals who are most culturally, ethnically, and racially dissimilar.
2. Compare and contrast the findings discovered in Exercise I. How were the beliefs about good health and poor health alike and different?
3. Compare and contrast the various home remedies identified in Exercise I. How were the home remedies across the cultural, ethnic, and racial groups alike and different?
4. Share your findings with the entire class.

Exercise III: Cultural Reflection

Purpose: Reflect on the health education needs of various cultural, ethnic, and racial groups.
Directions:

1. Individually reflect on the new knowledge you gained from participating in Exercises I and II. What are the implications for health education? How will this impact you in your role as an educator? Take about 15 minutes for reflection.
2. As a group, share your thoughts and conclusions with others in your class. Did others have similar thoughts and conclusions?
3. Using the Campinha-Bacote mnemonic, ASKED, described in this chapter, discuss how this exercise made you more culturally competent.

Exercise IV: Evidenced-Based Nursing Practice

Purpose: Apply evidence-based nursing research to client education.
Directions:

1. Search the literature for nursing research applicable to health education for the client whose racial/ethnic background differs from yours.
2. Describe how the findings could be applied in your practice to educating clients.

References

Agency for Healthcare Research and Quality. (2019). *2019 National healthcare quality and disparities report*. Retrieved from https://www.ahrq.gov/research/findings/nhqrdr/nhqdr19/index.html

American Medical Association. (1999). State-specific maternal mortality among black and white women: United States, 1987-1996. *The Journal of the American Medical Association*, 282(13), 1220–1222.

American Nurses Association. (2001). *Code for nurses*. Washington, DC: Author.

Anderson, L. M., Scrimshaw, S. C., Fullilove, M. T., Fielding, J. E., & Normand, J. (2003). Task Force on Community Preventive Services. Culturally competent healthcare systems: A systematic review [Suppl. 1]. *American Journal of Preventive Medicine*, 24(3), 68–79.

Andrews, M. M. (2012). Culturally competent nursing care. In M. M. Andrews & J. S. Boyle (Eds.), *Transcultural concepts in nursing care* (6th ed., pp. viii–xiii). Philadelphia, PA: Wolters Kluwer/Lippincott Williams & Wilkins.

Andrews, M. M., & Boyle, J. S. (2012). Andrews/Boyle transcultural nursing assessment guide for individuals and families. In M. M. Andrews & J. S. Boyle (Eds.), *Transcultural concepts in nursing care* (6th ed., pp. 451–455). Philadelphia, PA: Wolters Kluwer/Lippincott Williams & Wilkins.

Anft, Michael. (2017). Hispanic men often put off medical care, bringing bigger trouble. *Health News*, NPR. Retrieved from https://www.npr.org/sections/health-shots/2017/04/22/525076404/hispanic-men-often-put-off-medical-care-bringing-bigger-trouble

AORN Staff. (2021). Native American patients: 6 considerations for culturally sensitive care. AORN. Accessed https://www.aorn.org/article/2021-12-03-Considerations-for-Culturally-Sensitive-Care

Ariel Gelrud Shiro, A. G., & Reeves, R. V. (2023). Latinos often lack access to healthcare and have poor health outcomes. Here's how we can change that. *The Brookings Institute*. Retrieved from https://www.brookings.edu/articles/latinos-often-lack-access-to-healthcare-and-have-poor-health-outcomes-heres-how-we-can-change-that/

Beach, M. C., Price, E. G., Gary, T. L., Robinson, K. A., Gozu, A., Palacio, A., Smarth, C., Jenckes, M. W., Feuerstein, C., Bass, E. B., Powe, N. R., & Cooper, L. A. (2005a). Cultural competence: a systematic review of health care provider educational interventions. *Medical care*, 43(4), 356–373. https://doi.org/10.1097/01.mlr.0000156861.58905.96

Beach, M. T., Sugarman, J., Johnson, R., Arbelaez, J. J., Duggan, P. S., & Cooper, L. A. (2005b). Higher satisfaction, adherence, and receipt of preventive care? *Annals of Family Medicine*, 3(4), 331–338.

Berlin, E. A., & Fowkes, W. C., Jr. (1983). A teaching framework for cross-cultural health care. *Western Journal of Medicine*, 139, 934–938.

Esposito C. L. (2013). Provision of culturally competent health care: an interim status review and report. *The Journal of the New York State Nurses' Association*, 43(2), 4–10. PMID: 25109038.

Brach, C., & Fraser, I. (2000). Can cultural competency reduce racial and ethnic disparities? A review and conceptual model. *Medical Care Research and Review*, *57*(1), 181–217.

Burchum, J. L. R. (2002). Cultural competence: An evolutionary perspective. *Nursing Forum*, *37*(4), 5–15.

Campinha-Bacote, J. (1998). *The process of cultural competence in the delivery of healthcare services: A culturally competent model of care* (3rd ed.). Cincinnati, OH: Transcultural C.A.R.E. Associates.

Campinha-Bacote, J. (2002). The process of cultural competence in the delivery of healthcare services: A model of care. *Journal of Transcultural Nursing*, *13*(3), 181–184.

Campinha-Bacote, J. (2003). Many faces: Addressing diversity in health care. *Online Journal of Issues in Nursing*, *8*(1), Manuscript 2.

Campinha-Bacote, J. (2008). People of African American heritage. In L. D. Purnell & B. J. Paulanka (Eds.), *Transcultural health care* (3rd ed., pp. 56–74). Philadelphia, PA: F. A. Davis.

Campinha-Bacote, J., & Narayan, M. (2000). Culturally competent health care in the home. *Home Care Provider*, *5*(6), 213–219.

Centers for Disease Control and Prevention. (2023). Working together to reduce Black maternal mortality. Accessed at https://stacks.cdc.gov/view/cdc/127833

Cherry, B., & Giger, J. N. (2008). African-Americans. In J. N. Giger & R. E. Davidhizar (Eds.), *Trans-cultural nursing: Assessment and intervention* (5th ed., pp. 190–238). St. Louis, MO: Mosby Elsevier.

Cross, T., Bazron, B., Dennis, K., & Isaacs, M. (1989). *Towards a culturally competent system of care: A monograph on effective services for minority children who are severely emotionally disturbed: Volume I*. Washington, DC: Georgetown University Child Development Center.

Culhane-Pera, K. A., Reif, C., Egli, E., Bake, N. J., & Kassekert, R. (1997). A curriculum for multicultural education in family medicine. *Family Medicine*, *29*(10), 719–723.

Daniel-Ulloa, J., Reyes, J. A., Morales-Campos, D. Y., Villareal, E., López Cevallos, D. F., Hernandez, H., & Baquero, B. (2023). Rural Latino men's experiences and attitudes toward health: A pilot photovoice study. *American Journal of Men's Health*, *17*(2), 15579883231158525. https://doi.org/10.1177/15579883231158525

Davidhizar, R. E., & DeLapp, T. D. (2008). American Eskimos: The Yup'ik and Inupiat. In J. N. Giger & R. E. Davidhizar (Eds.), *Transcultural nursing: Assessment and intervention* (5th ed., pp. 323–356). St. Louis, MO: Mosby Elsevier.

Department of Health and Human Services. Office of Minority Health. (2021). *Hispanic/Latino health*. Retrieved from http://minorityhealth.hhs.gov/omh/browse.aspx?lvl=3&rlvlid=64

DeRosa, N., & Kochurka, K. (2006). Implement culturally competent healthcare in your workplace. *Nursing Management*, *37*(10), 18–26.

Falvo, D. R. (2011). *Effective patient education: A guide to increased adherence* (4th ed.). Sudbury, MA: Jones & Bartlett Learning.

Giger, J. N., & Davidhizar, R. E. (2008). *Transcultural nursing: Assessment and intervention* (4th ed.). St. Louis, MO: Mosby Elsevier.

Gonzalez, E. W., Owen, D. C., & Esperat, C. R. (2008). Mexican Americans. In J. N. Giger & R. E. Davidhizar (Eds.), *Transcultural nursing: Assessment and intervention* (5th ed., pp. 239–275). St. Louis, MO: Mosby Elsevier.

Goode, T., Brown, M., Mason, J., & Sockalingam, S. (2006). *A guide for using the cultural and linguistic competence policy assessment instrument*. Washington, DC: National Center for Cultural Competence, Georgetown University Center for Child and Human Development. Retrieved from http://www.clcpa.info

Goode, T., & Jones, W. (2006). *Definition of linguistic competence*. Washington, DC: National Center for Cultural Competence, Georgetown University Center for Child and Human Development.

Hanley, C. E. (2008). Navajos. In J. N. Giger & R. E. Davidhizar (Eds.), *Transcultural nursing: Assessment and intervention* (5th ed., pp. 276–299). St. Louis, MO: Mosby Elsevier.

Harvard Medical School. (2009). *Culturally competent care online resource center*. Retrieved from https://www.hms.harvard.edu/cccec/about/index.htm

Healthy People 2010. (2009). *Health communications. (Definition of health literacy.)* Retrieved from http://www.healthypeople.gov/document/html/volume1/11healthcom.htm#_Toc490471359

Healthy People 2020. (2016). *Social determinants of health*. Retrieved from https://www.healthypeople.gov/2020/topics-objectives/topic/social-determinants-of-health

Heiman, H. J., & Artiga, S. (2015). *Beyond health care: The role of social determinants in promoting health and health equity*. The Henry J. Kaiser Family Foundation. Retrieved from http://www.census.gov/newsroom/releases/archives/population/cb12-243.html

Hoang, G. N., & Erickson, R. V. (1985). Cultural barriers to effective medical care among Indochinese patients. *Annual Review of Medicine*, *36*(2), 229–239.

Hook, J., Davis, D., Owen, J., Worthington, E., & Utsey, S. (2013). Cultural humility: Measuring openness to culturally diverse clients. *Journal of Counseling and Psychology*, *60*(3), 353–366.

Institute of Medicine. (2002). *Unequal treatment: Confronting racial and ethnic disparities in health care*. Washington, DC: National Academies Press.

Iwamasa, G.Y. (2012). Recommendations for the treatment of Asian-American/Pacific Islander populations. *Psychological Treatment of Ethnic Minority Populations* produced by the Council of National Psychological Associations for the Advancement of Ethnic Minority Issues. Retrieved from https://www.apa.org/pi/oema/resources/ethnicity-health/asian-american/psychological-treatment

Juckett G. (2013). Caring for Latino patients. *American Family Physician*, *87*(1), 48–54.

Juckett, G., Nguyen, C., & Shahbodaghi, S. D. (2014). Caring for Asian immigrants: Tips on culture that can enhance patient care. *The Journal of Family Practice*, *63*(1), E1–E9 https://pubmed.ncbi.nlm.nih.gov/24475470/.

Kaiser Family Foundation. (2001). *Generation Rx.com: How young people use the Internet for health information.* Retrieved from http://www.kff.org/entmedia/20011211a-index.cfm

Kim, J., & Tummala-Narra, P. (2022). Rise of anti-Asian violence and the COVID-19 pandemic for Asian Americans. *Asian American Journal of Psychology*, *13*(3), 217–219. https://doi.org/10.1037/aap0000301

King, M. (2014). The importance of cultural diversity in healthcare. *UVM Out Reach*. Retrieved from https://www.uvm.edu/publichealth/cultural-diversity-in-healthcare/

Kleinman, A. (1980). *Patients and healers in the context of culture.* Berkeley, CA: University of California Press.

Lee, J. H. (2021). Combating anti-Asian sentiment—A practical guide for clinicians. *The New England Journal of Medicine*, *384*, 2367–9. doi:10.1056/NEJMp2102656. http://www.ncbi.nlm.nih.gov/pubmed/33761204

Leininger, M. (1991). *Culture care diversity and universality: A theory of nursing.* New York, NY: National League for Nursing.

Maurer, F., & Smith, C. (2004). *Community/public health nursing practice: Health for families and populations.* St. Louis, MO: Elsevier Health Sciences.

Nelson, K., Brockie, T., & Him, D. A. (2020). What nurses need to know: Missing and murdered indigenous women and girls. *Johns Hopkins Nursing Magazine*. Retrieved from https://magazine.nursing.jhu.edu/2020/11/what-nurses-need-to-know-missing-and-murdered-indigenous-women-and-girls/#:~:text=As

Patient Protection and Affordable Care Act. (2010). *One Hundred Eleventh Congress of the United States of America at the Second Session Begun and held at the City of Washington on Tuesday, January 5, 2010.* Retrieved from http://www.gpo.gov/fdsys/pkg/BILLS-111hr3590enr/pdf/BILLS-111hr3590enr.pdf

Peters-Mosquera, A., Bingham-Hendricks, C., Woods, C., & Aronowitz, T. (2023). The role nurses can play in addressing and preventing the prevalence of missing or murdered indigenous women and girls (MMIWG). *Journal of Transcultural Nursing: Official Journal of the Transcultural Nursing Society*, 10436596231198274. Advance online publication. https://doi.org/10.1177/10436596231198274

Purnell, L. D. (2013). *Transcultural health care: A culturally competent approach* (4th ed.). Philadelphia, PA: F. A. Davis.

Putch, R. W. (1985). Cross-cultural communication: The special case of interpreters in health care. *Journal of the American Medical Association*, *254*(23), 3344–3348.

Schim, S. M., Doorenbos, A., Benkert, R., & Miller, J. (2007). Culturally congruent care: Putting the puzzle together. *Journal of Transcultural Nursing*, *18*(2), 103–110.

Smith, W. R., Betancourt, J. R., Wynia, M. K., Bussey-Jones, J., Stone, V. E., Phillips, C. O., Fernandez, A., Jacobs, E., & Bowles, J. (2007). Recommendations for teaching about racial and ethnic disparities in health and health care. *Annals of Internal Medicine*, *147*(9), 654–665.

Stewart, M., Brown, J. B., Boon, H., Galajda, J., Meredith, L., & Sangster, M. (1999). Evidence on patient–doctor communication. *Cancer Prevention and Control*, *3*(1), 25–30.

Tervalon, M., & Murray-Garcia, J. (1998). Cultural humility versus cultural competence: A critical distinction in defining physician training outcomes in multicultural education. *Journal of Health Care for the Poor and Underserved*, *9*, 117–125.

The Joint Commission. (2014). *Hospitals (CAMH).* Retrieved from https://www.jointcommission.org/standards/

U.S. Census Bureau. (2012). *U.S. Census Bureau projections show a slower growing, older, more diverse nation a half century from now.* Retrieved from http://www.census.gov/newsroom/releases/archives/population/cb12-243.html

U.S. Department of Health and Human Services. (2010). *Healthy People 2020.* Washington, DC: Author

U.S. Department of the Interior Indian Affairs. (2023). Missing and murdered indigenous people crisis violence against Native Americans and Alaska Natives far exceed national averages. Retrieved from https://www.bia.gov/service/mmu/missing-and-murdered-indigenous-people-crisis

U.S. Department of Justice Office of Justice Programs Office of Juvenile Justice and Delinquency Prevention. (2023). *When your child is missing: A family survival guide* (5th ed.). Accessed at https://ojjdp.ojp.gov/publications/family-survival-guide.pdf

Weaver, H. N. (1999). Transcultural nursing with Native Americans: Critical knowledge, skills, and attitudes. *Journal of Transcultural Nursing*, *10*(3):197–202. https://doi.org/10.1177/104365969901000310

Yee, B., Mokuau, N., & Kim, S. (Eds.). (1999). *Developing cultural competence in Asian and Pacific Islander communities: Opportunities in primary health care and substance abuse prevention* (Publication No. SMA 98-3193). Washington, DC: U.S. Department of Health and Human Services.

Zoucha, R., & Zamarripa, C. A. (2003). People of Mexican heritage. In L. D. Purnell & B. J. Paulanka (Eds.), *Transcultural health care* (3rd ed., pp. 309–324). Philadelphia, PA: F. A. Davis.

CHAPTER 9

Nurse Educator as Learner

OBJECTIVES

Upon completion of this chapter, you will be able to do the following:

- Describe the continuum of learning for nurse educators.
- Review the role of the nurse as educator in the Miller–Stoeckel Client Education Model.
- Review the advanced role of nurse educators.
- Discuss nurse educators in the academic environment.
- Discuss nurse educators in the practice environment.
- Examine how nurses learn to become effective educators.
- Examine the role of nurse educators as lifelong learners.
- Describe self-care coping strategies when dealing with physical, social, mental, spiritual, and emotional stressors.

CHAPTER OUTLINE

Introduction

This chapter focuses on the nurse as educator in the Miller–Stoeckel Client Education Model. The nurse educator is first and foremost a registered nurse who initiates and applies the concepts of the model. It is through the embedded concepts of cultural caring, communication, negotiation, and collaboration that the nurse–client relationship is established. The relationship evolves through integration of the nursing process, the teaching and learning process, clinical judgment, and evidence-based nursing practice. The nurse educator is also responsible for the client formative and summative education outcomes.

Entering the healthcare field as a member of the interprofessional team is the first step on the continuum of learning. New learning occurs, and awareness develops, as the nurse sees the scope of the role and responsibilities and how to best fulfill them in service of their clients. It is this growth through time that this chapter addresses. At some point, the nurse may desire further education, whether formal or informal. The nurse may want to experience different practice settings, whether in clinical specialties or academia. How the nurse takes on advanced roles is important. This chapter addresses the process of becoming an effective educator, the importance of lifelong learning, and self-care for nurse educators.

Overview of the Continuum of Learning

This overview presents a holistic picture of how the nurse educator learns. The nurse learns on a continuum that begins with the nurse's basic educational program. Teaching and learning principles are part of the general nursing curriculum, and student nurses are expected to learn how to teach clients as part of their clinical experience.

The next step along the continuum is to practice client teaching in the workplace. The workplace is a learning environment (Skar, 2010). It is where the nurse first experiences the give and take of teaching clients in different settings such as at the bedside, or in the community. The expectation is that the nurse will gain the skills and knowledge to meet clients' health education needs.

It is also in the workplace that the nurse recognizes that teaching clients involves an interprofessional collaboration. Interprofessional client education refers to the teaching and learning of clients by different professions working together as part of a practice team. Physicians, pharmacists, and others collaborate with the nurse in developing teaching plans for clients.

The nurse may find that they enjoy a specialty area and receives personal satisfaction from providing client education. This may come as a result of successful experiences in teaching or perhaps from taking a role in clinical teaching. The decision to become a nurse educator beyond the expected role usually involves achieving an advance degree or certification.

Upon completing advanced degrees, options for teaching positions increase. The nurse now enters a new learning environment in either the practice area or academic setting. The academic world of teaching is different from the hospital-based acute care environment. With the choice of these options, the nurse educator learns new skills.

The continuum of learning proceeds by the nurse educator participating in formal and informal continuing education as a part of lifelong learning. The experienced nurse educator in all settings passes on skills to the next generation of nurses as part of succession planning. Specific points along this continuum are discussed in the rest of this chapter. See **Figure 9-1**.

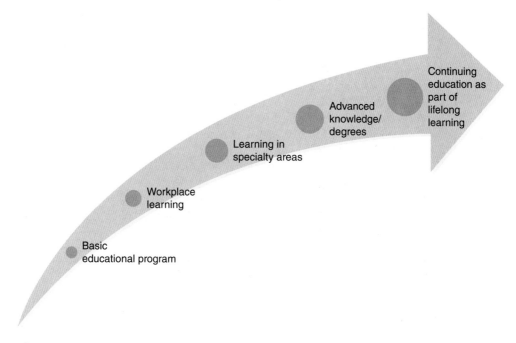

Figure 9-1 Continuum of Learning for Nurse Educators

Role of the Nurse as Educator

All nurses must maintain basic competency for educating patients and families as their professional obligation and responsibility to performing the core functions of nursing. According to the American Nurses Association (ANA) *Nursing: Scope and Standards of Practice,* Standard 5B: Health Teaching and Health Promotion states in part that "The registered nurse employs strategies to promote health and a safe environment" (ANA, 2010). By your licensure as a professional nurse, you are obligated to these standards. The nurse, "Promotes health teaching that addresses such topics as healthy lifestyles, risk-reducing behaviors, developmental needs, activities of daily living and preventive self-care" (ANA, 2010, p. 41).

The nurse "Uses health promotion and health teaching methods appropriate to the situation and the healthcare consumer's values, beliefs, health practices, developmental level, learning needs, readiness and ability to learn, language preference, spirituality, culture and socioeconomic status" (ANA, 2010, p. 41). The bedside nurse is with the patient more than any other discipline and plays the critical role in observing, detecting, advocating, and ensuring patients receive high-quality care (Agency for Healthcare Research and Quality [AHRQ], 2015, para. 1). **Figure 9-2** shows nurse educators.

Application of the Miller–Stoeckel Client Education Model

The Miller–Stoeckel Client Education Model encompasses the core competencies of teaching clients established by the ANA. The skills of communication, collaboration, cultural caring, and negotiation develop along with skill in clinical practice as novice nurses gain experience. Teaching

Figure 9-2 Nurse Educators Serve in a Variety of Health Care Settings When Teaching Individuals, Families, Groups and Communities, and Health Team Members

© Monkey Business Images/Shutterstock

clients requires clear verbal and nonverbal communication and collaboration with interprofessional team members. The concept of cultural caring joins client-centered care with awareness of the cultural context of clients.

Providing cultural care means basing teaching and learning on the totality of beliefs and practices of a group of people to incorporate a population health approach to client education (Kaprielian et al., 2013). This means addressing not only race, religion, and ethnicity but also the basic beliefs and practices of culture. It is within each nurse–client encounter that nurse educators strive to accurately assess clients' information and negotiate mutually acceptable and culturally relevant goals and plans.

The skill of negotiation means to acknowledge that it may be beneficial to include selected aspects of the client's culture when teaching and to strive to find mutually acceptable options to problems. It is through this process that the nurse confronts cross-cultural conflict that requires negotiation. The desired outcome is that the client feels valued, respected, and supported (Campinha-Bacote, 2011).

Workplace Learning

The nurse with basic preparation may gain advanced clinical training in the workplace. Nurses provide health education to clients in areas that have evolved as "specialties" through personal experience or certification in areas such as medical surgical, community health, cardiac rehabilitation, and pediatrics. Certification is the formal process by which a certifying agency such as the American Nurses Credentialing Center (ANCC, 2017) validates a nurse's knowledge, skills, and abilities in a defined role and clinical area of practice based on predetermined standards. Nurses achieve certification through specialized education, a specific level of experience in a specialty area, and a qualifying exam. Benefits of certification include professional recognition and creditability, and certification may provide a means of career advancement and promotion in the workplace.

Levels of Proficiency in Teaching

We believe there are levels of proficiency in teaching that nurse educators experience along the continuum of learning. The levels assume that nurses learn in their nursing programs the importance of the teaching role and the basic components of a client education plan. The levels of proficiency in teaching advance as the nurse gains experience. **Table 9-1** shows the advancement in teaching proficiency from novice to expert, adapted based on Benner's Model of Clinical Proficiency (Benner, 1982).

In today's dynamic healthcare environment, with its constant changes and new initiatives, nurses and healthcare team members often get lost in the shuffle of competing responsibilities. Nurses must remember their essential role as educator. Common barriers that keep nurses from teaching clients include the perception of lack of time, lack of knowledge about how to teach, and

Table 9-1 Levels of Proficiency in Teaching

Novice	▪ No experience teaching clients ▪ Follows rules and guidelines and provides client teaching using standardized teaching plans ▪ Provides teaching without individualization ▪ Needs supervision and assistance
Advanced Beginner	▪ Has some experience teaching clients ▪ Uses rules and guidelines, but there are new contextual insights about the teaching situation ▪ Operates on general guidelines and is beginning to perceive recurrent meaningful patterns while teaching clients ▪ Needs role models and mentors
Competent	▪ Has 2 to 3 years of experience teaching clients ▪ Perceives the long-range teaching goals for the client but has limited ability to individualize standardized teaching plans ▪ Has a feeling of growing mastery and the ability to address clients' learning needs ▪ Benefits from in-service education
Proficient	▪ Continued experience teaching clients ▪ Perceives the teaching situation as a "whole" and recognizes expected outcomes ▪ Recognizes events and modifies plans in response to the events based on a deeper understanding of what is more or less important to the situation ▪ Further learning gained through case studies
Expert	▪ Extensive clinical experience teaching clients ▪ No longer uses rules or guidelines but relies on an "intuitive grasp" of the situation and can focus on teaching needs without wasting time on unimportant variables. ▪ Has advanced clinical analytical skills that guides teaching ▪ Shares knowledge of goals and possible outcomes of client teaching that expand the scope of practice.

Data from Benner, P. (1982). From novice to expert. *American Journal of Nursing, 82*(3), 402–407.

lack of investing effort into client education (Carpenter & Bell, 2002). Efforts should be made to overcome these barriers.

Advanced Role of Nurse as Educator

Finding your niche in the healthcare system may be a motivator to acquire advanced education. Nurses choose a teaching career based on their knowledge of specialty areas. This section reviews things to consider when choosing a full-time teaching position.

Teaching is a rich and rewarding career path for nurses looking to share their clinical expertise with those entering nursing or advancing. One of the strongest motivators to teach is that it provides an opportunity to influence student and staff success and shape the next generation of nurses. Nurse educators typically express a high degree of satisfaction with their work. Benefits include access to cutting-edge knowledge and research, opportunities to collaborate with health professionals, and an intellectually stimulating workplace with a flexible work environment. Educators model professional values and skills and ultimately influence the quality of care provided by nurses (Penn, Wilson, & Rosseter, 2008.)

There is a shortage of nurse educators in academia in the United States. It is particularly important to address these issues as the shortage of nurse faculty limits the nation's ability to produce more nurses (National Council of State Boards of Nursing [NCSBN], 2006/2007; National League for Nursing [NLN], 2014; Yordy, 2006). The shortage of nurse educators may actually enhance the career horizon for new recruits since it affords a high level of job security and opportunities to advance quickly up the career ladder. Reasons for the shortage include:

- Recruitment challenges
- Difficulties in attracting and retaining qualified nurse faculty
- Challenges in achieving demographic diversity within nursing faculty
- A lack of awareness on the part of the public and among nurses that the faculty role is a viable career objective
- Problems in providing adequate nurse educational preparation specific to teaching
- Obstacles to sustaining and funding nurse faculty programs
- The aging and imminent retirement of current nurse faculty

The self-assessment in **Table 9-2** is offered to determine if the role of nurse educator beyond the role at the bedside is a good fit for you. These personal attributes are supported by research as a way to determine your aptitude for the role (Penn et al., 2008).

Nurse Educators in the Academic Environment

Nurses may continue their education and practice as faculty in colleges, universities, hospital-based schools of nursing, technical schools, or as staff development educators in the practice setting. In the academic setting, nurses work with recent high school graduates studying nursing for the first time, students entering nursing with other degrees, nurses pursuing advanced degrees, and practicing nurses interested in expanding their knowledge and skills.

Academic title or rank of full-time faculty is determined by the "track" to which one is appointed and the criteria for a specific track. Tenure is described as a permanent job contract within the academic institution. Faculty may be appointed to tenure versus nontenure track and part-time versus full-time positions (Penn et al., 2008). Titles range from adjunct, part-time clinical

Table 9-2 **Am I a Good Fit for the Advanced Role of Nurse Educator?**

Personal Attribute	Yes	No
Strong interpersonal communication skills		
Love of teaching		
Intellectual curiosity		
Works collegially with others		
Enjoys teaching others		
Has an approachable attitude		
Is flexible and adaptable		
Sense of humor		
Enjoys being independent		
Wants to be creative and innovative		
Genuine interest in helping learners		
Strong clinical skills		
Skillful listener		

faculty to deans of nursing. Other rank positions include nursing instructor, assistant professor, associate professor, and professor.

Educational Preparation

At a minimum, nurse educators who work in academic settings, at both community college and senior colleges and universities, must hold a master's degree in nursing and should have additional training in the science of teaching (NCSBN, 2006/2007). Graduate education in nursing programs is generally the expected preparation for full-time faculty roles. Faculty are expected to have advanced expertise in the areas of content they teach (AACN, 2008). In many schools, faculty are expected to teach at multiple levels so that additional educational preparation and clinical experience results in greater versatility.

When choosing to pursue graduate education in nursing, it is important to select a college or university that is accredited. Three agencies accredit nursing programs: Commission on Collegiate Nursing Education (CCNE), the National League for Nursing Commission for Nursing Education Accreditation (NLNCNEA), and the Accreditation Commission for Education in Nursing (ACEN). Each organization maintains a list of accredited programs that can be accessed online. Accreditation ensures that quality standards have been met.

Funding graduate education can be accomplished through the Nurses Higher Education and Loan Repayment Act of 2008, which provides graduate student loan reimbursement, and the Nurse Education Expansion and Development Act, which provides capitation grants to schools of nursing to recruit more faculty (Bartels, 2005). Many federal and private sources of funding exist to assist students looking to pursue graduate nursing education. The Nurse Reinvestment Act includes a student loan repayment program for nurses who agree to serve in faculty roles after graduation (Nursing World, 2002). Similar programs also are available through the National Health Service Corps and the Bureau of Health Professions.

The American Association of Colleges of Nursing (AACN, 2008) supports the achievement of the doctoral degree as the preferred preparation for nurse educators, mirroring the expectations of other disciplines in higher education. In order to be promoted to the upper academic ranks and be granted tenure, the academic faculty typically must hold an earned doctoral degree.

Role and Responsibilities

Academic positions offered by large academic health centers are different from those offered by smaller teaching and service-oriented institutions. The school's mission influences the expectations regarding the scope of the educator role and faculty responsibilities. The following lists the responsibilities of academic nurse educators:

- Facilitate learning
- Facilitate learner development and socialization
- Use assessment evaluation strategies
- Participate in curriculum design and evaluation of program outcomes
- Prepare class and clinical experiences
- Advise and mentor students
- Grade student assignments
- Serve on committees for nursing school and college/university
- Attend faculty meetings
- Engage in scholarly work such as writing/publishing/research
- Write grant proposals and secure extramural funding
- Participate in professional organizations, including seeking elected positions
- Present at conferences
- Maintain certification and/or clinical competence
- Engage in peer review
- Serve as an advisor to student groups
- Participate in community service and volunteer work

(Halstead, 2007; Penn et al., 2008)

Philosophy of Teaching and Learning

Green (1973), an educational philosopher, encouraged educators to take a closer look at what they do when they teach and how they teach. Palmer (2007) spoke of the importance of knowing and connecting with learners. These admonishments form the basis for a teaching philosophy. A teaching philosophy is a self-reflective statement of beliefs about teaching and learning. It discusses how you put your beliefs into practice and has several purposes:

- It concisely gathers your beliefs so you can articulate them to clients, students, peers, and employers.
- It is part of a teaching portfolio.
- It demonstrates professional growth as an educator.

The following is a template for a teaching and learning philosophy statement adapted from Chism (1998):

1. Definition of learning. Ask yourself "What is meant by learning?" and "What happens in a learning situation?" Describe what you think occurs during a learning episode based on your observation and experience and based on current literature on teaching and learning.
2. Conceptualization of teaching. Ask yourself "What is meant by teaching?" and "How do I facilitate this process as a teacher?" Describe a teacher with respect to motivating and facilitating learning. Address such issues as how to challenge students intellectually and support them academically and how to respond to different learning styles, help students who are frustrated, and accommodate different abilities.
3. Goals for students. Ask yourself "What skills do I expect my students to obtain as the result of learning?" Address such issues as class goals, rationale behind them, activities to implement the goals in class, and changes in the goals over time.
4. Implementation of the philosophy. Ask yourself "How do I operationalize my philosophy of teaching in the classroom?" and "What personal characteristics in myself or my students influence the way I approach teaching?" Address how you present yourself and course materials; what activities, assignments, and projects you implement; how you interact with students in and outside class and the consequences.
5. Professional growth plan. Ask yourself "What future goals have I set for myself as a teacher?" and "How will I accomplish these goals?" Address how you have grown professionally over the years, what challenges exist at the present, what long-term development goals you have projected, and what you will do to reach these goals.

Chism, N. V. N. (1998). Developing a philosophy of teaching statement. Essays on teaching excellence. *Professional and Organizational Development Network in Higher Education, 9*(3), 1–2.

Nurse Educators in the Practice Environment

Nurses who want to be nurse educators in practice settings and do not have advanced degrees may be hired as staff development program coordinators in their agencies. Nurses at the competent level of proficiency can share particular clinical expertise with staff or may be clinical instructors or clinical preceptors for schools of nursing. See Table 9-1.

Nurses in the practice setting work with staff nurses and provide continuing education, in-services, skill updates, and clinical assessments. The role also includes planning and coordinating patient and family education. Nurse educators who work in the clinical settings must hold the minimum of a baccalaureate degree in nursing, as institutions are increasingly requiring the master's degree.

Nurse educators in the practice environment may have the professional titles of Clinical Nurse Educator, Staff Development Officer, or Continuing Education Specialist, among others. Practice settings include hospitals, community health agencies, home care agencies, long-term care facilities, and education associations.

Role and Responsibilities

The responsibilities of nurse educators in the practice setting follow (WHO, 2016):

- Design curricula
- Apply theories and principles of adult learning

- Develop courses/programs of study
- Orient staff
- Evaluate staff/assess abilities of nurses in practice
- Collaborate with staff and their nurse managers to design learning experiences that will continually strengthen abilities
- Document outcomes of the educational process
- Engage in clinical research
- Plan and coordinate patient education
- Participate in professional associations
- Apply ethical and legal principles and professionalism
- Speak/present at nursing conferences
- Maintain clinical competence

Becoming an Effective Nurse Educator

This section looks to other factors beyond the personal attributes of nurse educators. These include the characteristics of effective educators, choosing a workplace, transition issues, evaluation process, and professional behaviors. A discussion of these factors follows.

Characteristics of Effective Nurse Educators

A study by Dattilo, Brewer, and Streit (2009) described the participants' views of being an experienced nurse educator. The study revealed the importance of being passionate about what you do, being harmonious with others, and fitting with the organization. Nurse educators were successful by being invested in student relationships and by maintaining boundaries. They were confident in themselves and their ability to make the right decisions.

Deans of nursing identified essential faculty skills: teaching skills, knowledge, experience, and preparation for the faculty role; curriculum/course development skills; evaluation and testing skills; and positive personal attributes (Penn et al., 2008). Of particular importance was the nurse educators' ability to help students learn how to master essential skills and knowledge. The most effective teachers engaged learners in seeking answers, finding meaning, and applying new information, rather than simply transmitting a vast amount of content.

Research revealed that effective educators looked beyond their own courses to view themselves as part of a larger whole. They took a broad understanding of the curriculum (Gardner, 2014). Most studies were conducted in academia but apply to practice settings. The characteristics of effective educators include:

- Confidence
- Acknowledgment that educators do not know all the answers
- Flexibility
- Engagement with learners
- Willingness to go the extra mile
- Willingness to support and help colleagues
- Multiple teaching approaches
- Willingness to change for, and accommodate to, different learners

Choosing a Workplace

Once you have decided to become a nurse educator, you will want to identify a workplace that meets your goals and aspirations. In making this choice, examine the institutional workplace to determine if it is a good fit for you, as well as its orientation program, mentoring program, and professional development opportunities. These four considerations are discussed in the next sections.

Institutional Fit

Determining organizational fit is an important part of being a successful nurse educator. When choosing a position, consider what you want and what the institution needs. Carefully assess expectations in advance, which will increase the chances of a good fit with your skills and priorities. Also check the accreditation status of the institution and by what agencies and in what specialty areas.

Nurse educators need to have knowledge of the institution's role, mission, and philosophy (Zambroski & Freeman, 2004). This information is a framework that guides how the institution serves its clients and community and if it is faith-based or public. This also clarifies whether the priority is placed on practice, teaching, research, service, or a combination of these activities. Ask if a nursing theory guides the curriculum.

Personal contact with faculty recruiters or human resource personnel often aids in securing a teaching position. Dattilo et al. (2009) noted that the initial interview for a nurse educator often involves being asked their philosophy of teaching, learning, and nursing in determining the fit with the organization. The interviewer looks for passion and enthusiasm when discussing clients, nursing, and teaching. Be aware of your verbal and nonverbal communication during the interview.

Orientation

Ask about the institution's orientation program. Formalized nurse educator orientation is an evidence-based strategy used to introduce academic and practice roles that increase job satisfaction and retention (Baker, 2010). An important component of orientation programs is introduction to the institution overall, and to specific departments. Orientation reviews the institution's role, mission, philosophy, organizational structure, policies, and procedures. The faculty handbook or the practice institution's policy and procedures are introduced.

Novice educators are introduced to the needed instructional skills, support, and socialization into the teaching role (Baker, 2010). New educators may need additional information related to instructional processes, including development of syllabi, lesson plans, lectures, clinical teaching, evaluating, and handling learner issues.

The formal and informal knowledge needed to be successful in practice or academic settings can be overwhelming. Novice educators need intense orientation to their teaching assignments and clinical responsibilities with frequent feedback (Dattilo et al., 2009). They need concrete guidelines about client management and expectations. Ask about the orientation time line. To ensure that needed information is integrated, the orientation program is best conducted over an extended period of time (Hessler & Ritchie, 2006). Educators should be provided with information on how to access teaching resources. They should also be informed of specific evaluation requirements for their departments.

Support groups are a valuable part of orientation. In academe, the formation of a new faculty orientation group provides an instant learning community and informal support group. These groups benefit novice educators by reducing stress, increasing collegiality, and providing a safe sounding board to air concerns and ask questions (Billings & Halstead, 2009). Such a support group is equally valuable to nurse educators in the practice setting.

Mentoring Opportunities

Mentoring new educators is important. When making a workplace choice, ask if mentoring will be provided. Schoening (2013) found that a combination of short and long-term mentoring assignments, using both formal and informal peer mentors, fit the information and social needs of novice educators. If formal mentoring is unavailable, informal mentoring and support are crucial. There is also value in the novice observing experienced nurse educators. It is essential for educators to examine their own values, beliefs, and assumptions about teaching before becoming a mentor. They should receive training in the elements of effective mentorship.

Professional Development Opportunities

When choosing a workplace, consider opportunities for advancement. Professional development is a process of achieving increasingly complex levels of competency as an educator (see Table 9-1). Nurse educators should spend time in self-evaluation to identify their goals and expectations. Oermann and Gaberson (2009) suggest that nurse learners need to determine their strengths and weaknesses in order to develop a professional development plan.

A professional development plan is a descriptive tool, used to guide promotion and merit review. Nurse educators complete an annual professional development plan with their director or supervisor. Most plans are based on Boyer's model of scholarship (AACN, 2017). Boyer's model is used to clarify and describe the range of scholarship within the discipline of nursing. The four types of scholarship are discovery, teaching, application, and integration. "These areas support the values of a profession committed to both social relevance and scientific advancement" (AACN, 2017, p. 1). See **Table 9-3** for the scholarship types, definitions, and examples (Peterson & Stevens, 2013).

Transition Issues

Nurses should be aware that transitioning from clinical practice to a teaching role in academia can be a struggle. There are differences between the academic work environment and the nursing practice environment. This can be a rewarding journey, but the nurse should be conscious of the different values and skills needed to make the change.

Research reveals stages in the transition process. Locasto and Kochanek (1989) suggested that new nurse educators experience a honeymoon phase, a shock and rejection phase, and a resolution phase as they adapt to their new role. Ramage (2004) described negotiating multiple roles through a process of disassembling the nursing identity and then rediscovering and realizing the new self as educator (p. 292). Schoening (2013) identified the phases of anticipation/expectation, orientation, information seeking, and identity formation.

Anderson (2009) identified factors such as previous work experience and unrealistic expectations that facilitated and hindered the transition. Understanding the implications of making a role change to an educator in academe is important to your success.

Table 9-3 Types of Scholarship

Type of Scholarship	Definition	Examples
Discovery	Development of new knowledge through research	■ Peer-reviewed journal publications of research ■ Presentations of research
Teaching	Development and testing of learning theory and teaching strategies	■ Successful application of technology to teaching and learning ■ Presentations related to teaching and learning
Application	Addressing societal problems and partnering with the community	■ Establishing academic-service partnerships ■ Presentations related to practice
Integration	Interdisciplinary interconnection of ideas	■ Publishing books ■ Reports of interdisciplinary programs and service projects

Data from American Association of Colleges of Nursing. (2017). *Defining scholarship for the discipline of nursing.* Retrieved from https://www.aacnnursing.org/Portals/0/PDFs/Position-Statements/Defining-Scholarship.pdf?ver=SWHIav1tRNMfYL5xPvjklA%3d%3d

Evaluation Process

Nurse educators in academic and practice settings are required to evaluate their teaching and use the feedback to improve their practice. The evaluation process involves collecting and using information to determine if desired learning outcomes were achieved. Evaluation can take many forms and enables nurse educators to ascertain what impact they are making on student learning and what they need to do to improve their practice (Ramsden, 2003). To get the most out of evaluation, nurse educators need an understanding of the different forms and the pros and cons of each. Forms of evaluation include learner evaluation, self-evaluation, peer evaluation, single-person evaluation, and multisource evaluation (Besing, 2011; Parkinson, 2016). A review of this information is presented in **Table 9-4**.

Learner evaluations are gathered by asking questions about how the educator taught using questionnaires, surveys, focus groups, or one-to-one discussion. The learner is asked to give information about the achievement of learning objectives, teaching strategies, teacher effectiveness, and the overall learning experience. Evaluations may be formative while the teaching is occurring or summative at the conclusion of the teaching session.

Self-evaluation helps educators reflect upon how they have met performance expectations and whether their teaching was effective. Many self-evaluation tools have a range for evaluation that includes *needs improvement, performs satisfactorily, performs above expectations,* and *excels in performance* or similar terms. Videotaping yourself teaching assists with self-reflection about your teaching style and can be viewed in privacy.

Peer evaluation is conducted by colleagues when they observe educators actually teaching. It can be a formal requirement of the institution's performance evaluation process or an informal activity. The purpose is to act as colleagues to assess and improve teaching skill. The process should be supportive with clear expectations and guidelines.

Table 9-4 Spectrum of Evaluation

Form	Definition	Pros	Cons
Learner Evaluation	Feedback from the recipients of health education	Provides helpful feedback in assessing teaching effectiveness	Personal characteristics can influence how teachers are evaluated
Self-Evaluation	Nurse educator's personal appraisal of performance	Gives ownership of their performance and is less stressful	May be biased and unrealistic
Peer Evaluation	Evaluation by colleagues of same or greater status	Creates positive, supportive relationships	Can be stressful and may not be representative
Single-Person Evaluation	Review by a supervisor or person of higher status	Enhances relationship, promotes professional growth, builds career	Lack of trust and respect
Multisource Evaluation	Integrated approach using more than one evaluation method	Provides a broad perspective of performance	Time intensive and may cause evaluation fatigue

Data from Besing, K. (2011, September 6). Nursing performance appraisals: What purpose do they serve? *Advance Healthcare Network for Nurses*. Retrieved from http://nursing.advanceweb.com/Regional-Content/Articles /Nurse-Performance-Appraisals.aspx; Parkinson, B. (2016, August 22). Using evaluation to improve teaching. *Nursing Times*. Retrieved from https://www.nursingtimes.net/roles/nurse-educators/using-evaluation-to-improve-teaching/7010065.article

Single-person evaluation is that which is conducted by the dean/director in the academic environment or the supervisor in the practice environment. It addresses the performance expectations of the institution and specific department where you are employed. A supportive director or supervisor can be instrumental in giving advice and supporting professional growth.

Multisource evaluation, or the *360 evaluation* as it is often called, uses more than one approach to evaluation. It results in a more complete picture of teaching and learning. It combines feedback from learners, self-evaluation, various types of peer evaluation, and director/supervisor evaluation. This gives a broader impression of the skills and abilities of the educator, but can result in evaluation fatigue.

The forms of evaluation mentioned here are based on feedback from different sources (learners, peers, self, director/supervisor). It is important to understand how you will be evaluated. Attending to this feedback is the key to becoming an effective nurse educator. It depends on your awareness, listening skills, ability to be responsive, and a willingness to incorporate feedback into your behavioral repertoire.

Professional Behaviors

Clients expect to be cared for by nurses who are not only competent but also behave professionally. Nurse educators in both practice and academic settings have a responsibility to foster professional nursing accountability in the nurses they teach. *Professional nursing accountability* is defined as taking responsibility for one's actions, nursing judgments, actions, and omissions as they relate to lifelong learning, maintaining competency, and upholding both quality patient care outcomes and standards of the profession (Krautscheid, 2014). This underlies safe nursing practice and is an essential behavior supporting congruence between nursing actions and standards associated with quality and safety in patient care.

Practice and academic educators have an equal stake in educating nurses about professional accountability. They are viewed as role models to present and future nurses. Educators should exemplify behaviors and attitudes that directly influence the development of professionalism. They need to nurture professional growth through positive learning environments. Opportunities should be provided for learners to reflect and solve problems to develop their moral thinking. Positive learning environments are needed to provide opportunities for learners to understand and experience the link between ethics, professionalism, and nursing practice (Solomon & Denatale, 2000). Every opportunity must be taken, in both classroom and clinical settings, to discuss ethical behavior and the rules that guide professional practice.

It is particularly important that nurse educators nurture expectations of civility between nurses and others for professionalism to occur. The Joint Commission (2009) stated that incivility is a serious threat to patient safety and the overall quality of care. As nurse educators, we have a responsibility to ensure that we are preparing competent, autonomous, ethical practitioners who can provide quality nursing care in a civil manner.

Lifelong Learning

The beginning of this chapter introduced the continuum of learning for nurse educators. Learning is a lifelong process that takes place for nurses at all stages of the life cycle and extends from formal schooling to the workplace, the home, and the community. Lifelong learning has been clearly identified as essential for professional nursing. The Institute of Medicine (IOM, 2010) recommended that nurses engage in lifelong learning and that healthcare organizations and schools of nursing create a culture of lifelong learning. The AACN (2009) and the NLN (2011) also identify lifelong learning as an expectation for professional nursing practice.

Lifelong learning is defined as the "development of human potential through a continuously supportive process which stimulates and empowers individuals to acquire all the knowledge, values, skills and understanding they will require throughout their lifetimes and to apply them with confidence, creativity, and enjoyment in all roles, circumstances, and environments (Longworth & Davies, 1996, p. 22). It is a dynamic process which includes both the personal and professional life of nurse educators. Eason (2010) states that it allows for development of critical thinking and supports introspection and detail in client care.

Essential characteristics of lifelong learners are reflection, questioning, enjoying learning, understanding the dynamic nature of knowledge, and engaging in learning by actively seeking learning opportunities (Davis, Taylor, & Reyes, 2014). Self-direction is an important attribute of successful lifelong learners. The competencies you will need include knowledge of how to acquire and retrieve current research related to education through literature searches, as well as how to implement change into practice.

The process of learning can be both formal and informal. Types of *formal learning* may occur through an organized structured framework designed to lead to a diploma or certificate. Achieving advanced degrees and continuing education (CE) fit into this formal structure. For nurse educators who teach nurses, the challenge is to create continuing education that is personally meaningful, engaging, and built on previous knowledge. CE should also be interactive, relevant, and based on current evidence-based knowledge.

Informal learning consists of learning embedded in planned activities that are not explicitly designed as learning, such as vocational skills acquired at the workplace. This type of learning includes workshops, journal clubs, and required skills updates. Other forms of informal learning result from daily life activities related to family, work, or leisure that are viewed as experiential learning. It is essential to recognize and value all forms of learning because we live in a world where people must have the skills to understand, interpret, and process different information.

It is imperative for nurse educators to focus on and model the development of skills and attitudes for lifelong learning. Nurses should actively seek out opportunities to continue personal and professional learning. As a nurse educator, it is important to display a commitment to lifelong learning, exercise leadership, and be concerned with the scholarly development of the discipline.

Self-Care for Nurse Educators

Being a nurse educator is a professionally rewarding career. Nurses enter the profession with altruistic motives to care for others with compassion. Nurses who teach at the bedside bring their clinical knowledge of evidence-based practice to promote health, prevent disease, and help clients cope with illness. In educational settings, nurse educators mentor and teach other nurses and students entering the profession. The best care is provided when nurses are functioning at optimal levels of their own wellness. Wellness is the act of practicing healthy habits on a daily basis to attain better physical and mental health outcomes. A nurse educator who is practicing wellness is not just surviving, they are thriving!

Linton and Koonman (2020) found that nurses frequently place client wellness above their own. Some nurses even regard concern about their personal wellness as selfish. When nurses neglect their own needs, the profession is affected and may result in nurses providing sub-optimal care or they may leave the profession. Nurses may also experience compassion fatigue due to lack of self-care. Cocker and Joss (2016) defined compassion fatigue as the psycho-emotional distress that originates from long-term exposure to self-sacrifice, coupled with prolonged exposure to difficult and challenging situations. Many codes of ethics, including the American Nurses Association Code of Ethics, state clearly that nurses must adopt self-care as a duty to self in addition to their duty to provide care to clients (ANA, 2015).

The World Health Organization defines self-care as: "the ability of individuals, families, and communities to promote health, prevent disease, maintain health, and cope with illness and disability with or without the support of a health worker" (accessed July 5, 2023, at https://www. who.int/health-topics/self-care#tab=tab_1). According to this definition, self-care includes everything related to staying physically healthy including hygiene, nutrition, and seeking medical care when needed. This includes all the steps an individual can take to manage stressors in their life and take care of their own health and well-being. Self-care is a process of practicing activities to preserve one's own health in an effort to nurture or restore physical, mental, and spiritual well-being.

Nursing is regarded as a stressful occupation. Stress is an important cause of job dissatisfaction in nursing and can contribute to disease (Blum, 2014). Linton and Koonman (2020) identified the types of stress that nurses experience on a daily basis as: environmental, psychological, and biological. Environmental stress includes work conditions, management and organizational features, technologies, distance from the workplace, and lack of continuing education. Psychological stress can be caused by conflicting duties, lack of autonomy, interpersonal relationships, dealing with death, fear of loss, fear of making errors, job dissatisfaction, dealing with families and patients, work overload, conflicting roles, and staff

Table 9-5 The Brief Nursing Stress Scale (BNSS)

Item Number	Item Content Please Indicate How Frequently You Suffer...
1	stressful situations derived from the process of dying or death
2	stressful situations derived from conflicts with doctors
3	stressful situations derived from lack of support
4	stressful situations derived from conflict between nurses
5	stressful situations derived from workload
6	stressful situations derived from the uncertainty of the treatment

Modified from Sansó, N., Vidal-Blanco, G., Galiana, L. (2021). Development and validation of the brief nursing stress scale (BNSS) in a sample of end-of-life care nurses. *Nursing Reports*, 11, 311–319. https://doi.org/10.3390/nursrep11020030

shortages (Linton & Koonman, 2020). Biological stress includes double shifts, fatigue, and pain (Linton & Koonman, 2020). Nurse educators in academic settings may experience work overload due to a shortage of faculty. They may also lack resources to complete their work and lack time to build student relationships.

Nurses must find ways to combat work stressors. The Brief Nursing Stress Scale (BNSS) (see **Table 9-5**) is an instrument to help nurses assess stressors and is based on 6 dimensions of stress (Sansó et al., 2021). These 6 dimensions are stressful situations derived from: (1) the process of dying or death; (2) conflicts with doctors; (3) lack of support; (4) conflict between nurses; (5) workload; and (6) uncertainty of the treatment. The scale uses a 0–3 point score, with 0 being no stress and 3 being the most stressful. This stress assessment can be a starting point for nurses to examine major career stressors (Sansó et al., 2021).

Nurses are encouraged to identify work stressors and take the time to discover coping strategies through addressing types of self-care. There are 5 types of self-care: physical, social, mental, spiritual and emotional (Scott, 2024). These are described in **Table 9-6** with descriptions of activities and questions to help identify coping strategies.

Nurse self-care looks different from one person to another so an individualized plan is necessary. An effective self-care plan should be tailored to the nurse's life and needs. It needs to be something created by you, for you. Customizing your own self-care plan can act as a preventive measure to make sure you do not get overwhelmed, overstressed, and burned out. Assess which areas of your life need some more attention and self-care. And reassess your life often. As your situation changes, your self-care needs are likely to shift, too. As you build your self-care plan, the steps in **Table 9-7** can be helpful.

Employers are aware that nurses who engage in self-care activities are more likely to be productive and motivated at work. Workplace models of self-care designed to decrease stress and incorporate self-care for nurses have been implemented and evaluated (Kravits et al., 2008; Blum, 2016). These programs highlight the impact of stress on health, and encourage program participants to develop a personalized wellness plan. Administrators are in an excellent position to build and support nurses' professional well-being. Establishing effective workplace policies, procedures, and valuable programs, such as resilience training, can help achieve this

Table 9-6 Types of Self-Care

Type of Self- Care	Description	Specific Activities	Personal Questions to Assess Coping
Physical	Caring for your physical needs, attending healthcare appointments, taking medication as prescribed, and managing your health	Eating, sleeping, physical activity	■ Are you getting adequate sleep? ■ Is your diet meeting your body's needs? ■ Are you taking charge of your health? ■ Are you getting enough exercise?
Social	Socialization and relationships	Cultivating and maintaining relationships	■ Are you getting enough face-to-face time with your friends? ■ What are you doing to nurture your relationships with friends and family?
Mental	Ways of thinking and the ideas filling the mind	Doing things that keep your mind sharp such as reading books or watching movies, doing things that help you stay mentally healthy. Practicing self-compassion and acceptance	■ Are you making enough time for activities that mentally stimulate you? ■ Are you doing proactive things to help you stay mentally healthy? ■ Do you treat yourself with kindness, patience, empathy, and forgiveness when you experience pain and failure, rather than being harshly critical or self-judgmental?
Spiritual	Religion and spirituality	Nurturing your spirit, anything that helps you develop a deeper sense of meaning, understanding, or connection with the universe, such as meditation, attending a religious service, or praying	■ What questions do you ask yourself about your life and experience? ■ Are you engaging in spiritual practices that you find fulfilling?
Emotional	Dealing with uncomfortable emotions such as anger anxiety and sadness	Talking or leisure activities that help you acknowledge and express your feelings regularly and safely	■ Do you have healthy ways to process your emotions? ■ Do you incorporate activities into your life that help you feel recharged?

Data from Scott, E. (2024). *5 self-care practices for every area of your life.* Verywell Mind. Retrieved from https://www.verywellmind.com/self-care-strategies
-overall-stress-reduction-3144729

(Jehloh & Zolkefli, 2022) When seeking employment, prospective nurse educators should in-quire into what self-care programs are available. Nurse educators are advocates for their clients and their families, so we need to be physically and emotionally available to care for our clients to the best of our ability. This means insuring our own well-being through self-care.

Table 9-7 Steps in Building a Self-Care Plan

Steps	Self-Care Plan
1. Assess your needs	Take some time to evaluate different aspects of your life and daily activities. This could include work, school, relationships, and family. Make a comprehensive list of these areas to gain a better understanding of your priorities.
2. Identify sources of stress	Reflect on the specific aspects of these areas that cause you stress. By recognizing your stressors, you can begin to develop strategies to address and manage them effectively.
3. Create self-care strategies	Brainstorm activities that promote self-care and well-being in each area of your life. For example, spending quality time with friends or setting healthy boundaries by learning to say "no" can foster healthy social connections.
4. Prepare for challenges	Anticipate potential obstacles that may hinder your self-care efforts. Develop a plan to overcome these challenges and ensure that you remain committed to your well-being.
5. Take small steps	Remember that change doesn't happen overnight. Start by implementing small, achievable steps towards self-care. These incremental changes can have a significant impact on your overall well-being.
6. Prioritize self-care time	Even during busy periods or when you don't feel motivated, make self-care a priority. Schedule dedicated time to focus on your needs and ensure that you are taking care of all aspects of yourself. This will enhance your ability to function effectively and efficiently in other areas of your life.

Modified from Scott, E. (2021). *5 self-care practices for every area of your life. Verywell Mind*. Retrieved July 5, 2023, from https://www.verywellmind.com/self-care-strategies-overall-stress-reduction-3144729#citation-7

Summary

This chapter addresses a major concept of the Miller–Stoeckel Client Education Model: the Nurse as Educator. The basic definition of the nurse as educator, as stated in Chapter 1, is a nurse who plans, organizes, teaches, and directs health education to promote, retain, and restore health in a variety of settings. This chapter looks deeper into the role and expands upon what it means to be an effective nurse educator. Nurse educators are on a continuum of learning, beginning with basic nursing education and continuing through the nursing career. All nurses are educators at the bedside and are at different levels of proficiency. A guide is provided to gauge your progress as a nurse educator.

Nurses may choose different paths depending on their goals and ambitions. Some may remain as an important part of the interprofessional team by providing client education at the bedside. Others may seek out advanced roles as educators. Generally, this involves attaining further education or receiving certification. A self-assessment and description of the educational preparation and roles and responsibilities is provided to help determine your fit for an advanced role as a nurse educator in the practice or academic setting.

Once the decision is made to move to an advanced role, there are issues to consider when choosing a workplace. These include institutional fit, orientation process, mentoring opportunities, professional development opportunities, transition issues, and evaluation process. Thoughtful preparation can enhance the chances of being successful.

Finally, the chapter concludes by describing the nurse educator's commitment to professional nursing accountability, lifelong learning, and self-care for nurse educators. Clients expect nurses to demonstrate professional and civil behavior. It is also expected that nurse educators will nurture these qualities in the nurses they teach. Lifelong learning is part of the continuum of learning for nurse educators and is about commitment to improving care for the clients and students we serve.

Exercises
Exercise I: Becoming a Teacher

Purpose: Self-Evaluation
Directions: Think about your initial efforts at teaching something to a client or colleague. How did you feel? Were you awkward? Nervous? Do you think the client understood your message? How would you assess your efforts?

Exercise II: Philosophy Statement

Purpose: Self-Examination
Directions: Review the questions posed in the discussion of philosophy, and prepare a written statement describing your beliefs about nursing, clients as learners, nurses as educators, the nature of teaching, the nature of learning, and the role of knowledge in the teaching/learning process. Write "I believe" statements that honestly represent what you believe. Then reflect on what you have written. Are you more aware of what you truly believe? Are your beliefs and actions consistent and compatible? What goals have you set for yourself as a teacher? How will you accomplish these goals?

Exercise III: Levels of Proficiency in Teaching

Purpose: Self-Evaluation
Directions: Review Table 9-1, Levels of Proficiency in Teaching. Reflect on your experience thus far, and then assess the level at which you would place yourself. Provide a rationale.

Exercise IV: Peer Evaluation

Purpose: Gain experience and confidence in teaching
Directions: Select a teaching opportunity, and invite a trusted colleague(s) to observe you while teaching. Establish the criteria upon which you wish to be evaluated prior to teaching. Criteria may include how clearly you presented the material and answered questions, the teaching environment you established, and how well you achieved the learning objectives.

Exercise V: Identify Self-Care Needs

Purpose: Addressing personal self-care needs
Directions: Thinking about your current situation, answer the questions in The Brief Nursing Stress Scale. Then customize your own self-care plan. Identify specific activities to nurture yourself and restore your physical, social, mental, spiritual, and emotional well-being.

Exercise VI: Evidence-Based Nursing Practice

Purpose: Apply evidence-based nursing research to client education
Directions:

1. Search the literature for nursing research applicable to the role of nurse as learner.
2. Describe how the findings could be applied in your practice.

References

Agency for Healthcare Research and Quality, U.S. Department of Health and Human Services. (2015). *Nursing and patient safety*. Retrieved from https://www.ahrq.gov/sites/default/files/wysiwyg/professionals/quality-patient-safety/patientsafetyculture/hospital/resourcelist/hospitalresourcelist.pdf

American Association of Colleges of Nursing. (2008). *Nursing workforce development programs: Supporting the next generation of nurses and faculty who educate them*. Retrieved from http://www.aacn.nche.edu/government-affairs/TitleVIII.pdf.

American Association of Colleges of Nursing. (2009). *Lifelong learning in medicine and nursing final conference report*. Retrieved from http://www.aacn.nche.edu/education-resources/MacyReport.pdf

American Association of Colleges of Nursing. (2017). *Defining scholarship for the discipline of nursing*. Retrieved from http://www.aacn.nche.edu/publications/position/defining-scholarship

American Nurses Association. (2010). *Nursing: Scope and standards of practice* (2nd ed.). Silver Spring, MD: Author.

American Nurses Association. (2015). *Code of ethics for nurses with interpretive statements* (p. 9). Silver Spring, MD: Author.

American Nurses Credentialing Center. (2017). *Choose your certification*. Retrieved at http://www.nursecredentialing.org/certification.aspx

Anderson, J. K. (2009). The work-role transition from expert nurse clinician to novice nurse educator in a baccalaureate nursing program. *Journal of Nursing Education, 48*(4), 203–208.

Baker, S. L., (2010). Nurse educator orientation: Professional development that promotes retention. *The Journal of Continuing Education in Nursing, 41*(9), 413–417.

Bartels, J. E. (2005, January). Your career as a nurse educator. *NSNA IMPRINT*.

Benner, P. (1982). From novice to expert. *American Journal of Nursing, 82*(3), 402–407.

Besing, K. (2011). Nursing performance appraisals: What purpose do they serve? *Advance Healthcare Network for Nurses*. Retrieved from http://nursing.advanceweb.com/Regional-Content/Articles/Nurse-Performance-Appraisals.aspx

Billings, D., & Halstead, J. (2009). *Teaching in nursing: A guide for faculty* (3rd ed.). St. Louis, MO: Saunders.

Blum, C. (2014). Practicing self-care for nurses: A nursing program initiative. *OJIN: The Online Journal of Issues in Nursing, 19*(3), Manuscript 3.

Campinha-Bacote, J. (2011). Delivering patient-centered care in the midst of a cultural conflict: The role of cultural competence. *OJIN: The Online Journal of Issues in Nursing, 16*(2), Manuscript 5.

Carpenter, J., & Bell, S. (2002). What do nurses know about teaching patients? *Journal for Nurses in Staff Development, 18*(3), 157–161.

Chism, N. V. N. (1998). Developing a philosophy of teaching statement. Essays on teaching excellence. *Professional and Organizational Development Network in Higher Education, 9*(3), 1–2.

Cocker, F., & Joss, N. (2016). Compassion fatigue among healthcare, emergency and community service workers: A systematic review. *International Journal of Environmental Research and Public Health, 13*(6), 1–18.

Dattilo, J., Brewer, M. K., & Streit, L. (2009). Voices of experience: Reflections of nurse educators. *The Journal of Continuing Education in Nursing, 40*(8), 367–370.

Davis, L., Taylor, H., & Reyes, H. (2014). Lifelong learning in nursing: A Delphi study. *Nurse Education Today, 34*, 441–445.

Eason, T. (2010). Lifelong learning: Fostering a culture of curiosity. *Creative Nursing, 16*(4), 155–159.

Gardner, S. S. (2014). From learning to teach to teaching effectiveness: Nurse educators describe their experiences. *Nursing Education Perspectives*, 106–111.

Greene, M. (1973). *Teacher as stranger: Educational philosophy in the modern age*. Belmont, CA: Wadsworth.

Halstead, J. A. (2007). *Nurse educator competencies: Creating an evidence-based practice for nurse educators*. New York, NY: National League for Nursing.

Hessler, K., & Ritchie, H. (2006). Recruitment and retention of novice faculty. *Journal of Nursing Education, 45*(5), 150–154.

Institute of Medicine. (2010). *The future of nursing: Leading change, advancing health*. Washington, DC: National Academies Press. Retrieved from http://books.nap.edu/openbook.php?record_id=12956&page=R1

Jehloh, L., & Zolkefli, Z. (2022). Compassion fatigue in nurse educators. *International Journal of Care Scholars, 5*(2), 133–134.

Joint Commission, The. (2009). *Behaviors that undermine a culture of safety*. Retrieved at https://www.jointcommission.org/podcast.aspx?CategoryId=1&F_All=y

Kaprielian, V. S., Silberberg, M., McDonald, M. A., Koo, D., Hull, S. K., Murphy, G., . . . Michener, J. L. (2013). Teaching population health: A competency map approach to education. *Academic Medicine, 88*(5), 626–637.

Krautscheid, L. (2014). Defining professional nursing accountability: A literature review. *Journal of Professional Nursing, 30*(1), 43–47.

Kravits, K., McAllister-Black, R., Grant, M., & Kirk, C. (2008). Self-care strategies for nurses: A psycho-educational intervention for stress reduction and the prevention of burnout. *Applied Nursing Research, 23*, 130–138. https://doi.org/10.1016/j.apnr.2008.08.002

Linton, M., & Koonmen, J. (2020). Self-care as an ethical obligation for nurses. *Nursing Ethics*, 27(8), 1694–1702. https://doi.org/10.1177/0969733020940371

Locasto, L. W., & Kochanek, D. (1989). Reality shock in the nurse educator. *Journal of Nursing Education*, 28(2), 79–81.

Longworth, N., & Davies, W. K. (1996). *Lifelong learning: New vision, new implications, new roles for people, organizations, nations and communities in the 21st century*. London, England: Kogan Page Publishing.

National Council of State Boards of Nursing. (2006/2007). *Practice, regulation, and education (PR&E) committee faculty shortage survey in nursing faculty qualifications and roles*. Retrieved from https://ncsbn.org/Final_08 _Faculty_Qual _Report.pdf

National League for Nursing. (2011). *Academic progression in nursing education: A living document*. New York, NY: Author.

National League for Nursing. (2014). *Nurse educator shortage fact sheet*. Retrieved from http://www.nln.org/docs/default -source/advocacy-public-policy/nurse-faculty-shortage-fact-sheet-pdf.pdf?sfvrsn=0

Nursing World. (2002). *Nurse Reinvestment Act*. Retrieved from http://www.nursingworld.org/NurseReinvestmentAct .aspx

Oermann, M., & Gaberson, K. (2009). *Evaluation and testing in nursing education* (3rd ed.). New York, NY: Springer.

Palmer, P. (2007). *The courage to teach: Exploring the inner landscape of a teacher's life*. San Francisco, CA: Jossey-Bass.

Parkinson, B. (2016). Using evaluation to improve teaching. *Nursing Times*. Retrieved from https://www.nursingtimes.net /roles/nurse-educators/using-evaluation-to-improve-teaching/7010065.article

Penn, B. K., Wilson, L. D., & Rosseter, R. (2008). Transitioning from nursing practice to a teaching role. *OJIN: The On-line Journal of Issues in Nursing*, 13(3), Manuscript 3. Retrieved from https://ojin.nursingworld.org/table-of-contents /volume-13-2008/number-3-september-2008/nursing-practice-to-teaching-role/

Peterson, K., & Stevens, J. (2013). Integrating the scholarship of practice into the nurse academician portfolio. *Nursing Faculty Publications*, Paper 1. Retrieved from http://digitalcommons.brockport.edu/cgi/viewcontent .cgi?article=1000&context=nursing_facpub

Ramage, C. (2004). Negotiating multiple roles: Link teachers in clinical nursing practice. *Journal of Advanced Nursing*, 45(3), 287–296.

Ramsden, P. (2003). *Learning to teach in higher education*. New York, NY: Routledge Falmer.

Sansó, N., Vidal-Blanco, G., Galiana, L. (2021). Development and validation of the Brief Nursing Stress Scale (BNSS) in a sample of end-of-life care nurses. *Nursing Reports*, 11, 311–319. https://doi.org/10.3390/nursrep11020030

Schoening, A. M., (2013). From bedside to classroom: The nurse educator transition model. *Nursing Education Research*, 34(3), 167–172.

Scott, E. (2021). *5 self-care practices for every area of your life*. Verywell Mind. Retrieved July 5, 2023, from https://www .verywellmind.com/self-care-strategies-overall-stress-reduction-3144729#citation-7

Scott, E. (2024). *5 self-care practices for every area of your life*. Verywell Mind. Retrieved January 26, 2022, from https:// www.verywellmind.com/self-care-strategies-overall-stress-reduction-3144729

Skar, R. (2010). How nurses experience their work as a learning environment. *Vocations and Learning, 3*, 1–18.

Solomon, M. R., & Denatale, M. L. (2000). Academic dishonesty and professional practice: A convocation. *Nurse Educator*, 25, 270–271

World Health Organization. (2016). *Nurse educator core competencies*. Retrieved from https://www.who.int/publications/i /item/nurse-educator-core-competencies

Yordy, K. D. (2006). *The nursing faculty shortage: A crisis for health care*. Robert Wood Johnson Foundation. Retrieved from http://www.rwjf.org/en/library/research/2006/04/the-nursing-faculty-shortage.html

Zambroski, C., & Freeman, L. (2004). Faculty role transition from community college to a research-intensive university. *Journal of Nursing Education*, 43(3), 104–106.

PART IV

Planning and Implementing Client Education

© Peter Cade/Stone/Getty Images

CHAPTER 10

Client Education Plan

OBJECTIVES

Upon completion of this chapter, you will be able to do the following:

- Identify the importance of the client education plan.
- Discuss how an institutional mission impacts the client education plan.
- Distinguish between different methods of developing short-term and long-term goals, including the SMART method.
- Develop learning outcomes using gap analysis and develop learning objectives using the ABCD method.
- Select the appropriate hierarchical levels for Bloom's three learning domains when writing learning objectives.
- Select appropriate content, teaching strategies, and evaluation methods for the client education plan.
- Use the client education plan template in preparation for teaching clients.

CHAPTER OUTLINE

Introduction

In this chapter, we illustrate the development of the client education plan, with further explanation in subsequent chapters. Developing the client education plan helps to see the totality of the approach to client education and how to implement it. The chapter identifies the sections of the plan and gives a case study example. To optimize learning, we suggest you identify a client for whom you wish to provide health education and begin to develop a client education plan that is appropriate for that client.

Client Education Plan

The *client education plan* is a tool that nurse educators use to compile activities to meet clients' learning needs. The Miller–Stoeckel Client Education Model is the framework for building the client education plan. The model identifies clients as individuals, families, groups/communities, and health team members with different learning needs. Developing a plan keeps you on track to reach your goals of educating clients. The plan includes: (1) goals/learning outcomes, (2) learning objectives, (3) content outline, (4) teaching strategies/instructional materials, (5) time, and (6) evaluation.

The essential steps of building the client education plan are comprised of terminology that lacks consensus in the literature. The concepts of goals, outcomes, and objectives have a range of definitions and are often used interchangeably. A reason for differences in terminology is due to changes in approaches to education that include shifts from objective-based to outcomes-based learning.

Objective-based learning is a process driven by specific, detailed hierarchical objectives that describe intended results or consequences of instruction (Mager, 1997). *Outcome-based learning*, in contrast, has a broad-based focus on the outcomes of learning (Miller, 1997). These changes have resulted in confusion of terms, because you will see both approaches in practice. This chapter prepares you to use both approaches and presents key concepts in the client education plan. Mission, goals, learning outcomes, and learning objectives will be defined and integrated into a client education plan template that can be used to optimize client learning.

Mission

A *mission statement* is a formal, broad summary of the aims, philosophy, and values of an institution, organization, or individual. Mission statements guide priorities, activities, and responsibilities of organizations and individuals that provide education. An inverted pyramid structure shows how the client education process flows from the broad emphasis on mission to goals, learning outcomes, and learning objectives. See **Figure 10-1**.

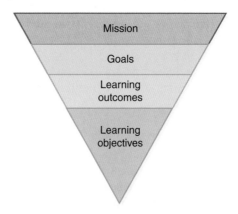

Figure 10-1 Broad to Narrow Focus of the Client Education Plan

It is important to be aware of the mission of the organization because goals, outcomes, and objectives should be in harmony. The mission statement is written as a concise, one-sentence statement that guides the purpose and practice of an entity. An example is the mission statement of the American Heart Association: To build healthier lives, free of cardiovascular diseases and stroke.

Goals

Goals describe broad educational outcomes and concepts and provide a framework for more specific learning outcomes. A single goal may have more than one learning outcome and many specific learning objectives. Goals are broad, general statements that express what an individual, program, course, or activity intends to accomplish. They are not measurable and can be both short and long term. For example, a short-term goal for a client with diabetes would be to self-administer insulin. A long-term goal would be to keep blood sugars under control.

Individuals can set specific individual career goals using the *SMART method* developed by George Doran (1981). This approach helps improve the chances of an individual achieving personal goals in a business setting and is not a format for learning objectives in the client education plan. The meaning of the acronym is:

S–Specific (Who, what, when, where, which, why?)

M–Measurable (How will it be measured?)

A–Achievable (Is it attainable?)

R–Relevant (Does it align with mission and goals?)

T–Time-bound (What is the target date for achievement?)

Learning Outcomes

Learning outcomes identify what the learner will know and be able to do by the end of a teaching activity, course, or program. They reflect the essential, specific abilities (knowledge, skills, or practice/performance) that meet learning needs of clients. Learning outcomes generally have multiple learning objectives.

The process of writing learning outcomes begins with an assessment of clients' learning needs. The identification of an individual client's needs may be accomplished through interviews, observation, self-reflection, or referral from other professionals. The learning needs of a group can be identified through a gap analysis, focus groups, or critical incident review.

A *gap analysis* or root cause analysis is a determination of the current state of clinical practice and the desired state of clinical practice. By determining the learning needs of a group through a gap analysis, the nurse educator gains a clearer picture of the behavior that is needed and what learning is required. To perform a gap analysis (American Nurses Credentialing Center, 2016):

* Determine the current state and ask, "What is currently happening? What evidence supports that there is a learning need or practice gap?"
* Determine the desired state and ask, "What should be happening?"
* Determine if the need or gap is due to lack of knowledge, skill, and or practice/performance and ask, "Why do you think the current state exists? What is the underlying or root cause?"
* Determine the method of evaluation and ask, "How is the change going to be measured?"

Once the need or practice gap is determined, the learning outcome is written using the following format:

- "The client will . . . ."
- Use an action verb to identify the performance to be demonstrated.
- Specify what learning will be demonstrated in the performance.
- Broadly identify the criterion or standard for acceptable performance.
  - Example of a learning outcome statement:
  - Knowledge: The client will demonstrate knowledge of evidence-based treatment for hypertensive patients by passing a post-test with a score of 80% or higher.
  - Competence/Skill: The client will correctly identify required actions to manage patients in hypertensive crisis by analyzing a case study.
  - Performance: The client will be observed using an evidence-based protocol.

Learning Objectives

Learning objectives are specific actions to achieve learning outcomes and are the intended results of instruction, programs, or learning activities. They are generally extensive, detailed, and specific. Learning objectives reflect teaching intentions and typically indicate the subject content that the teacher intends to cover in the learning activity. Learning objectives guide the parts of the client education plan: teaching content, strategies, instructional materials, and evaluation methods. They are composed of four parts in the ABCD format adapted from Mager (1997):

- *Audience* (who the learner is, "The client will . . .").
- *Behavior* (what the learner is to do using action verbs).
- *Conditions* (the conditions under which the learner is to perform).
- *Degree* (how well the learner will perform; includes the quality and level of performance).

A summary of the parts of the ABCD approach to writing learning objectives is shown in **Table 10-1**. Poorly and clearly stated objectives are shown in **Table 10-2**.

Reordering of the ABCD Components

The order of the *ABCD components* can be changed to make the most comprehensive and clear statement of the objective. **A**udience + **B**ehavior + **C**ondition + **D**egree can be altered to **C**ondition + **A**udience + **B**ehavior + **D**egree. For example: Given a syringe and a basin, the client will perform a colostomy irrigation without verbal guidance from the nurse. **A** + **B** + **D** + **C** can also be stated: The client will perform a colostomy irrigation without verbal guidance from the nurse when given a syringe and a basin. The order of the components should be carefully thought through to help the learner understand the learning expectations.

Domains of Learning

Verbs that are used to describe behavior in the ABCD approach to writing learning objectives are categorized by the domains of learning and hierarchies within the domains (Bloom, Englehart, Furst, Hill, & Krathwohl, 1956). The domains of learning help make clear what is expected of different levels of intellectual behavior. The three domains are:

- Cognitive domain, which emphasizes thinking.
- Affective domain, which emphasizes attitudes and feelings.
- Psychomotor domain, which emphasizes doing and performing skills.

Table 10-1 The ABCD Approach to Writing Learning Objectives

Objective Part	Description	Example
Audience	To whom is the objective applied?	**The client will**
Behavior	What will the client do? What is the action verb? What learning domain is addressed?	The client will **create a time line of the main events that occur with hypoglycemia**.
Conditions	How will the action be accomplished? What specifics about the situation must be met?	The client will create a time line of the main events that occur with hypoglycemia **by drawing a diagram of the process using a list of items provided by the teacher**.
Degree	Describe the minimum criteria for acceptable student performance. ■ How often? ■ How well? ■ How many? ■ How much? Define expectations regarding accuracy, quality, and speed.	The client will create a time line of the main events that occur with hypoglycemia by drawing a diagram of the process using a list of items provided by the teacher **showing the order that the events normally occur**.

Table 10-2 Poorly and Clearly Stated Objectives

Poorly Stated Objectives	Clearly Stated Objectives
The client will *know* the symptoms of diabetes.	The client will *verbally state* the three signs and symptoms of hyperglycemia and state why they occur to the nurse.
The client will *understand* the distinction between hypoglycemia and hyperglycemia.	The client will *correctly identify the signs and symptoms* of hypoglycemia from a list on a written exam.
The client will *know how* to test their blood sugar.	The client will *demonstrate the proper use* of a glucometer to test their blood sugar to the nurse during a home visit.

Nurses must be knowledgeable about how to structure, write, and evaluate learning objectives that can be written in all three domains. It is important to choose the correct verb to illustrate the domain for which you are writing objectives. Avoid verbs with many interpretations such as appreciate, believe, enjoy, feel, know, learn, think, and understand. In writing learning objectives, you will soon realize that many behaviors do not fall exclusively in one of the three domains. Learners learn as an integrated whole; however, you must isolate the particular behavior of concern. For example, irrigating a colostomy is not only a psychomotor activity; it also requires cognition and an affective response. Thus, learning objectives may involve more than one domain.

Cognitive Domain

The *cognitive domain* is concerned with knowledge, beliefs, and reasoning. The cognitive levels are remembering, understanding, applying, analyzing, evaluating, and creating (Anderson et al., 2001).

Table 10-3 **Cognitive Categories with Sample Objectives**

Cognitive Category	Description	Verb	Sample Objective
Remembering	Client recalls information	Define	The client will define the terms *hypoglycemia* and *hyperglycemia*.
Understanding	Client explains ideas and concepts	Describe	The client will describe the signs and symptoms of insulin shock.
Applying	Client grasps ideas and concepts	Interpret	The client will interpret their blood sugar level to determine if more insulin is needed.
Analyzing	Client distinguishes among different parts	Compare, contrast	The client will compare and contrast the signs and symptoms of hypoglycemia and hyperglycemia.
Evaluating	Client justifies a stand or takes a position	Support	The client will support the need to keep blood sugar within normal limits.
Creating	Client creates a new product or point of view	Design	The client will design a calendar to keep track of daily blood sugar levels.

The levels are presented from the lowest (remembering) to the highest level (creating) of cognitive complexity (**Table 10-3**) and a detailed list of verbs (Table 10-7). Table 10-8 identifies sample verbs for affective objectives.

Affective Domain

The *affective domain* addresses the client's attitudes, interests, attention, awareness, and values. The levels of the affective domain are receiving, responding, valuing, and organization in increasing order of depth (Krathwohl, Bloom, & Masia, 1964). Affective objectives are more difficult to isolate and express accurately; consequently, they are difficult to evaluate through measurement. See **Table 10-4**.

Psychomotor Domain

Psychomotor skills are concerned with physical movement and coordination which are easier to identify and measure because they are readily observable. We adapted and abbreviated the hierarchy of skills developed by Simpson (1972) because it appears to have the most relevance for client education. The levels are perception, set, guided response, mechanism, complex overt response, and adaptation, which move from the lowest to highest level. See **Table 10-5** and Table 10-9.

Conditions

The third step in the ABCD process of writing learning objectives is to define the *conditions* under which the client will perform the desired task. This includes specifying situations and restraints during which the objective must be met, or describing important conditions under which the *performance* is expected to occur. The statement of conditions is not always necessary to a clear

Table 10-4 Affective Categories and Sample Objectives

Affective Category	Description	Verbs	Sample Objective
Receiving	Client is aware of or attending to something in the environment	Listen to	The client will listen to a presentation on colostomy care and share the information with family members.
Responding	Client shows new behaviors as a result of experience	Choose	The client will choose to discuss their feelings about caring for the colostomy in a support group.
Valuing	Client shows involvement or commitment	Express	The client will express agreement with the guidelines for maintaining sterile technique in wound care.
Organization	Client integrates a new value, ranking it among priorities	Select	The client will select foods that meet the requirements of a diabetic diet.
Characterization by value	Client acts consistently with the new value	Display	By taking medication, the client will demonstrate acceptance that they have a chronic illness.

Table 10-5 Psychomotor Categories and Sample Objectives

Psychomotor Category	Description	Verb	Sample Objective
Perception	Client attains sensory awareness of clues associated with the task to be performed	Watches	The client watches the nurse perform a colostomy irrigation.
Set	Client exhibits readiness to take action through verbal expressions or body language	Expresses	The client expresses willingness to try to do part of the colostomy irrigation.
Guided response	Client exerts efforts to imitate observed behavior; attempts to comply with directions and coaching	Performs	The client will perform colostomy irrigation with assistance.
Mechanism	Client achieves the ability to perform the skill, which is becoming a habit	Demonstrates	The client will demonstrate how to irrigate a colostomy without assistance.
Complex overt response	Client performs the skill easily and independently in sequence with attention to details	Coordinates	The client coordinates complete colostomy care and makes adjustments as needed in the process.
Adaption	Client achieves the ability to alter the skill to suit conditions and performs the skill automatically as needed	Adapts	The client adapts skill knowledge and performs colostomy care while on a camping trip.

Data from Gronlund, N. E., & Brookhart, S. M. (2009). *Gronlund's writing instructional objectives* (8th ed.). Upper Saddle River, NJ: Pearson Education; Gronlund, N. E. (2004). *Writing instructional objectives for teaching and assessment* (7th ed.). Upper Saddle River, NJ: Pearson Education.

Table 10-6 Audience, Behavior, Condition, Degree

Audience	Behavior	Condition	Degree
The client will	perform a colostomy irrigation	given a syringe and a basin	without verbal guidance from the nurse
The client will	verbally tell the pulse rate under which they should not take digoxin	when asked by the nurse	correctly before discharge from the hospital

statement of objectives, but it should be included when pertinent. As demonstrated in **Table 10-6**, conditions might be stated with the following phrases:

- given a list of . . .
- when provided with . . .
- without using . . .
- by the end of this lesson . . .
- the learner will be denied . . .
- under special conditions of . . .
- within 15 minutes . . .
- as measured against a checklist . . .

Degree

Degree refers to the quality or level of performance that is considered acceptable and should be specified or implied when writing objectives. The degree may be based on practice standards, which the nurse should be aware of. The degree defines what level the client must perform at so you can determine if learning is successful. The *criteria* might include concepts such as amount, quality, and speed. For instance, clients may be considered successful if they are able to slow their pulse by 5 beats per minute during relaxation training or identify 2 out of 3 causes of hypertension. Accuracy is an important criterion when a client is preparing an insulin injection. The degree might specify without error or correctly. Other criteria might be without any verbal guidance or from memory. **Table 10-7** identifies sample verbs appropriate for cognitive objectives. **Table 10-8** identifies sample verbs appropriate for affective objectives. **Table 10-9** identifies sample verbs appropriate for psychomotor objectives and summarizes how the parts of the ABCD method of writing learning objectives come together to give a complete picture of client expectations.

Selection of Content

The time has come to select appropriate content to add to your client education plan. *Content* is based on learning outcomes and objectives and is drawn from your review of current literature to provide the most up-to-date information to clients. Information about various age groups and health problems is provided in the chapters on the child, adult, and older learners in this text. Use current research and clinical guidelines to prepare the client education plan.

Format content in outline form and make it succinct and clear. Keep in mind the amount of time you have to present the information and the amount of time the learner will need to grasp the information.

Table 10-7 Sample Verbs for Cognitive Objectives

Remembering	Defines	Lists	Recalls	Reproduces	Tells
	Identifies	Matches	Records	Selects	Underlines
	Indicates	Names	Repeats	Shows	
	Labels	Points	Reports	States	
Understanding	Describes	Explains	Identifies	Paraphrases	Rewrites
	Discusses	Expresses	Increases	Reiterates	Summarizes
	Draws	Generalizes	Locates	Restates	Translates
	Estimates	Gives example	Outlines	Reviews	
Applying	Applies	Draws	Investigates	Predicts	Selects
	Calculates	Eliminates	Manipulates	Prepares	Shops
	Changes	Formulates	Measures	Produces	Shows
	Computes	Illustrates	Modifies	Proposes	Solves
	Demonstrates	Implements	Negotiates	Relates	Uses
	Designs	Infers	Operates	Revises	
	Develops	Interprets	Orders	Schedules	
Analyzing	Analyzes	Calculates	Criticizes	Distinguishes	Relates
	Appraises	Categorizes	Debates	Identifies	Selects
	Arranges	Classifies	Diagrams	Illustrates	Separates
	Assigns	Compares	Differentiates	Infers	Subdivides
	Breaks down	Contrasts	Discriminates	Outlines	Tests
Evaluating	Appraises	Contrasts	Distinguishes	Interprets	Selects
	Assesses	Criticizes	Estimates	Judges	Summarizes
	Calibrates	Debates	Evaluates	Justifies	Supports
	Compares	Defends	Explains	Measures	Values
	Computes	Describes		Relates	
	Concludes	Discriminates		Revises	
Creating	Arranges	Compiles	Devises	Orders	Reorganizes
	Assembles	Composes	Estimates	Organizes	Revises
	Blends	Constructs	Formulates	Paraphrases	Rewrites
	Categorizes	Contrasts	Generates	Plans	Simplifies
	Classifies	Correlates	Integrates	Prepares	Summarizes
	Collects	Creates	Manages	Rearranges	Teaches
	Combines	Defends	Mixes	Reconstructs	Writes
	Compares	Designs	Modifies	Relates	

Data from Gronlund, N. E., & Brookhart, S. M. (2009). *Gronlund's writing instructional objectives* (8th ed.). Upper Saddle River, NJ: Pearson Education; Gronlund, N. E. (2004). *Writing instructional objectives for teaching and assessment* (7th ed.). Upper Saddle River, NJ: Pearson Education.

Selection of Evaluation Methods

Determine carefully how you will measure learning that takes place in the client education plan, as this is the purpose of your efforts. Outcomes and objectives are written so they are measurable. This implies that the nurse educator will be able to show evidence that learning has been successful. Learning is assessed in the areas of knowledge, attitude formation, and performance. Examples of measuring learning include:

Table 10-8 Sample Verbs for Affective Objectives

Receiving	Accepts	Focuses	Names
	Admits	Follows	Observes
	Allows	Heeds	Pays attention
	Asks	Identifies	Replies
	Attends	Listens	Stays
	Describes	Looks	Uses
Responding	Agrees	Discusses	Replies
	Answers	Explains	Reports
	Assists	Labels	Selects
	Attempts	Participates	Shows
	Chooses	Performs	States willingness
	Complies	Practices	Tries
	Conforms	Reacts	Verbalizes
Valuing	Asks	Differentiates	Justifies
	Asserts	Disagrees	Proposes
	Assists	Explains	Reports
	Attempts	Follows	Selects
	Chooses	Gives	Volunteers
	Completes	Helps	Works
	Defends	Initiates	
	Describes	Joins	
Organization	Adheres	Completes	Modifies
	Alters	Defends	Orders
	Arranges	Explains	Organizes
	Chooses	Expresses	Relates
	Combines	Generalizes	Resolves
	Compares	Integrates	Synthesizes
Internalizing values (characterization)	Acts	Describes	Performs
	Adheres	Discriminates	Practices
	Asserts	Displays	Revises
	Assists	Endures	Solves
	Commits	Explains	Uses
	Defends	Influences	

Data from Gronlund, N. E., & Brookhart, S. M. (2009). *Gronlund's writing instructional objectives* (8th ed.). Upper Saddle River, NJ: Pearson Education; Gronlund, N. E. (2004). *Writing instructional objectives for teaching and assessment* (7th ed.). Upper Saddle River, NJ: Pearson Education.

- Assessing knowledge can be done through testing in a variety of ways such as multiple choice, essay, or short answer.
- Skills can be assessed through case studies, case presentations, discussion, and written questions.
- Applying knowledge can be assessed through simulation and observation in the home, clinical setting, or lab.

An example of a client education plan template follows, which can be adapted to fit any learning situation (**Exhibit 10-1**). The template is used to develop the plan in stages. The example of Mrs. Rosa Lopez illustrates the first three columns of the client education plan. The remaining columns will be developed in subsequent chapters.

Table 10-9 Sample Verbs for Psychomotor Objectives

Perception	Attends	Contrasts	Distinguishes	Looks	Selects
	Chooses	Describes	Focuses on	Observes	Separates
	Compares	Detects	Identifies	Perceives	
	Concentrates	Differentiates	Isolates	Relates	
Set	Aims	Begins	Gets ready	Reacts	Starts
	Aligns	Copies	Positions	Responds	Tries
	Asks	Displays	Prepares	Shows	Volunteers
	Attempts	Expresses	Proceeds	Stands up	
Guided response	Aligns	Combs	Holds	Presses	Solves
	Applies	Compiles	Inserts	Produces	Splints
	Arises	Connects	Joins	Pulls	Spreads
	Arranges	Constructs	Leans	Pushes	Squeezes
	Assembles	Cools	Lifts	Raises	Stands
	Attaches	Coordinates	Locates	Reassembles	Starts
	Attempts	Counts	Lowers	Reclines	Sticks
Mechanism	Auscultates	Covers	Makes	Removes	Stimulates
	Avoids	Crawls	Manipulates	Repairs	Stoops
	Balances	Cuts	Mends	Replaces	Stops
	Bathes	Demonstrates	Molds	Restores	Synchronizes
	Boils	Disconnects	Navigates	Rubs	Tears
	Breathes	Discriminates	Opens	Runs	Tests
Complex overt response	Brushes	Dissects	Operates	Scrubs	Ties
	Builds	Examines	Palpates	Secures	Transfers
	Calibrates	Fastens	Parts	Separates	Turns
	Catheterizes	Finds	Picks up	Sews	Types
	Changes	Folds	Pinches	Shakes	Ventilates
	Chooses	Grasps	Pivots	Sharpens	Walks
	Cleans	Guides	Places	Shortens	Washes
	Cleanses	Heats	Pours	Simulates	Weighs
	Closes	Hops	Practices	Slides	Wipes
Adaptation	Adapts	Creates	Modifies	Reverses	Substitutes
	Alters	Designs	Rearranges	Revises	Swaps
	Changes	Diverts	Reformulates	Rotates	Switches
	Composes	Exchanges	Remodels	Shifts	Varies
	Converts		Reorganizes		
	Corrects		Replaces		

Data from Gronlund, N. E., & Brookhart, S. M. (2009). *Gronlund's writing instructional objectives* (8th ed.). Upper Saddle River, NJ: Pearson Education; Gronlund, N. E. (2004). *Writing instructional objectives for teaching and assessment* (7th ed.). Upper Saddle River, NJ: Pearson Education.

Case Example: Mrs. Rosa Lopez

The example we are using is Mrs. Rosa Lopez, a 40-year-old Hispanic woman. She is a single mother who is supporting and raising two teenage children, a son and a daughter, who live at home. She is a teacher's aide in kindergarten at a public school and experiences the stress of working with young children at work. Her diet is mainly Mexican cuisine, but she admits to

Exhibit 10-1 Client Education Plan Template

Short-Term Goal: _____

Long-Term Goal: _____

Learning Outcomes	Learning Objectives	Content	Teaching Strategies and Instructional Materials	Time	Evaluation

snacking from machines at work. She was recently diagnosed with hypertension. The doctor prescribed an antihypertensive medication and recommended she limit her sodium intake to 2,000 mg per day.

Mrs. Lopez has a family history of hypertension, but she is reluctant to take medication to treat it. She stated that the hypertension is not bothering her, and she does not understand why it is necessary to take medication for it. Her behavior emphasizes the fact that hypertension is an invisible disease with multiple factors contributing to its etiology and treatment, including medications, nutrition, weight management, and stress reduction. The long-term goal for Rosa would be to maintain her blood pressure in a safe range. For this teaching session, the short-term goal is focused on making Rosa aware of how salt intake affects her blood pressure. We determined that she has educational needs in the three domains of learning: cognitive, affective, and psychomotor. Although there are many things our client needs to learn about hypertension, for the purposes of illustrating a client education plan related to her nutritional needs, we will provide an example of one learning objective in each domain. This plan gives the nurse educator a guide on what to teach and how to teach it.

Our client education plan has six columns (**Table 10-10**). The first column contains the learning outcome, which in this case would be maintenance of blood pressure within normal limits. The second column is the learning objectives, which for this client includes examples from Bloom's three domains, addressing nutritional concerns. The third column identifies the content in outline form. The fourth column lists the teaching strategies and instructional materials. The fifth column lists the time for each teaching strategy. The sixth column is the choice of evaluation methods to meet the learning outcome and individual objectives. Each component of the plan prepares the nurse for instructing Rosa in an organized and deliberate way. In this chapter, we review the first three columns: the learning outcome, learning objectives, and the content. The final three shaded columns will be added in the next chapter.

Table 10-10 Sample Client Education Plan for Mrs. Rosa Lopez

Learning Outcome	Learning Objectives	Content Outline	Teaching Strategies and Instructional Materials	Time	Evaluation
Maintenance of client blood pressure within normal limits	1. The client will correctly verbally explain to the nurse from memory how excessive salt intake affects blood pressure (cognitive).	1. Review factors that contribute to high blood pressure: • Family history • Overweight/obesity • Excessive alcohol intake • Inactive lifestyle/lack of exercise • A high-salt and/or a high-fat diet • High intake of caffeine • Smoking • Stress 2. Effect of Na/salt on B/P: • A blood pressure of 140/90 or above is high. • The amount of salt has a direct effect on BP. • Salt makes the body hold water, which raises BP. • The more salt, the higher the BP. 3. Signs and symptoms of excess salt intake: • Thirst • Dehydration, including dry mouth and skin, dizziness, sleepiness, constipation, and headache			

(continues)

Table 10-10 Sample Client Education Plan for Mrs. Rosa Lopez

(continued)

Learning Outcome	Learning Objectives	Content Outline	Teaching Strategies and Instructional Materials	Time	Evaluation

	2. The client will choose to limit sodium intake by preparing a low-sodium dietary plan for 1 week (affective).	Components of dietary plan for hypertension:
		1. Explanation of the DASH diet:
		  a. Eat more fruits, vegetables, and low-fat dairy foods.
		  b. Cut back on foods high in saturated fat, cholesterol, and trans fats.
		  c. Eat more whole-grain foods, fish, poultry, and nuts.
		  d. Limit sodium, sweets, sugary drinks, and red meats.
		2. Level of salt that can be consumed safely:
		  a. 1,500 milligrams of sodium per day (about 2/3 teaspoon).
		3. Tips to decrease salt
		  a. Remove shaker from table.
		  b. Instead of snacking on chips or sweets, eat unsalted pretzels or nuts, raisins, low-fat and fat-free yogurt, frozen yogurt, unsalted plain popcorn with no butter, and raw vegetables.
		  c. Read food labels to choose products that are lower in sodium.
		  d. No salt in cooking.
		  e. Avoid canned or processed foods that are high in sodium.
		  f. Use low-sodium seasonings, such as herbs and spices.			

	3. The client will demonstrate how to accurately obtain her own blood pressure using digital monitor without guidance from the nurse (psychomotor).	Techniques for obtaining blood pressure: 1. Read equipment directions. 2. Locate brachial artery. 3. Place arm in cuff. 4. Inflate cuff. 5. Release air in cuff. 6. Record findings.			

Summary

This chapter explains the components of the client education plan. Learning goals and outcomes are defined, and the gap analysis process is explained. Learning outcomes focus on what the learner is expected to know or accomplish at the end of the teaching session. Learning objectives are defined as precise, measurable, and attainable statements that describe what should be learned as a result of participating in the learning activity. A four-part process for writing objectives was presented: Audience, Behavior, Conditions, and Degree (ABCD). Examples of outcomes and objectives were given in the three domains: cognitive, affective, and psychomotor. The correct choice of verbs for each domain was emphasized. The chapter concluded with the introduction of the case example of Mrs. Rosa Lopez and a template for creating the client education plan.

Exercises

Exercise I: Writing Learning Objectives in Each Learning Domain

Purposes:
- Differentiate among cognitive, affective, and psychomotor learning domains.
- Write clear statements to describe client learning outcomes in each domain.

Directions: Review the incorrectly written learning objectives and complete the following tasks:

1. State the learning domain or domains and **level of complexity** inferred by each objective.
2. Correct the objectives using the ABCD method of Audience, Behavior, Conditions, and Degree. Use verbs with few meanings (listed in this chapter).

The incorrectly written learning objectives are as follows:

- The client will demonstrate how to weigh herself at the conclusion of the teaching session without assistance from the nurse.
  - What ABCD component is missing?
  - What are the learning domain and level of complexity?
- After completing the learning module, the client will correctly identify foods from a list of foods provided by the nurse.
  - What ABCD component is missing?
  - What are the learning domain and level of complexity?
- After meeting with the nurse, make the association between physical activity and weight control from memory in a personal written reflection.
  - What ABCD component is missing?
  - What are the learning domain and level of complexity?

Exercise II: Writing Learning Objectives for Clients

Purpose: Write learning objectives using the ABCD method of Audience, Behavior, Conditions, and Degree.

Directions: Divide into small working groups and (1) write at least one learning objective using the ABCD method in each one of the three domains, cognitive, affective, and psychomotor; and (2) identify appropriate teaching content.

1. John Martinez is a 50-year-old farm worker who was admitted to the coronary care unit 4 days ago. This is his first myocardial infarction, and he states that he has never been ill a day in his life. He lives with his wife and their four teenaged children. He speaks very little English.
2. Suzie Scofield is a blind 6-year-old African American girl who has been admitted to the pediatric unit in preparation for a tonsillectomy tomorrow. Suzie lives with her mother, one older brother, and one younger sister. Her mother is a licensed practical nurse at the hospital.
3. Delores Johnson is a 30-year-old woman with a stormy 10-year history of ulcerative colitis. She has been hospitalized again for medical treatment. The doctors are trying to persuade Ms. Johnson to accept surgery, an ileostomy. She is a buyer for a large department store and travels in her work. She is married and has no children, but she would like to become pregnant sometime in the near future.

References

American Nurses Credentialing Center. (2016). *CE Workshop Continuing Education WMSD.* Arizona Nurses Association workshop, Phoenix, AZ.

Anderson, L. W., Krathwohl, D. R., Airasian, P. W., Cruikshank, K. A., Mayer, R. E., Pintrich, P. R., . . . Wittrock, M. C. (Eds.). (2001). *A taxonomy for learning, teaching, and assessing: A revision of Bloom's taxonomy of educational objectives.* New York, NY: Longman.

Bloom, B. S., Englehart, M. D., Furst, E. J., Hill, W. H., & Krathwohl, D. R. (1956). *Taxonomy of educational objectives: The classification of educational goals. Handbook I: Cognitive domain.* New York, NY: David McKay.

Doran, G. T. (1981). There's a S.M.A.R.T. way to write management's goals and objectives. Management Review. *AMA FORUM, 70* (11): 35–36.

Gronlund, N. E. (2004). *Writing instructional objectives for teaching and assessment* (7th ed.). Upper Saddle River, NJ: Pearson Education.

Gronlund, N. E., & Brookhart, S. M. (2009). *Gronlund's writing instructional objectives* (8th ed.). Upper Saddle River, NJ: Pearson Education.

Krathwohl, D. R., Bloom, B. S., & Masia, B. B. (1964). *Taxonomy of educational objectives: The classification of educational goals. Handbook II: Affective domain.* New York, NY: David McKay.

Mager, R. F. (1997). *Preparing instructional objectives* (3rd ed.). Atlanta, GA: CEP Press.

Miller, G. E. (1990). The assessment of clinical skills/competence/performance. *Academic Medicine.* Sep;65(9 Suppl): S63–67.

Simpson, E. J. (1972). *The psychomotor domain* (Vol. 3). Washington, DC: Gryphon House.

CHAPTER 11

Teaching Strategies

OBJECTIVES

Upon completion of this chapter, you will be able to do the following:

- Define the term *teaching strategy*.
- Compare and contrast teacher-directed, teacher-facilitated, and learner-directed teaching strategies according to their advantages and disadvantages.
- Describe a teachable moment.
- Contrast formal and informal teaching.
- State at least two examples of teaching strategies for achieving learning objectives in each of the following domains: cognitive, affective, and psychomotor.
- Identify three factors that affect the choice of teaching strategies.
- Demonstrate selected teaching strategies when implementing a client education plan.

CHAPTER OUTLINE

Introduction

Teaching is an active process in which information is shared with others to provide them with the information needed to make behavioral changes. *Learning* is the process of assimilating information with a resultant positive change in behavior. The purposes of client teaching are to promote, retain, and restore health. Learning needs related to health education include three *levels of prevention*: primary prevention (health maintenance), secondary prevention (diagnosis and treatment), and tertiary prevention (follow-up). Health teaching in these areas is used to prevent disease and provide nurses with starting points in making effective, positive changes in the health status of clients. The challenge for nurses as educators is to choose teaching strategies that nurture health-promoting habits, values, and attitudes.

This chapter looks at the use of teaching strategies when preparing client education plans for health education. A *teaching strategy* is defined as an instructional method that presents content in a way that is designed to bring about specific changes in learners. Teaching strategies include activities that are done by learners as well as teachers. They are a part of the teaching and learning process, which is a planned interaction that promotes a behavioral change. An important distinction in the current nurse's role as educator includes *facilitating learning* rather than being a source of all knowledge. The nurse helps learners construct their own knowledge rather than telling them things they are expected to memorize. The client as learner is the center of all teaching, and as a result, no one single teaching strategy is effective all the time for all learners (Killen, 2000).

Types of Teaching Strategies

Different teaching strategies are simply different ways of helping clients achieve learning objectives. The choices range from a totally teacher-dominated approach in which clients are passive recipients of information, to totally independent learning in which the teacher plays no active role. In between these extremes are several major strategies and numerous variations of each strategy. No single teaching strategy is better than another in all circumstances. Your choice of teaching strategy is influenced by the outcome you want for the client. Different types of learning can be facilitated by different strategies. There is an array of teaching strategies from which to choose. This chapter discusses different teaching strategies and factors to consider in selecting them. We discuss teaching strategies under three broad headings: *teacher-directed strategies, teacher-facilitated strategies,* and *learner-directed strategies.*

Teacher-Directed Strategies

Teacher-directed strategies are those in which the teacher presents information in a highly structured format and directs the activities of learners. These strategies include one-to-one individualized instruction, lecture format, lecture with discussion and questions and answers, demonstration and return demonstration, and team teaching. These strategies are described here, the necessary preparation is identified, and the advantages and disadvantages are discussed.

One-to-One Individual Instruction

One-to-one individual instruction is either formal or informal and includes clients alone or clients and family members as appropriate. Formal one-to-one individual instruction occurs when nurses meet individually with clients at a planned time for the purpose of providing health education. A common clinical example is preoperative teaching. The nurse selects the meeting location and time, and the content to be covered based on the client's schedule for surgery. Meeting face to face allows the nurse to give clients personalized attention. This is a good initial format to provide basic knowledge in an atmosphere that gives the client an opportunity to ask questions and get immediate feedback. Individual teaching allows clients to share confidential information and problems. This format is adaptable to the needs of clients with low health-literacy skills, physical impairments, or emotional difficulties (Rankin, Stallings, & London, 2005).

Plan *formal one-to-one individual instruction* ahead of time. Planning involves creating an outline of the content that sequences learning and choosing supplemental materials specific to the client's background and experiences. When sequencing information, teach basic concepts first and then variations and adjustments. Clients are more interested in learning what is meaningful to them, so it is helpful to begin with what clients have identified as a need or concern. To assess teaching effectiveness, ask the client to restate the information in their own words.

The most frequent type of teaching is *informal one-to-one individual instruction* that occurs at the bedside while interacting with clients for other reasons. These interactions turn into teachable moments, those unplanned moments when nurses recognize a client's readiness to learn and capture the opportunity to facilitate learning. Romano states that "the reality of the complex environment we practice in requires us to do much of our teaching on the fly, which can be effective if done right and done often" (2009, p. 141). Watch for teachable moments during your interactions with clients, and use clinical judgment to determine when teaching is appropriate. Opportune times to teach are before procedures, after a doctor's visit, while transporting a client, or when you are waiting for test results. Other opportune times to teach include the following circumstances:

- The client asks questions and shows a facial expression of curiosity or puzzlement.
- The client voices concerns about specific issues.
- The client makes innocent comments that indicate misunderstanding.
- The client shows nonverbal signs of confusion, frustration, or discouragement.
- The family voices concerns.

During *teachable moments*, constantly assess the clients' knowledge by listening and developing what Lowenstein and Reeder identify as "meta-cognitive empathy" (2009). In other words, be aware of what the client does and does not understand by evaluating their responses to pointed questions. Ask what they know about the illness, what they consider positive lifestyle behaviors, and what lifestyle changes are needed to improve health. Avoid starting your conversation by telling clients what you think they need to know. Listen carefully to identify thoughts that may need strengthening or reinforcing. This also includes correcting misunderstandings, adding knowledge, or referring the client to appropriate resources (Lowenstein & Reeder, 2009). Information that you glean from informal conversations helps you construct a mini–client education plan with appropriate teaching strategies on the spot to address client concerns. Although informal client education takes place spontaneously, you still need to present information in a clear, organized manner based on the client's level of need (Falvo, 2011). Present information to clients when they are ready to receive it and in amounts they are able to comprehend. Use the teach-back method to evaluate your teaching by asking the client to restate in their own words what you have taught. Using this strategy, you can assess how well the client comprehended your message (Tamura-Lis, 2013).

Another form of one-to-one individual instruction is telehealth, which is the use of electronic and telecommunication technologies to support long-distance clinical health care. This strategy is used for client care and health-related education. It uses video conferencing to connect the nurse and the client. Some of the technologies used in telehealth include videoconferencing, Internet access, streaming media, and wireless communications. These approaches hold great potential for health education for homebound clients and clients in remote areas. There continues to be, however, significant barriers in making this a part of daily health practices. One barrier is the mindset of health professionals who continue to focus on face-to-face care based on tradition and fragmented delivery systems. Clients want care based in their communities, but providers today wrestle with financial, regulatory, and operational challenges. The slow adoption of electronic health records (EHRs) and information sharing is another barrier. In addition, reimbursement models need to be modified with less focus on fee-for-service and face-to-face visits so clinicians and healthcare organizations get paid for the care delivered via telehealth. It is anticipated that the adoption of telehealth will accelerate as an understanding of cultural changes develops (Rogove, McArthur, Demaerschalk, & Vespa, 2012).

The advantages of one-to-one individual instruction are the personal approach to the client, the active learner role in a give-and-take relationship with the nurse, and the flexible format in an informal atmosphere. Individualized teaching also is done through phone calls, email, and telehealth. The disadvantages include lack of sharing with, and support from, other clients and their families. This strategy exacts a high cost in terms of staff time for instruction (Rankin et al., 2005).

Lecture

A *lecture* is an oral presentation of a given subject delivered before an audience or class for the purpose of instruction. Lectures are given in person or are televised, and they can be delivered as audio recordings such as podcasts. The nurse presents information on a topic that is divided into three major segments: introduction (5 minutes), body, and conclusion (5 minutes) (Woodring & Woodring, 2007). Usually in health education, the lecture is short, lasting from 15 to 20 minutes. The introduction is your opportunity to gain the attention of the audience and state what clients should gain from the lecture. The body of the lecture should explain the main concepts and convey the critical information clients need to know. The conclusion summarizes the information that was presented and makes a link between what was taught and what the clients will be able to practically use. The lecture format is an efficient, versatile, and economical teaching strategy that can be used when time is limited or when a group of clients and family members can benefit from core factual information (Bucher & Kotecki, 2014).

Preparation for giving a lecture requires planning ahead and includes knowing the learners, clarifying learning objectives, knowing the topic, and organizing and sequencing the content. Visual reinforcement, such as a PowerPoint presentation or handouts, is used to emphasize the key points. Keep in mind that an individual's optimal attention span is approximately 1 minute per year of age up to 45 years. For example, a 5-year-old has a 5-minute attention span, whereas a 21-year-old has a 21-minute attention span (Woodring & Woodring, 2007). This illustrates the importance of varying the presentation pace and including other supplemental strategies to add interest. The effectiveness of the lecture strategy depends on the skill of the speaker. **Table 11-1** offers suggestions for how to successfully prepare a lecture and avoid pitfalls.

The advantage of a lecture is that you can address a large number of clients in one setting. It is also useful for people who cannot read well, it allows auditory learners to receive succinct information quickly, and it allows you to make facts more interesting and understandable by clarifying confusing points. Disadvantages of lectures are that clients are in a passive learner role and they provide few feedback opportunities for clients. Eighty percent of lecture information is forgotten

Table 11-1 Suggestions for the Lecturer

Stage of Lecture Preparation	Suggestions	Avoid
Preparation stage (weeks in advance)	■ Specify the date, time, and location of the lecture. ■ Visit the lecture venue if possible. ■ Clarify the purpose and objectives of the lecture. ■ Cover only three to five main points. ■ Gather evidence-based research on the topic. ■ Analyze the audience. Consider age, culture, socioeconomic factors, and language. ■ Make sure your tone and examples are appropriate to the audience. ■ Prepare an outline and notes for the presentation. ■ Practice giving the lecture. ■ Choose appropriate attire. ■ Check to be sure technology is working and accessible. ■ Prepare handouts in advance. ■ Prepare in advance for questions.	■ Procrastinating ■ Lack of preparation ■ Trying to wing it at the last minute
Giving the presentation (introduction)	■ Introduce yourself. ■ State the purpose and objectives of the lecture. ■ Get the attention of the audience. ■ Remain calm and cope with anxiety. ■ Place a glass of water on the podium in case of a dry throat. ■ Gain learner attention by showing enthusiasm and self-confidence. ■ Smile and look at the audience frequently. ■ Speak clearly, strongly, and loudly; use a microphone if needed. ■ Use a conversational pace when speaking. ■ Use natural gestures. ■ Use language and expressions appropriate to the audience. ■ Provide handouts with an outline of the presentation if appropriate.	■ Distracting mannerisms or gestures, such as pacing, clearing the throat ■ Saying you are nervous ■ Apologizing ■ Looking down at your notes
Giving the presentation (body of the lecture)	■ Define the main concepts and principles. ■ Provide smooth transitions between topics. ■ Do not try to provide every detail pertaining to your topic. ■ Talk from notes; do not read from notes. ■ Use humor, stories, analogies, or metaphors to make a point. ■ If appropriate, move from behind the podium to engage the audience. ■ Use appropriate audiovisuals. ■ Provide a change of pace in longer presentations; combine strategies. ■ Provide 15-minute breaks if the lecture is longer than 20 minutes.	■ Repeating phrases or expressions such as "umm" or "you know" ■ Turning your back on the audience ■ Reading from notes ■ Talking down to the audience

(continues)

Table 11-1 Suggestions for the Lecturer   *(continued)*

Stage of Lecture Preparation	Suggestions	Avoid
Giving the presentation (conclusion)	■ Stay within the allotted time. ■ Review the key points and emphasize practical learning aspects. ■ Provide the opportunity for learners to ask questions if time allows. ■ Admit when you do not know an answer. ■ Thank the audience for their attention.	■ Stopping abruptly and leaving the podium ■ Speaking longer than the specified time

within 1 day (Woodring & Woodring, 2007). A modification of the lecture strategy that addresses the disadvantages is the interactive lecture, in which the nurse gives clients something to do during the lecture. This strategy includes segments of lecture combined with segments in which clients are interacting with each other and the teacher. An example is a lecture followed by clients answering questions using clickers, or clients interacting in pairs or small groups to answer questions.

Guest Lecture

Guest lecturers are a good choice for teacher-directed learning because they provide role models with whom clients can identify. An example of an appropriate guest speaker is to invite a person who has quit smoking to talk with a group of clients who are trying to stop smoking. The testimony of a guest lecturer can have a powerful effect on clients and be a source of motivation. It should be noted that guest lecturers can be invited into online environments as well. Some important aspects of the guest lecturer strategy are as follows:

- The guest lecturer should be chosen carefully and be fully informed of the learning objectives they are expected to cover.
- If possible, attend a presentation, or talk with someone who has attended a presentation, by the guest lecturer to determine if the presentation is appropriate.
- Provide the guest lecturer with exact information about time, place, and location, including the URL for online sessions. Plan to have someone meet or call the guest lecturer to orient the person to the learning format or venue.
- Check with the guest lecturer to identify what equipment, special tools, and web links will be needed.

Lecture with Discussion and Questions and Answers

A lecture is most effective when used with a discussion that involves clients. Discussion is a two-way verbal interaction that involves talking, listening, asking questions, and answering questions. The discussion strategy is sometimes referred to as *teach back* when it encourages the client to verbalize what was learned. The use of discussion or an exchange of points of view helps clients become active participants in the learning process. This strategy is a good choice when clients have previous experience with a subject and have information to share. It promotes understanding and application of knowledge. It also fosters the development of desirable attitudes (Bucher & Kotecki, 2014; Rankin et al., 2005).

There are several different types of discussions. Open discussions occur when clients determine the topic, and the role of the nurse is to ask questions that lead learners to consider various ideas. With this format, the nurse needs to define terms and encourage different points of view. Planned discussion occurs when the nurse determines the content of the discussion, plans questions in advance, and guides clients toward a predetermined goal or conclusion. Formal debate is a type of discussion in which clients present opposing viewpoints, usually in a structured format.

Nurses play a big part in the discussion strategy by choosing the type of discussion and forming focus questions that guide clients toward the learning outcomes that are the focus of the lesson. *Questions* serve many purposes in the teaching and learning process. They help to assess what clients already know, stimulate interest in a new topic, discern whether or not clients grasped the main points, explore ideas, and promote higher levels of thinking. It is important to prepare questions ahead of time and modify them as needed.

As the teacher, you shape the discussion by the manner in which contributions are treated. If clients feel that their contributions are valued and used, they experience the freedom to express themselves. Do not dominate the discussion; use the time to identify and correct inaccurate information and guide the discussion. Encourage participation by all clients; do not let the conversation be dominated by a few group members. It is important to maintain a nonthreatening environment that encourages informal sharing. A disadvantage is that this strategy takes more time, depending on the topic and the number of participants.

An important skill is the ability to manage the discussion and facilitate learning. This requires thought and preparation. The first task in leading a discussion is to get the discussion started. It is often helpful to begin by reviewing the objectives of the session with the group. Another approach is to summarize past information and then ask group members their opinions. Sometimes a skilled teacher will make a controversial statement to stimulate the group's participation. After the discussion is in progress, there are several ways to keep it on track by focusing, refocusing, changing the focus, and recapping what has been said (deTornyay & Thompson, 1982).

Focusing is keeping the group discussion centered on the learning objectives. One way to focus the group is to ask questions that specifically direct the group's attention to the point or points you wish to make. This can be done by asking open-ended questions, such as "What do you find is the most interesting part of . . ."

Refocusing is getting the group discussion back on the topic when it has strayed from the original topic. Sometimes groups bring interesting but irrelevant information into the discussion. You can refocus the group by saying something such as, "Let's get back to our topic." There may be times the group has deviated from the topic and you must choose whether or not to refocus the discussion. This is a judgment call because the new topic may be important to discuss. Group members may need to deal with the new topic before they can focus on anything else. When a group has discussed a topic sufficiently and no new information or ideas are forthcoming, then it is time to change the focus of the discussion. You might say, "Now that we've discussed the . . . let us examine another aspect of . . ." Recapping is summarizing the discussion to help clients see relationships and draw conclusions.

Using Questions as a Teaching Strategy

Questioning is a useful teaching strategy to stimulate thinking. Types of questions that are useful in client education are remembering/factual, understanding/describing, clarifying, and higher order. Remembering/factual questions begin with words such as who, what, where, or when. For example, "What is the normal range for blood pressure?" Understanding/describing questions require clients to organize their thoughts in a logical relationship and respond with a longer answer. For example, "Describe the signs and symptoms of insulin shock." Clarifying questions help clients clarify an idea based on their own statements and go beyond a superficial response. For example, "I don't quite understand what you mean; please tell me more."

Higher-order questions help clients think critically and require considerable thought. They have a place in health education in group discussions and when working individually with clients who are confronted with complex health decisions. Higher-order questions help clients compare and contrast (find similarities and differences), analyze (examine the parts and elements), and evaluate (determine the value of) information. Examples of these types of questions are provided in **Table 11-2**.

Questions also prompt clients to examine their assumptions (a fact or statement taken for granted) and make inferences (drawing conclusions and deducing) (*Webster's*, 2013). A sample question to identify assumptions is, "Why must a surgery consent form be signed before your operation?" A sample question to make inferences is, "After reading this pamphlet about the risk of heart attacks in people with high cholesterol, what would you infer about the foods you usually eat?"

Clients often find themselves in situations where there are few right and wrong answers. They simply must make the best decision in difficult circumstances. There is a danger of not thinking

Table 11-2 Examples of Types of Questions

Sample Question	Type of Question
What is your . . . ?	Remembering/factual
Who is your . . . ?	Remembering/factual
Describe the signs of . . .	Understanding/describing
Describe how you do this at home . . .	Understanding/describing
Tell me what you mean when . . .	Clarifying
Describe how you . . .	Clarifying
How does . . . compare with . . . ?	Comparing/contrasting
How are . . . and . . . alike and different?	Comparing/contrasting
Give me an example of . . .	Applying
How will you manage . . . at home?	Applying
How would . . . work for you?	Analyzing
What can you infer from . . . ?	Analyzing
How does . . . relate to . . . ?	Synthesizing
How has your past experience . . . ?	Synthesizing
Which . . . will work best for you and why?	Evaluating
What are the pros and cons of . . . ?	Evaluating
How will you design . . . ?	Creating
How would you create . . . ?	Creating

critically about the consequences of these decisions (Browne & Keeley, 2007). Clients often hear contradictory opinions when they are under the care of specialists, and sorting through this information requires thought. As educators, encourage clients and their families to think through all aspects of a situation. For example, "Your family doctor and the surgeon told you different opinions about treatment. What are the pros and cons of each? What are the long-range results of having open-heart surgery or taking medication and changing your lifestyle?" **Table 11-2** can help you use questioning as a teaching strategy.

Problems with the Discussion Strategy

A disadvantage of the discussion strategy is that it requires additional time, depending on the topic and the number of participants. When using this strategy, you give up some control because you allow clients to share some of the leadership. At times, this means clients diverge on a topic that is very different from what you had in mind and you need to decide whether or not to refocus the group.

Another problem with the discussion strategy occurs if the participants lose interest. This is evident when they start side conversations, yawn, become restless, and look glassy eyed. At this point, you should consider changing your strategy. For instance, you could conduct a group activity and have the participants move their chairs into a new arrangement that is more appropriate for the activity. Or you could have everyone stand up and stretch or perhaps call for a 15-minute break. Another option is to change the topic of the discussion.

Other problems with the discussion strategy are nonparticipants, overparticipants, and rude participants. When the participants know each other and are comfortable being together, most clients will participate. If you have a very quiet nonparticipant in the group, you can encourage that person to speak up. For example, after some participants have commented, you can say, "What do some of the rest of you think about this?" It rarely helps to call on a specific participant unless the learning objective is to learn to be verbally assertive. Keep the environment welcoming, and usually quiet people will eventually share their thoughts.

Handling an overly talkative participant can be a challenge. This is a client who is outgoing, has lots of ideas, and likes to talk. There are several ways to handle this situation. For example, you can say to the overparticipant, "That is a great idea. Now, what do some of the rest of you think?" or "Do you all agree with . . .?" or "Does . . . speak for all of you?" It helps when you look away from the overparticipant and look at other members of the group. If the overparticipant continues to talk, you can say, "Now I'd like to hear from some others in the group." If the person persists, you may need to have a private conversation with the person away from the group. This is also true for a rude participant.

Demonstration and Return Demonstration

Demonstration is performing a practical activity to teach skills. It is also called the show-back method, which asks clients to verbalize and demonstrate what they learned from the nurse educator. This strategy requires that clients have an adequate sense of sight and manual dexterity. Demonstration is useful for cognitive and psychomotor learning (Bucher & Kotecki, 2014; Rankin et al., 2005). An example of the demonstration strategy is teaching child care skills to parents of an ill child. Demonstration can be done in person or by video. It involves a single client or small or large groups.

Begin by informing the clients about the learning objectives and the purpose of the demonstration. It is important for you to understand the procedure before attempting to perform it for others. Gather the essential equipment at the beginning of the demonstration to avoid fumbling and false starts when your clients are present. Be sure that all clients are positioned so they can see the demonstration and hear your comments. Provide a running commentary throughout the demonstration to focus the attention of clients on the relevant components. If possible, hold the demonstration in the actual place where clients will carry out the procedure. Clarify and repeat your demonstration as needed; then have each client return the demonstration. Be sure to define unfamiliar terms and have a discussion period after the demonstration to answer questions. The entire process should last no more than 15 to 20 minutes. If clients are learning motor skills, provide time for clients to practice as soon as possible after the demonstration. **Table 11-3** reviews the steps to follow when performing a demonstration.

Team Teaching

Team teaching occurs when two or more teachers with different preparation, abilities, and skills cooperate and share with one another the responsibilities for planning, teaching, and evaluating client learning. In team teaching, teachers combine their strengths to make the presentation stronger. Refer to the guidelines for effective team teaching found in **Box 11-1**.

Table 11-3 Demonstration Guidelines

Phase	Guidelines
Predemonstration phase	■ Assess client needs. ■ Identify learning objectives. ■ Become familiar with the procedure. ■ Choose the location. ■ Gather essential equipment and supplies.
Demonstration phase	■ Inform clients of objectives and purpose. ■ Define unfamiliar terms. ■ Be sure clients can see and hear. ■ Give commentary about the procedure. ■ Clarify and repeat as needed.
Postdemonstration phase	■ Provide time for discussion and questions. ■ Limit time to 20 minutes. ■ Provide time for practice as soon as possible.

Box 11-1 Guidelines for Effective Team Teaching

1. All team members participate in formulation of the objectives.
2. All team members contribute to the specific planning of each member's presentation.
3. All team members should be conversant with the specific plans of the other team members.
4. All team members should carry on teaching functions in the presence of others whose roles might be to assist, observe client reactions, and offer constructive criticism in subsequent discussion.
5. All team members participate in periodic evaluation of the class.
6. Conflicts should be viewed as opportunities for growth. They should be addressed before the team encounters the clients.

Teacher-Facilitated Strategies

Teacher-facilitated strategies are a bridge between teacher-directed strategies and learner-directed strategies. The teacher takes the role of facilitator rather than directing the process of learning. The strategies in this group include group activities and teaching, role-play, simulation, and web-based delivery of health education.

Group Activities and Teaching

Teaching in groups occurs when two or more clients work together on an activity. All approaches to group work have the distinguishing feature that clients are working together without direct intervention by the teacher at least some of the time (Killen, 2000). The principal reason to use this teaching strategy is to offer greater active learning opportunities. Cognitive and affective learning objectives are addressed through group activities. Community-based group interventions offer a cost-effective approach to developing a network of social support based on principles of social learning theory to affect change (Todd et al., 2010). Some examples of situations in which group work might be an appropriate teaching strategy are as follows (Killen, 2000):

- When you want to increase clients' depth of understanding of the course content by having them explore it and discuss their understanding with other learners
- When you want clients to exchange ideas and learn from one another by exploring issues from many perspectives, such as with parent education interventions
- When you want to enhance clients' motivation and increase their active participation in learning

You facilitate the group process by making the learning objectives clear and explaining the directions for the group activities. You should also develop guidelines to help clients participate productively in the group process. Some disadvantages of group activities and teaching are that clients who are accustomed to teacher-directed strategies may have difficulty changing their expectations. Some clients may find the activities a waste of time. Also, you may find it difficult to assess individual clients fairly when they have worked within a group. Group work requires preparation and an adequate room arrangement to accommodate the planned activities. High-ability learners may lose their incentive to learn when placed in mixed-ability groups (Curry, as cited in Killen, 2000).

Nurse educators may need to plan for teaching a group of people. Interested groups are found in hospitals, long-term care and assisted-living facilities, schools, worksites, and community settings. We recommend that nurse educators review teaching priorities, goals, objectives, and content with a representative at the facility before the presentation. Careful assessment of the educational needs and communication with a representative at the facility will help bring about a successful educational offering. See **Table 11-4**.

Role-Play

In *role-play*, clients act out their own situation or that of another person. Role-playing requires maturity, confidence, and flexibility on the part of clients. This strategy is effective in meeting cognitive, affective, and psychomotor learning objectives. It is most often used when clients need to examine their attitudes and behaviors, when they need to understand the viewpoints and attitudes of others, and when they need to practice carrying out ideas or decisions. For example, a

Table 11-4 Strategies for Teaching Groups

Assessment Steps	Action Steps
Identify the educational need	1. Assess group members' perceptions and knowledge base through surveys and focus groups. 2. Examine and clarify educational needs.
Identify group characteristics	1. Determine the group size. 2. Determine the group's educational level. 3. Determine the group's pertinent cultural aspects. 4. Determine the group's other pertinent characteristics.
Identify current evidence-based practice research	1. Review the literature for evidence-based research on the topic. 2. Evaluate the current evidence-based practice research that is applicable to the educational need.
Identify goals, objectives, and content	1. Formulate goals and objectives based on educational need. 2. Prepare a content outline.
Determine facility support	1. Does the facility agree with the educational need? 2. Does the facility support the content you are proposing in the educational offering? 3. Will the facility provide space and resources for the educational offering? 4. Are facilities and resources available to hold the class? 5. Does the facility have a plan to ensure that group members can participate in the educational offering?

parent may want to rehearse how they will talk to a son or daughter about drug use (Bucher & Kotecki, 2014).

Assertiveness training is an example of a situation in which role-playing works well. Your role is that of facilitator; you give instructions and provide time for feedback and evaluation. It is important to remember that this strategy takes extra time, and some clients may feel uncomfortable and inhibited with this method.

Simulation

A major challenge for nurse educators is to coordinate theory and practice when teaching nursing. An educational technique that accomplishes this goal is simulation. Simulation uses technology to replace or enhance real experiences with guided practice that replicates real-world situations in an interactive manner (Gaba, 2004). A simulator is a "device" that mimics a real patient or a part of the human body, and that is capable of interaction with the learner (Gaba, 2004). A simulated event helps to develop different scenarios requiring the use of both clinical skills and critical thinking skills by nurses, in order to solve problems (see **Figure 11-1**). Participation in simulation allows students to learn skills, develop clinical reasoning abilities, and to become competent in caring for patients and families in a safe environment. An advantage of simulation is that students can practice skills confidently without the concern of making errors in patient care.

Reasons for the need for simulation are the nursing shortage, fewer nurse educators, and the decrease in number of clinical sites (American Colleges of Nursing, 2017). Simulation is increasingly needed to fill required clinical hours. Research shows simulation-based learning is effective

Figure 11-1 Simulation in a Learning Situation
© Tyler Olson/Shutterstock

Table 11-5 Kolb's Theory Applied to Simulation Activity

Kolb's Steps	Simulation Activity
Concrete experience	■ Engage in the simulation ■ Care for the simulated patient
Reflective observation	■ Debrief and reflect on performance ■ Identify gaps in care
Abstract conceptualization	■ Facilitator creates new mental models ■ Learning occurs
Active experimentation	■ New clinical situations arise ■ Incorporate learning into practice

in supporting student learning. A study conducted by the National Council of State Boards of Nursing (NCSBN) was a randomized, controlled trial looking at the effectiveness of simulation. It showed students who had either 25% or 50% of their hours replaced with simulation had no difference in NCLEX pass rates or end-of-program educational outcomes (Hayden, Smiley, Alexander, Kardong-Edgren, & Jeffries, 2014).

Kolb's Experiential Learning Theory (Kolb, 1984), introduced in Chapter 2, serves as a foundational theory for simulation. The four steps of Kolb's theory include concrete experience, reflective observation, abstract conceptualization, and active experimentation. **Table 11-5** describes Kolb's theory applied to simulation activity.

Box 11-2 Criteria for a Standard Debriefing

1. It should be conducted by an authorized individual.
2. It should be conducted in a learning and supportive environment with reliable, open communication, allowing self-assessment, feedback, and reflective thinking.
3. It should be facilitated by individuals who can effectively manage the duration of the simulation.
4. It should be based on a theoretical purpose-driven framework.
5. It should be consistent with the goals and learning outcomes of the simulation-based experience.

Data from INACSL Standards Committee. (2016). INACSL standards of best practice: SimulationSM simulation design. *Clinical Simulation in Nursing, 12*(Supplement), S5–S12. https://doi.org/10.1016/j.ecns.2016.09.005

When applying Kolb's Theory to simulation, an essential part of the reflective stage is debriefing. "Debriefing" is an activity that follows a simulation experience led by a facilitator who encourages participants' reflective thinking (Sahin, & Basak, 2021). It is at this stage that facilitators provide feedback to students regarding performance. This requires an experienced and knowledgeable facilitator. With feedback and new mental models gained in the debriefing, it is proposed that students incorporate the new learning into future nursing practice. **Box 11-2** lists the criteria for a standard debriefing as defined by the International Nursing Association for Clinical Simulation and Learning (INACSL) Standards Committee (2016).

There are a variety of simulators and different simulation methods. The most common methods utilize role-play, computerized mannequins, standardized or simulated patients, and virtual simulations (Galloway, 2009). Although a sophisticated, computerized mannequin can produce a high-fidelity simulation, so can an actor who is playing a role. "Fidelity" refers to realism or the ability to replicate the real "thing" that the simulator or actor is representing (Abersold, 2018).

Types of Simulation and Benefits/Disadvantages

Simulation can be used in a variety of teaching situations. Undergraduate nursing programs integrate simulation into the curriculum to support student learning in pediatrics, maternal health, mental health, medical surgical nursing, and leadership. Simulation is increasingly used by continuing education and in-service educators for staff development and to improve nurse expertise as they move into new settings. Other health-related areas that use simulation include end-of-life care, recognition and response to the rapidly deteriorating patient, and mass causality training (Aebersold, 2018). An innovative use of simulation is that of teamwork training where multiple providers train and collaborate together. Virtual simulations are used in multiple healthcare settings to assess competency. The use of simulation is predicted to continue to expand in years to come. See **Table 11-6** for a description of common types of simulation methods, including the benefits and disadvantages of each.

We know it is imperative that new and present nurse educators be prepared to be active participants in simulation. This involves understanding what simulation is, how it is administered, and how faculty are adequately trained. As a nurse educator that seeks employment at an organization in either an academic, community, or hospital setting, you should be prepared to ask specific questions about your anticipated role in simulation. Questions to ask are included in **Box 11-3** based on the National Council of State Boards of Nursing (NCSBN)

Table 11-6 Common Types of Simulation Methods

Types	Description	Benefits/Disadvantages
Role-play	Learners act out a close replication of real-life, human clinical situations to help students react as they would in a real-life clinical situation.	Low-cost low fidelity good for team training and changes in attitude.
Computerized mannequins	Integrated simulators are whole-body mannequins (adult, child, or infant) with technology to respond in real time to care interventions and treatments.	High degrees of realism, Fidelity can range from low to high with cost rising as the fidelity increases. Can be used in complex situations that involves teams.
Standardized or simulated patients	Standardized patients are actors that use a script to present real-life situations that require communication and clinical skills.	Helps students gain personal awareness and clinical strengths. Disadvantages are recurring cost and rescheduling of actors.
Virtual simulations	Re-creation of reality depicted on a computer screen. Can be used to evaluate learning by using decision- making, motor control, and communication skills	Improves knowledge retention and clinical reasoning and increases the satisfaction with learning. High cost.

Box 11-3 Questions to Ask about Simulation Programs

- Is there commitment to budgetary support and provision of adequate facilities for the simulation program?
- Are there objectives for integrating simulation into the curriculum and evaluating the simulation program?
- Are there adequate qualified personnel to conduct simulation who were trained using International Nursing Association of Clinical Simulation and Learning (INACSL) Standards?
- Does the program provide a means for faculty to be oriented and trained in simulation?
- Is ongoing simulation education provided, such as webinars, conferences, journal group discussions, readings, and certifications such as Certified Healthcare Simulation Educator (CHSE)?

Data from Alexander, M., Durham, C. F., Hooper, J. I., Jeffries, P. R., Goldman, N., Kardong-Edgren, S. "Suzie," Kesten, K. S., Spector, N., Tagliareni, E., Radtke, B., & Tillman, C. (2015). NCSBN simulation guidelines for prelicensure nursing programs. Journal of Nursing Regulation, 6(3), 39–42. https://doi-org.dml.regis.edu/10.1016/S2155-8256(15)30783-3

Simulation Guidelines (2017). Alexander, M., Durham, C. F., Hooper, J. I., Jeffries, P. R., Goldman, N., Kardong-Edgren, S. "Suzie," Kesten, K. S., Spector, N., Tagliareni, E., Radtke, B., & Tillman, C. (2015).

The role of an educator in simulation is different from being a traditional educator. Faculty in the simulation role need to learn to effectively design, facilitate, and debrief simulation-based experiences. Nurse educators can seek out simulation preparation courses available to nurse educators that use International Nursing Association for Clinical Simulation and Learning (INACSL) Standards of Best Practice (INACSL Standards of Best Practice, 2016).

A nurse educator may apply to take the Certified Healthcare Simulation Educator (CHSE) exam to become certified if they demonstrate meeting the following criteria (Handbook for the Certification Process, 2021):

- Participate in healthcare simulation in an educational role.
- Demonstrate focused simulation expertise with learners in undergraduate, graduate, allied health, or healthcare practitioners.
- Possess a bachelor's degree or an equivalent combination of education and experience.
- Document 2 years continued use of simulation in healthcare education, research, or administration.

Educators play a significant role in the successful implementation of simulation programs. Teaching using simulation must be done as carefully as any other new teaching method. Poor facilitator preparation and poorly designed scenarios may result in negative learning. Teaching with simulation requires a careful, thoughtful approach to ensure success for both students and facilitators.

Web-Based Delivery of Health Education

Technology is changing the way health education is provided to clients because 81% of American adults now use the Internet (Fox, 2013). Web-based delivery of health education is a cooperative activity between the teacher and clients. The teacher is responsible for preparing the health education materials, facilitating periodic interaction with clients, and measuring learning outcomes. Clients engage with the health education materials at their own pace, interact with the teacher periodically, and participate in evaluation of their learning. Nurse educators are developing web-based health education programs for clients with diabetes literacy (Moussa, Sherrod, & Choi, 2013). Other educators have found web-based education effective for parent training (Breitenstein & Gross, 2013) and nutrition education (Neuenschwander, Abbott, & Mobley, 2013). Web-based health education programs are flexible, convenient, easy for clients to use, and more efficient in terms of cost and time for nurse educators.

Learner-Directed Strategies

Learner-directed strategies focus on clients as the initiators and designers of the learning process. These strategies include the use of e-health interactive tutorials, games, self-directed instruction (technology-assisted strategies and program instruction), and peer counseling groups.

E-health Interactive Tutorials

Many websites are available for clients to learn about health. Last year, 56% of American adults reported searching the Internet for health information (Fox, 2013). Many were looking for specific information for themselves or a family member. Excellent health tutorials can be found on MedlinePlus, a service of the U.S. National Library of Medicine, and the Mayo Clinic website. The abundance of web-based health information facilitates self-education for large segments of the population.

Many clients are health conscious and track health parameters and monitor their progress in achieving health-related goals. For example, 60% of adults track their weight, diet, or exercise routines, and 33% of adults track their blood pressure, blood sugar, headaches, or sleep patterns.

To track this information, 21% use some form of technology, such as a spreadsheet, a website, a device, or an app (Fox & Duggan, 2013). Teaching clients to track their health parameters helps motivate them by monitoring their progress in achieving their health goals.

In addition, 91% of adults report owning some kind of cell phone, 56% report their phone operates on a smartphone platform (Smith, 2013), and 60% access the Internet on their phone (Duggan, 2013). Multiple *health apps* are available for the iOS and Android platforms. For example, apps are offered by health organizations (such as Kaiser Permanente and Aetna), the Centers for Disease Control and Prevention, and commercial vendors (such as Lose It! and Weight Watchers for weight loss, and Strava and Fitbit for activity and calorie tracking). In addition to smartphones, tablet ownership has increased. According to Zickuhr (2013), 34% of adults now own a tablet computer such as an iPad, Samsung Galaxy Tab, Google Nexus, or Kindle Fire, all with Internet access to health information.

Games

A *game* is an organized, active competition or contest engaged in by players who act individually or collectively as a team. The objective of a game is winning. Rules define the method of play and the criteria for winning. Instructional games use a body of knowledge or set of skills that must be drawn on as resources. Games provide a pleasurable structure for providing information, testing the level and application of skills and knowledge, and offering practice in simulated situations. They are often used with pediatric patients for preoperative teaching that introduces them to hospital procedures, the environment, and the staff before surgery (Rankin et al., 2005). During a game, clients take a course of action and view the consequences in a nonthreatening way. Problem solving can be incorporated into the game. Clients should succeed, yet be challenged in the exercise. Gaming has become increasingly sophisticated. Players can adopt avatars that allow them to live in and interact with the virtual or game-based environment. Bauman (2012) believes that gaming can be used to enhance patient education. He describes a learning environment that has been specifically engineered to replicate actual existing environments that allow for "suspension of disbelief." This encourages clients to learn within a social context. Today's learners have an advanced degree of technical and digital literacy with expectations of how information should be disseminated, presented, and transferred. To engage these learners, consider virtual environments as a learning tool. Games may use flash cards, pictures, or computer applications. They may be modifications of popular games such as Bingo, Scrabble, or crossword puzzles. A benefit is that games can be inexpensive to purchase or make. Before introducing a game, evaluate its appropriateness for each specific client. An important aspect of games is that they should be entertaining because there is a clear relationship between learning and fun (Baranich & Currie, 2004).

Self-Directed Learning (Technology-Assisted Strategies and Programmed Instruction)

Self-directed learning is the process of clients engaging in learning activities that they, rather than the teacher, define (Schmidt, 2000). Clients who use this strategy identify their learning needs, formulate goals, identify resources, select and implement learning strategies, and evaluate learning outcomes. Clients demonstrate the initiative and consciously accept responsibility for their own learning. This involves searching out information and resources. Clients focus on information gathering. When used effectively, this strategy has many advantages over teaching-directed strategies. Some of the advantages of this strategy are as follows (Killen, 2000):

- It encourages clients to ask questions and investigate, discover, and create answers for themselves, rather than waiting for someone to provide answers for them.
- It enables clients to develop a deeper level of understanding of the subject than would be possible if other teaching strategies, such as lectures, were used.
- It shows clients that their existing knowledge is valuable and can form the basis for future learning.

Clients use this strategy when they access the Internet and resource centers in libraries and hospitals to find information about health and illness. Personal computer competency is a necessary skill for clients who want to search online. They need to be taught how to identify reliable and accurate information. Encourage them to use websites from the government, universities, or reputable medical or health associations.

Programmed instruction is another self-directed learning strategy that comes prepackaged from a book or computer software company. All the steps necessary to systematically learn the information are presented sequentially. The information is broken into small steps called frames. Clients are required to make frequent responses as they work through the information. Immediate feedback is given about the correctness or accuracy of responses. Programmed instruction is particularly useful for clients who are independent learners and who learn better when they have no time constraints.

Peer Counseling

Peer counseling is a self-help activity that is learner directed. The members of a peer counseling group provide support for one another by giving information, sharing experiences, and accepting and understanding each other. Peer counseling also provides useful suggestions about a problem or concern. Support groups help clients improve their coping skills, provide motivation to get further help, or take a more active role in their treatment. Participation gives clients hope and the knowledge that they are not alone. Peer counseling groups exist for clients with virtually all health-related problems, such as cancer, diabetes, and disabilities. You can refer clients or family members to a peer counseling group to help with follow-up care after initial treatment. Research indicates that attending support groups is beneficial. Studies indicate that clients who participate in support groups, in addition to their medical treatments, report less anxiety and depression and live longer than those who did not attend (Campbell, Phaneuf, & Deane, 2004). It is speculated that having the social support of others in the group boosts the immune system by reducing anxiety and psychological stress. Support groups take place in person, on the Internet, or by phone. Peer counseling helps clients connect with others who share the same problem. It helps people improve their coping skills, motivates them to get further help, or encourages them to take a more active role in treatment. Support groups give hope.

Selecting the Right Teaching Strategy

We now review important factors to take into consideration when selecting teaching strategies to implement the client education plan. There are many factors to consider, but the most important is to choose a strategy based on what you want clients to be able to do as a result of your teaching. To help you select appropriate teaching strategies, the following factors are briefly reviewed: the

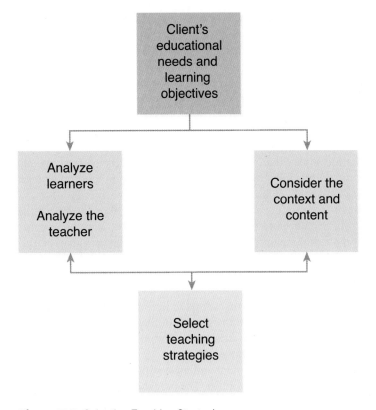

Figure 11-2 Selecting Teaching Strategies

client's educational needs and learning objectives, characteristics of the client and the teacher, the learning context, and the content to be taught. **Figure 11-2** illustrates these factors.

The first factor to consider in selecting teaching strategies is to *determine the client's educational needs and learning outcomes and objectives.* Carefully listen to what clients want to know and determine what they need to know. Determine their current health knowledge and if they have misinformation or a history of health problems. Consider readiness to learn, ability to learn, motivation to learn, and barriers to learning. Each of these impacts how you state the learning objectives and your choice of teaching strategies. Most client education plans have learning objectives in each of the three domains: cognitive, affective, and psychomotor. When you are clear about the client's expected learning objectives, appropriate teaching strategies can be considered. When choosing teaching strategies, it is important to consider whether the client has the necessary abilities, including intellectual, emotional, and physical, to learn the skill (Onega & Devers, 2008).

Keep in mind that the client's age, developmental stage, sensory impairments, educational background, nature of the illness, and culture should be taken into consideration. Teaching strategies should match the client's strengths and needs and help them reach the level of mastery you set for them. For example, a client with hearing loss does not respond well to a lecture format. A client with limited vision does not learn through the use of demonstration. Also consider the time frame available for teaching. Choose a strategy that allows you to achieve the objectives within the available time frame. If you need to present information as quickly as possible to a group, a lecture is the best choice.

The second factor to consider in selecting teaching strategies is the *characteristics of the client and the teacher*. Knowing clients' learning styles is particularly important when selecting teaching strategies. Learning styles are characteristic ways that clients perceive, interact with, and respond to their environment. They are the clients' preferred mode of gaining knowledge. Styles are *auditory* (through hearing), *visual* (through seeing), *kinesthetic* (through the whole body), or a combination of these. As the teacher, you should also be aware of your preferred teaching and learning styles. Your clients will achieve learning objectives more quickly if your teaching style is compatible with their learning style. Based on this information about styles, choose from the teacher-directed, teacher-facilitated, or learner-directed approaches. Selecting among these approaches is more complex than just choosing one. A variety of teaching strategies helps to maintain clients' attention and increases achievement. For example, supplement the lecture with a group activity (Kindsvatter, Wilen, & Ishler, 1988).

The third factor to consider in selecting teaching strategies is *the learning context*. Learning context refers to the circumstances surrounding teaching and learning and includes both the physical and psychological environment. The physical environment may be the hospital, long-term care or assisted-living facility, private home, school, work site, or community. Consider the need for privacy and how much space is needed. Ensuring privacy and minimizing extraneous noises and interruptions are important.

If you are teaching a group of clients using the lecture strategy, assess the physical environment. Arrive at the location ahead of time to confirm that the environment is adequate and the seating is sufficient, comfortable, and arranged to support learning. Environmental factors are important and affect client learning (Dunn, 1983).

The psychological context is important and must support the teaching strategies. Be actively involved in creating the psychological context. The psychological environment should be relaxed, nonthreatening, and inviting to clients. Maintain a respectful, warm, and enthusiastic attitude.

The fourth factor to consider in selecting teaching strategies is the *content to be learned*. Content is the basic information you want to teach. You should choose teaching strategies to facilitate the efficient and successful accomplishment of learning objectives. Your task is to structure learning experiences that encourage clients to think in particular ways about the things you want them to learn (Killen, 2000). Choose the simplest, clearest, and most succinct manner of presentation (Onega & Devers, 2008). Focus first on must-know content and save nice-to-know information if time allows. Be aware of and take into consideration the client's current knowledge and previous experiences related to the content. Emphasize the relevance of the content to the client's age and lifestyle. You will find that certain content lends itself to specific strategies. For example, children will respond well to teaching strategies that permit them to participate actively. Would a lecture be an appropriate strategy to teach hand washing to a class of 6-year-olds? Probably not. A hands-on demonstration better meets the needs of this group.

Schedule and pace learning according to the clients' needs and abilities. When giving information, use simple but accurate words. Avoid using medical jargon and periodically check for understanding and interpretation of the information. Avoid information overload; repetition helps to emphasize important points. Using more than one teaching strategy enhances learning. Written materials clarify information and give clients something to refer to at home. Verbal and written communication should complement each other (Falvo, 2011). Finally, remember that interactive teaching strategies are more effective than those that are not (Killen, 2000).

Table 11-7 lists the various teaching strategies and their learning domains and gives a description of each strategy.

Table 11-8 summarizes this information to help you choose strategies that fit the learning needs and objectives.

Table 11-7 Teaching Strategy, Learning Domain, and Description

Teaching Strategy	Learning Domain	Description
Teacher Directed		
Lecture	Cognitive	■ Teacher-directed content and pace ■ Feedback determined by teacher ■ Use with individuals or groups ■ Encourages retention of facts
One-on-one discussion	Affective Cognitive	■ Teacher-directed content and pace ■ Encourages participation by clients ■ Permits reinforcement and repetition at client's level ■ Supports introduction of sensitive subjects
Guest lecturer	Cognitive Affective	■ Teacher-directed content and pace ■ Modeling by an expert
Team teaching	Cognitive	■ Teacher-directed content and pace ■ Use with groups ■ Encourages retention of facts ■ Offers varied viewpoints ■ Members present based on their teaching strengths
Lecture with discussion and questions and answers	Cognitive Affective	■ Teacher controls most content and pace ■ Teacher must know the content and be prepared to answer questions ■ Use with individuals and groups ■ Teacher confirms understanding by asking questions
Demonstration	Cognitive Psychomotor	■ Teacher-directed content and pace ■ Modeling of skills and behaviors by teacher ■ Gives commentary with demonstration ■ Use with individuals and groups ■ Does not include hands-on experience
Demonstration, return demonstration, practice	Cognitive	■ Teacher-facilitated content and pace ■ Allows repetition and immediate feedback ■ Includes hands-on experience
Teacher Facilitated		
Group activities and discussion	Affective Cognitive	■ Teacher-facilitated content and pace ■ Clients obtain assistance from supportive group ■ Group members learn from one another
Role-playing	Affective Cognitive	■ Teacher-facilitated content and pace ■ Encourages expression of values, attitudes, and emotions ■ Assists in the development of communication skills ■ Involves active participation by client

(continues)

Table 11-7 Teaching Strategy, Learning Domain, and Description (continued)

Teaching Strategy	Learning Domain	Description
Simulation	Cognitive Affective Psychomotor	■ Teacher facilitated ■ Use with individuals and groups ■ Group members learn from one another ■ Encourages expression of values, attitudes, and emotions
Learner Directed		
Peer group	Affective Cognitive	■ Client directed ■ Support and modeling from clients with similar issues ■ Encourages expression of values, attitudes, and emotions
Games	Cognitive	■ Client directed ■ Permits reinforcement and repetition at client's level ■ Offers practice and application of skills ■ Fun, competitive ■ Individual or with a partner
Technology-assisted instruction	Cognitive	■ Client directed ■ Promotes individual initiative and responsibility for learning ■ Stimulates information gathering and questioning

Table 11-8 Teaching Strategies: Advantages and Disadvantages

Teaching Strategy	Advantages	Disadvantages
Lecture	■ Easy to organize ■ Predictable ■ Efficient ■ Good for large group ■ Allows teacher control	■ Lacks client feedback ■ Lacks client participation ■ Can create information overload
One-on-one individual instruction	■ Personalized attention ■ Provides basic knowledge ■ Immediate feedback ■ Clients can share confidential information ■ Adaptable to clients with low health-literacy skills, physical impairments, or emotional difficulties ■ Flexible and informal	■ Lack of sharing with and support from other clients and family ■ High cost in terms of staff time
Guest lecturer	■ Source of motivation ■ Role-modeling	■ May not follow learning objectives ■ May deviate from topic ■ May exceed the allotted time

Teaching Strategy	Advantages	Disadvantages
Lecture with discussion and questions and answers	■ Continual feedback ■ Attitude development and modification ■ Picks up confusion and helps resolve difficulties ■ Vehicle for clients to network with each other ■ Active learning process ■ Assess client's knowledge	■ Teacher can dominate the discussion ■ Takes more time ■ Nonparticipant ■ Overparticipant
Demonstration and return demonstration	■ Activates many senses ■ Clarifies the whys of principles ■ Correlates theory with practice ■ Commands interest	■ Takes a lot of time ■ Does not cover all aspects of cognitive learning ■ Must have adequate sight and manual dexterity ■ Practice is needed
Team teaching	■ Enhances teaching by using competencies of more than one teacher ■ Allows teachers to learn from each other ■ Accentuates divergent points of view	■ Lacks continuity and internal consistency ■ Requires more planning time ■ Makes group processing slower ■ Forces teachers to give up autonomy
Group activities and teaching	■ Increases depth of client understanding ■ Encourages clients to exchange ideas ■ Clients learn from one another ■ Increases active participation and learning	■ Clients may find activities a waste of time ■ Clients may have difficulties changing their expectations ■ Requires increased preparation time ■ Adequate room accommodations are needed ■ Some learners lose interest in mixed-ability groups
Role-play	■ Helps examine attitudes and behaviors ■ Helps examine viewpoints of others ■ A way to practice carrying out ideas or decisions	■ Requires maturity, confidence, and flexibility from clients ■ May embarrass clients ■ Requires some self-disclosure
Simulation	■ Mimics clinical situations ■ Requires hands-on participation ■ Learning without fear of harming a real person ■ Beneficial in evaluating competencies ■ Promotes the greatest transfer of learning	■ The cost of mannequins and support technology ■ Scenarios have to be developed and carried out ■ Time consuming ■ Requires teachers who are familiar with the technology and process

(continues)

Table 11-8 Teaching Strategies: Advantages and Disadvantages *(continued)*

Teaching Strategy	Advantages	Disadvantages
Games	■ Fun ■ Challenging ■ Competitive ■ Active learning ■ Encourages problem solving ■ Relatively inexpensive ■ Application of knowledge	■ Makes achievement of outcomes difficult to assess ■ Some clients may not like them ■ Cost and development of games ■ Not effective for presenting information
Computer-assisted learning and programmed instruction	■ Allows clients to go at their own pace ■ Repeat a section at will ■ Breaks material down into manageable increments ■ Saves teacher time	■ Depends on motivation of learner ■ Does not account for unplanned feedback, which can distract clients
Peer counseling	■ Clients provide support for each other ■ Useful suggestions about a problem or concern ■ Helps clients improve coping skills ■ Provides motivation ■ Gives hope	■ Challenge is for clients to stay in contact with the group ■ Information may be incorrect ■ May not be suitable for all clients

Case Example: Mrs. Rosa Lopez

In this case example, we are supplementing the educational plan for Mrs. Rosa Lopez (from the Chapter 10 Case Example) by adding the teaching strategies, instructional materials, and evaluation sections. Refer to **Table 11-9** to see the updated educational plan. Additional information on instructional materials and evaluation can be found in the chapters on instructional materials and formative and summative evaluation. The learning outcome continues to be the focus of all the objectives, which is for Rosa to maintain control of her blood pressure. The cognitive objective, "The client will correctly verbally explain to the nurse from memory how excessive salt intake affects blood pressure," is to increase knowledge. Because our example is an individual client, we would use the strategy of one-to-one discussion to increase her knowledge about the relationship between excessive sodium intake and hypertension. Discussion is a useful strategy for assessing what the client already knows and building on that knowledge. We identify specific questions to ask her during the evaluation section to assess her understanding of hypertension and to determine if the outcome was met.

The affective objective is, "The client will choose to limit sodium intake by preparing a low-sodium dietary plan for 1 week." This objective looks to see willingness on the part of Rosa to make dietary changes. We note that Mrs. Lopez is at the valuing level, so we would have her think through the steps of how she will prepare a dietary plan and put it into effect. This is important because she is not only cooking for herself but also for her two children. Teaching strategies to encourage this behavior include a video and pamphlets that review the DASH diet. We would assess her willingness to make these dietary changes by reviewing the dietary plan she created.

Table 11-9 Sample Client Education Plan for Mrs. Rosa Lopez

Learning Outcome	Learning Objectives	Content Outline	Teaching Strategies and Instructional Materials	Time	Evaluation
Maintenance of client's blood pressure within normal limits	1. The client will correctly verbally explain to the nurse from memory how excessive salt intake affects blood pressure (cognitive).	1. Review factors that contribute to high blood pressure: • Family history • Overweight/obesity • Excessive alcohol intake • Inactive lifestyle/lack of exercise • A high-salt and/or a high-fat diet • High intake of caffeine • Smoking • Stress 2. Effect of Na/salt on blood pressure (BP): • A blood pressure of 140/90 or above is high. • The amount of salt has a direct effect on BP. • Salt makes the body hold water, which raises BP. • The more salt, the higher the BP. 3. Signs and symptoms of excess salt intake: • Thirst • Dehydration including dry mouth and skin, dizziness, sleepiness, constipation, and headache	1. One-on-one discussion 2. Practice reviewing the content with the instructor. 3. Instructional handout reviewing causes of hypertension and signs and symptoms of excess salt intake	15 min	One-on-one questioning by correctly answering: What is a normal BP? How does salt affect your BP? What are the signs and symptoms of excess salt intake?
	2. The client will choose to limit sodium intake by preparing a low-sodium dietary plan for 1 week (affective).	Components of dietary plan for hypertension: 1. Explanation of the DASH diet a. Eat more fruits, vegetables, and low-fat dairy foods. b. Cut back on foods high in saturated fat, cholesterol, and trans fats. c. Eat more whole-grain foods, fish, poultry, and nuts. d. Limit sodium, sweets, sugary drinks, and red meats.	■ Technology-assisted instruction with use of video ■ One-on-one instruction reviewing a dietary plan using a DASH diet pamphlet	15 min	Observation of the written plan showing use of a low-sodium diet plan Verbalization of agreement with the plan

(continues)

Table 11-9 Sample Client Education Plan for Mrs. Rosa Lopez

(continued)

Learning Outcome	Learning Objectives	Content Outline	Teaching Strategies and Instructional Materials	Time	Evaluation

		1. Level of salt that can be consumed safely
		  a. 1,500 milligrams of sodium per day (about 2/3 teaspoon)
		2. Tips to decrease salt:
		  a. Remove shaker from table.
		  b. Instead of snacking on chips or sweets, eat unsalted pretzels or nuts, raisins, low-fat and fat-free yogurt, frozen yogurt, unsalted plain popcorn with no butter, and raw vegetables.
		  c. Read food labels to choose products that are lower in sodium.
		  d. No salt in cooking.
		  e. Avoid canned or processed foods that are high in sodium.
		  f. Use low-sodium seasonings, such as herbs and spices.			

	3. The client will demonstrate how to accurately obtain her own blood pressure using digital monitor without guidance from the nurse (psychomotor).	Techniques for obtaining blood pressure: 1. Read equipment directions. 2. Locate brachial artery. 3. Place arm in cuff. 4. Inflate cuff. 5. Release air in cuff. 6. Record findings.	■ Demonstration and return demonstration using checklist ■ Use of flip chart, models, and chart for recording	15 min	■ Return demonstration showing client's ability to take their own blood pressure accurately and record the findings

The psychomotor objective is, "The client will demonstrate how to accurately obtain her own blood pressure reading using digital monitor without guidance from the nurse." This objective is directed toward teaching the skill of using a digital blood pressure instrument. The strategy of demonstration and return demonstration would be used. Mrs. Lopez would refer to the checklist as the educator demonstrates how to take the blood pressure using the digital equipment. Mrs. Lopez would then perform a return demonstration and record the findings using the checklist to assess successful achievement of the outcome (Table 11-7). A column for time is included in the educational plan. It is important to have a comprehensive picture of the time allotted for implementing the client educational plan. Some aspects may require more time than others. Careful planning improves the chances of a successful outcome.

Summary

Teaching strategies involve much more than transmitting information. Teaching is the process of collaborating with clients to achieve learning outcomes and objectives. This chapter emphasized the importance of engaging clients in the teaching and learning process so they can benefit from the educational plan. The desired learning outcomes and objectives, characteristics of the client, the learning context, time, and the content must guide the choice of teaching strategies. When selecting teaching strategies, there are teacher-directed, teacher-facilitated, and learner-directed strategies from which to choose. Base your choice on the learning outcomes and objectives. Select instructional materials to complement your teaching strategies. It is important to vary your approach to instruction, keeping in mind that clients have different needs, abilities, and learning preferences.

Exercises
Exercise I: Choosing Learning Strategies

Purpose: Distinguish among teacher-directed, teacher-facilitated, and learner-directed teaching strategies.
Directions:

1. Make a list of various topics that require client health education.
2. Review the list and describe whether each topic should be addressed through teacher-directed, teacher-facilitated, or learner-directed teaching strategies.
3. Identify the specific type of teacher-directed, teacher-facilitated, or learner-directed teaching strategy you would use.
4. Discuss how each group member made their decision and why.

Exercise II: Develop and Implement a Client Education Plan

Purpose: Select appropriate strategies to teach a self-selected topic.
Directions:

1. Divide into groups of five or six members.
2. Identify topics about which each member wants to know more.

3. Each member should choose a topic and then independently do the following:
   a. Identify the learning outcome, and then prepare three learning objectives, one in each domain (cognitive, affective, and psychomotor), using the ABCD method.
   b. Prepare a client education plan that includes learning outcome, objectives, content outline, teaching strategies and instructional materials, time, and evaluation.
4. Have each member give a 15-minute presentation of the client education plan.
5. Share and reflect on the experience of presenting your educational plan.

Exercise III: Evidence-Based Nursing Practice

Purpose: Apply evidence-based nursing research to client education.
Directions:

1. Search the literature for nursing research applicable to health education strategies.
2. Describe how the findings could be applied to educating clients in your practice.

References

Aebersold, M., (2018). Simulation-based learning: No longer a novelty in undergraduate education. *OJIN: The Online Journal of Issues in Nursing, 23*(2).

Alexander, M., Durham, C. F., Hooper, J. I., Jeffries, P. R., Goldman, N., Kardong-Edgren, S. "Suzie," Kesten, K. S., Spector, N., Tagliareni, E., Radtke, B., & Tillman, C. (2015). NCSBN simulation guidelines for prelicensure nursing programs. *Journal of Nursing Regulation, 6*(3), 39–42. https://doi-org.dml.regis.edu/10.1016/S2155-8256(15)30783-3

American Association of Colleges of Nursing. (2017). *Fact sheet: Nursing shortage.* Retrieved from http://www.aacnnursing.org/Portals/42/News/Factsheets/Nursing-Shortage-Factsheet-2017.pdf?ver=2017-10-18-144118-163

Baranich, K. L., & Currie, C. C. (2004, September/October). Using games to teach motivate and engage. *The Games Journal*, 6–9.

Bauman, E. B. (2012). *Game-based teaching and simulation in nursing and healthcare.* New York, NY: Springer.

Beyea, S., & Kobokovich, L. (2004). Human patient simulation: A teaching strategy. *AORN Journal, 8*(4), 738–742.

Breitenstein, S. M., & Gross, D. (2013). Web-based delivery of a preventive parent training intervention: A feasibility study. *Journal of Child and Adolescent Psychiatric Nursing, 26*, 149–157.

Browne, M. N., & Keeley, S. M. (2007). *Asking the right questions: A guide to critical thinking* (8th ed.). Upper Saddle River, NJ: Pearson Prentice Hall.

Bucher, L., & Kotecki, C. N. (2014). Patient and caregiver teaching. In S. L. Lewis, S. R. Dirksen, M. M. Heitkemper, & L. Bucher (Eds.), *Medical-surgical nursing: Assessment and management of clinical problems* (9th ed., pp. 47–60). St. Louis, MO: Elsevier Mosby.

Campbell, H. S., Phaneuf, M. R., & Deane, K. (2004). Cancer peer support programs: Do they work? *Patient Education and Counseling, 55*(1), 3–15.

deTornyay, R., & Thompson, M. A. (1982). *Strategies for teaching nursing.* New York, NY: John Wiley and Sons.

Diener, E., & Hobbs, N. (2012). Simulated care: Technology-mediated learning in twenty-first century nursing education. *Nursing Forum, 46*(1), 34–38.

Duggan, M. (2013). *Cell phone activities 2013.* Retrieved from http://www.pewinternet.org/Reports/2013/Cell-Activities.aspx

Dunn, R. (1983). Can students identify their own learning styles? *Educational Leadership, 40*(5), 60–62.

Falvo, D. R. (2011). *Effective patient education: A guide to increased adherence* (4th ed.). Sudbury, MA: Jones & Bartlett Learning.

Fox, S. (2013). *Health online 2013.* Retrieved from http://www.pewinternet.org/Reports/2013/Health-online.aspx

Fox, S., & Duggan, M. (2013). *Tracking for health.* Retrieved from http://www.pewinternet.org/Reports/2013/Tracking-for-Health.aspx

Gaba D. M. (2004). The future vision of simulation in health care. *Quality & safety in health care, 13*(Suppl 1), i2–i10. https://doi-org.dml.regis.edu/10.1136/qhc.13.suppl_1.i2

Galloway, S. J., (2009). Simulation techniques to bridge the gap between novice and competent healthcare professionals. *OJIN: The Online Journal of Issues in Nursing, 14*(2), Manuscript 3.

Handbook for the Certification Process from the SSH Council for Certification (2021). Society for Simulation in Healthcare. Retrieved on June 14, 2023, from https://www.ssih.org/Certification/CHSE/Handbook

Hayden, J. K., Smiley, R. A., Alexander, M., Kardong-Edgren, S., & Jeffries, P. R. (2014). Supplement: The NCSBN National Simulation Study: A longitudinal, randomized, controlled study replacing clinical hours with simulation in prelicensure nursing education. *Journal of Nursing Regulation, 5*(2), C1-S64.

INACSL Standards Committee. (2016). INACSL standards of best practice: SimulationSM Debriefing. *Clinical Simulation in Nursing, 12*(S), 21–25.

INACSL Standards Committee. (2016, December). INACSL standards of best practice: Simulation^SM Simulation design. *Clinical Simulation in Nursing,* 12(S), S5-S12. http://dx.doi.org/10.1016/ j.ecns.2016.09.005.

Killen, R. (2000). *Effective teaching strategies: Lessons from research and practice* (4th ed.). Lansdowne, South Africa: Juta.

Kindsvatter, R., Wilen, W., & Ishler, M. (1988). *Dynamics of effective teaching.* New York, NY: Longman.

Kolb, D. A. (1984). *Experiential learning.* Englewood Cliffs, NJ: Prentice Hall.

Koukourikos, K., Tsaloglidou, A., Kourkouta, L., Papathanasiou, I. V., Iliadis, C., Fratzana, A., & Panagiotou, A. (2021). Simulation in Clinical Nursing Education. *Acta informatica medica: AIM: Journal of the Society for Medical Informatics of Bosnia & Herzegovina: casopis Drustva za medicinsku informatiku BiH, 29*(1), 15–20. https://doi.org/10.5455 /aim.2021.29.15-20

Lowenstein, A., & Reeder, J. A. (2009). Making learning stick. In A. Lowenstein, L. Foord-May, & J. C. Romano (Eds.), *Teaching strategies for health education and health promotion: Working with patients, families, and communities* (pp. 151–177). Sudbury, MA: Jones & Bartlett Learning.

Moussa, M., Sherrod, D., & Choi, J. (2013). An e-health intervention for increasing diabetes knowledge in African Americans [Suppl. 3]. *International Journal of Nursing Practice, 19*, 36–43.

Neuenschwander, L. M., Abbott, A., & Mobley, A. R. (2013). Comparison of a web-based vs in-person nutrition education program for low-income adults. *Journal of the Academy of Nutrition and Dietetics, 113*(1), 120–126.

Onega, L. L., & Devers, E. (2008). Health education and group process. In M. Stanhope & J. Lancaster (Eds.), *Public health nursing: Population-centered health care in the community* (2nd ed., pp. 290–315). St. Louis, MO: Mosby Elsevier.

Rankin, S. H., Stallings, K. D., & London, F. (2005). *Patient education in health and illness* (5th ed.). Philadelphia, PA: Lippincott Williams & Wilkins.

Rogove, H. J., McArthur, D., Demaerschalk, B. M., & Vespa, P. M. (2012). Barriers to telemedicine: Survey of current users in acute care units. *Telemedicine and e-Health, 18*(1), 48–53.

Romano, J. C. (2009). Teaching on the fly. In A. F. Lowenstein, L. Foord-May, & J. C. Romano (Eds.), *Teaching strategies for health education and health promotion: Working with patients, families, and communities* (pp. 139–150). Sudbury, MA: Jones & Bartlett Learning.

Sahin, G., & Basak, T. (2021). Debriefing methods in simulation-based education. *Journal of Education and Research in Nursing, 18*(3), 341. https://doi-org.dml.regis.edu/10.5152/jern.2021.57431

Schmidt, H. G. (2000). Assumptions underlying self directed learning may be false. *Medical Education, 34*(4), 243–245.

Smith, A. (2013). *Smartphone ownership 2013.* Retrieved from https://www.pewresearch.org/internet/2013/06/05/smartphone -ownership-2013/

Steward-Gelinas, D., & Romano, J. (2009). Individualized instruction. In A. Lowenstein, L. Foord-May, & J. C. Romano (Eds.), *Teaching strategies for health education and health promotion: Working with patients, families, and communities* (pp. 117–128). Sudbury, MA: Jones & Bartlett Learning.

Tamura-Lis, W. (2013). Teach-back for quality education and patient safety. *Urologic Nursing, 33*(6), 267–271.

Todd, S., Bromely, J., Ioannou, K., Harrison, J., Mellor, C., Taylor, E., & Crabtree, E. (2010). Using group-based parent training interventions with parents of children with disabilities: A description of process, content and outcomes in clinical practice. *Child and Adolescent Mental Health, 15*(3), 171–175.

Webster's All-in-One Dictionary & Thesaurus (2nd ed.). (2013). Springfield, MA: Federal Street Press.

Woodring, B. C., & Woodring, R. C. (2007). Lecture is not a four-letter word. In M. J. Bradshaw & A. J. Lowenstein (Eds.), *Innovative teaching strategies in nursing and related health professions* (4th ed., pp. 109–130). Sudbury, MA: Jones & Bartlett Learning.

Zickuhr, K. (2013). *Tablet ownership 2013.* Retrieved from https://www.pewresearch.org/internet/2013/06/10/tablet -ownership-2013/

CHAPTER 12

Instructional Materials

OBJECTIVES

Upon completion of this chapter, you will be able to do the following:

- State at least two purposes of instructional materials.
- Describe the importance of health literacy in evaluating instructional materials.
- Evaluate the readability and appropriateness of selected health education materials.
- Identify reliable sources for obtaining health-related pamphlets and brochures.
- List five criteria for evaluating the accuracy and reliability of websites.
- Critique the advantages and disadvantages of at least 10 types of media.

CHAPTER OUTLINE

Introduction

The purpose of instructional materials is to convey information. This chapter examines a number of instructional materials that supplement your teaching strategies to achieve the learning objectives. Underlying instructional materials is the assumption that the source of the information is both reliable and accurate.

Multiple sources of information are widely available in today's rich media environment that includes the traditional media outlets and social media platforms. While much accurate information is available, clients are often exposed to information that is false, inaccurate, or misleading. The consequences of the latter resulted in vaccine hesitancy/resistance/refusal, rejecting face masks and physical distancing, and using unproven treatments. As a trusted professional, your challenge is to distinguish between misinformation and disinformation.

The U.S. Surgeon General (2001) defined *misinformation* as "information that is false, inaccurate, or misleading according to the best available evidence at the time." It is not intentionally focused on misleading others. *Disinformation* is defined as information that is "created and spread with malicious intent" often with a financial motive. Both misinformation and disinformation spread rapidly during the COVID-19 pandemic. Nurses must be a reliable source of accurate, evidence-based information and curtail the spread of misinformation (Czerniak et al., 2023).

The recent COVID-19 pandemic revealed how serious a problem misinformation and disinformation became (Benoit & Mauldin, 2021). Vaccine usage became politicized as clients questioned the accuracy and validity of the statistics (Lewis, 2020). Nurses and other healthcare providers encountered clients who refused vaccinations believing they were harmful or even resulted in death. Some clients refused doctor-recommended treatments, preferring alternatives they read about in a disinformation source. Some clients simply distrust science and promote their own explanations for illness. Because people didn't know what to believe or the best source of reliable information, the consequences impacted vaccine acceptance, mask usage, physical distancing, and confidence in government.

Instructional materials are the actual matter or substance physically manipulated with the aim of promoting client learning. These materials are used by the teacher and the client. Instructional materials provide ways to use all senses to enhance learning. Some materials allow for the physical contact that kinesthetic learners need, whereas others enhance and reinforce cognitive knowledge. Still other materials invite emotional involvement, which is crucial for changing attitudes.

Instructional materials serve several purposes (Pohl, 1981). These purposes include extending the client's sensory experience, introducing variety into the teaching and learning process, giving meaning to abstractions, and making otherwise complicated explanations understandable. Pohl identified a number of factors to consider when determining which instructional materials to use. These factors include assessment of the topic being presented, the clients who are being addressed, and the available materials.

Instructional materials do not take the place of an effective teacher. Instructional materials enrich the learning experience of clients if they are appropriate to the learning objectives. Instructional materials must be carefully examined, evaluated, and selected on the basis of how they supplement the learning objectives to achieve the educational outcomes. The clinical judgment of nurses as educators is essential in this process.

Although instructional materials are available from a number of different sources, they may not be more effective than materials you develop yourself. By tapping into your creativity, you can develop materials that are specific to the health concerns of clients who are served by your employer or healthcare institution.

In this chapter, we discuss health literacy and examples of instructional materials such as print media, multimedia, and the Internet and World Wide Web (web). There are a variety of instructional materials available, and each has advantages and disadvantages for any specific teaching and learning situation. We discuss these advantages and disadvantages of selected materials, along with their purposes and helpful hints for using them.

Health Literacy

Health literacy is receiving increased attention by health professionals, and it has particular importance for nurses as educators. It is an important consideration in selecting instructional materials, especially printed materials given to clients in the form of pamphlets and handouts, and information downloaded from the Internet. To benefit from instructional materials, clients must be health literate, and nurse educators must be capable of assessing literacy and suitability of materials.

Literacy is defined as the ability to read and write (*Webster's*, 2013). Health literacy expands that definition by its focus on the client's abilities in the healthcare environment. The Patient Protection and Affordable Care Act (PPACA), Title V, defines health literacy as the degree to which an individual has the capacity to obtain, communicate, process, and understand basic health information and services to make appropriate health decisions (U.S. Government Publishing Office, 2010). The health literacy goal (HC/HIT-1) of Healthy People 2020 is to "improve the health literacy of the population." One of its subgoals (HC/HIT-1-1) is to "increase the proportion of persons who report their healthcare provider always gave them easy-to-understand instructions about what to do to take care of their illness or health condition" (HealthyPeople.gov, 2014).

A quick and accurate assessment tool called the Newest Vital Sign, introduced in Chapter 4, can determine a client's ability to read and apply information from a nutrition label. According to the National Assessment of Adult Literacy, in the United States in 2003, approximately 22% (47 million) of the population had basic health literacy skills, and 14% (30 million) had below-basic skills (National Center for Education Statistics [NCES], 2003). Combined, these groups represent 36% (77 million) of the population. Individuals in these groups have difficulty processing and understanding basic health information and services and making appropriate health decisions. According to Clancy (2008), those with basic or below-basic health literacy skills have now increased to almost 90 million. This latter figure is important and indicates a substantial health literacy problem that affects you in preparing client education plans.

Health literacy requires increased client engagement (McCormack et al., 2017) when you are teaching about medications, following treatment regimens, and preparing for diagnostic examinations. Health literacy is required for communicating with healthcare providers, describing symptoms, and understanding treatment recommendations. It is also required to critically evaluate newspaper and magazine advertisements and determine the credibility of information found on the Internet. It involves being able to fill out complex forms, understand insurance coverage, and navigate the healthcare system. It is fundamental to making informed decisions about promoting, retaining, and restoring health.

Low health literacy is observed across the demographic spectrum. However, it is more often seen in clients aged 65 years and older, clients with limited English-speaking skills, racial and ethnic minority populations, people with lower incomes, and clients who have not attended or completed high school (Mooney & Prins, 2013; NCES, 2003). It is easy to assume that clients who appear to be middle class, well groomed, and articulate are also health literate, but this is not always the case (Doak, Doak, & Root, 1996). Even clients who are well educated can have difficulty understanding health-related information. Consider a client with diabetes who does not understand how to use food exchanges, or a client on a fat-restricted diet who thinks pork is a white meat and is therefore low in fat.

Low health literacy has a financial impact. Clients with low literacy skills have poorer health outcomes and adhere less to medical recommendations than those with higher literacy skills. They have higher rates of hospitalization and use emergency services more, perhaps attributable to using fewer preventive and treatment services (Levy & Royne, 2009). The ramifications of low health literacy are particularly important in the treatment of clients with chronic illnesses who must manage their own health and implement lifestyle changes for success (Seligman et al., 2007).

Types of Instructional Materials

We are fortunate today to have an abundance of instructional materials to facilitate learning that appeal to all learning styles: *visual*, *auditory*, and *kinesthetic*. However, it is important to remember that they cannot substitute for good teaching. Instructional materials enrich and supplement the teaching and learning process. They do not replace the teacher. They help clients understand concepts and retain information when teachers use a variety of materials. Illustrations quickly bring to life concepts that may take many words to describe. A teacher is essential to assess client needs, develop the client education plan, provide guidance, answer questions, and evaluate teaching effectiveness. Take-home handouts remind clients about your teaching.

In selecting instructional materials, you are constrained by what is available where you are employed. Make use of what your employer has available and, if possible, recommend the purchase of new materials and equipment. Be sure the materials are current. Clients may be turned off by visual images of out-of-date clothing, hairstyles, and equipment, and they may consider the information irrelevant to their situation (Falvo, 2011). If what you need is not available, we encourage you to adapt and be creative. Is there some way to improvise or create illustrations? Healthcare institutions are cost conscious, and your employer may appreciate your creativity. In this section, we discuss printed materials, multimedia, and the Internet and World Wide Web.

Printed Materials

Printed material is the most widely used source of information given to clients. Examples of common printed materials include pamphlets, brochures, instructional handouts, and booklets. It is common for clients participating in health education classes to expect handouts and to leave with reading material that supplements and enhances their learning. Falvo (2011) recommends having a good supply of written materials on hand for the common health problems seen in clients who are served by your employer or healthcare institution.

There are multiple sources of printed material. Every voluntary healthcare organization, such as the American Cancer Society, is more than happy to supply you with printed materials. This is also true for local, state, and federal governments, depending on the type of information you request. Pharmaceutical firms and commercial sources also have printed materials you can distribute to clients. When you cannot find exactly what you want from these sources, consider preparing your own materials.

All printed materials are not equal. They need to be evaluated carefully to determine which ones best meet your purposes. You may want to have a committee help you evaluate the printed materials distributed to clients. Things to consider include the philosophy of your department, healthcare institution, or physicians; the clients and their needs; the availability of appropriate materials; and cost.

If you decide to prepare your own materials, consider the amount of *time* and *cost* it requires. You need to conceptualize and write the copy, then arrange for artistic design, layout, printing, and duplicating the material. This process can be lengthy and costly, and the effort needs to be worthwhile (Falvo, 2011). It may not be as cost effective to prepare your own materials as it first seems.

Selecting Printed Materials

As the educator, you are responsible for providing clients with understandable health information (Wood, Kettinger, & Lessick, 2007). Clients vary greatly in their ability to read and translate symbols on a piece of paper into information that is meaningful to them. You may be tempted to depend on printed materials to convey information to clients. This is especially true when you feel pressed for time and depend on reading materials to enhance the client's knowledge regarding the topic at hand. Brochures, written instructions, and consent forms are often sources of information. Many of them are written above the reading level of the average adult client, which is eighth-grade level (Winslow, 2001).

The essential issues in evaluating written materials are *readability* and *appropriateness* (Hasselkus, 2009). It is your responsibility to review all written materials before sharing them with clients. Select materials that are at a suitable reading level for clients and are appropriate to the learning objectives.

Readability

Readability of written materials refers to the language level (expressed in terms of grade level), layout, and design (Hasselkus, 2009). Readability involves examining the number of syllables in each word and the number of words in each sentence. Words with many syllables require a higher level of reading skill than words with fewer syllables. Short sentences are easier to read than long sentences.

In selecting written materials, consider the *client's background* and the *purpose of the materials*. The client's background and educational level provide clues to reading ability; however, most clients read at three to five grade levels below their educational attainment (Doak et al., 1996). Observe the reading materials in the client's room. If none are available, ask the client what their favorite reading materials are. Listen to the vocabulary clients use. How simple or complex are the individual words? If the client is employed, try to determine how much reading is required on the job. Answering these questions provides a quick overview of reading ability.

Next consider the purpose of the written materials. What information does the client need that the material is expected to provide? What must the material communicate? Is the purpose to supplement your teaching, fill in gaps that you did not have time to explain, or expand on a topic of interest? Is the material a set of instructions on how to do a procedure? Is the material designed to encourage or inspire?

Online software programs can quickly calculate readability. The Free Text Readability Consensus Calculator calculates the number of sentences, words, syllables, and characters in the sample (http://www.readabilityformulas.com/free-readability-formula-tests.php). Based on these numbers, it applies seven popular readability formulas to determine the reading level and grade level of the sample (Flesch Reading Ease, Gunning Fog, Flesch-Kincaid Grade Level, Coleman-Liau

Index, SMOG Index, Automated Readability Index, and the Linsear Write Formula). Other helpful websites are:

- WordsCount: http://www.wordscount.info/
- SAM (Suitability Assessment of Materials): http://www.beginningsguides.com/upload/sam-for-beginnings.pdf

When the written material is beyond the reading ability of the client, comprehension is decreased, and recall is sketchy and inaccurate. The client also may interpret the information differently than what was intended. As a result, the client's motivation to seek further instruction from written sources may be reduced. One way to assess a client's ability to make use of a pamphlet is to have them look it over and ask questions about the content. For example, you could say, "I want to give you a pamphlet that explains things clearly. Will you look at this and tell me if it appeals to you?"

Another way is to ask the client to read a pamphlet and report its comprehensibility. For example, you could say, "Tell me what this pamphlet says to you. Is it boring? Confusing?"

Look carefully at the client while they are reading. Does the client show signs of tension? Watch the client's eyes. Do their eyes move across and down the page in a systematic manner? These answers provide clues to both readability and appropriateness.

Appropriateness

The appropriateness of written materials focuses on the information itself. Is it suitable given the client's health problem and circumstances? Does the physician want the client to have this information? Is the information appropriate to the client's ethnic and cultural values and beliefs (Hasselkus, 2009)? Written materials should be age, gender, and culturally appropriate and respectful (Zarcadoolas, Pleasant, & Greer, 2006). Whatever written materials are provided, it is important to assess the client's ability to understand and use the information to improve health and well-being.

Generational differences may influence the type of printed material you give to clients. Something that a young person finds captivating may be insulting to an older client. Whatever the case, you do not want to offend clients by distributing materials they consider beneath their intelligence.

In the acute care setting, many clients who need instruction are affected by medications they are receiving. It is not unusual for certain drug-induced states and other postsurgical or disease conditions to blur vision and slow intellectual processing. Visual acuity may be a problem, and it may be affected by mundane problems, such as the need to put on eyeglasses. Fear and anxiety can reduce reading ability or even make it impossible for the client to grasp the meaning of printed words. Selecting an appropriate time to discuss and share written materials is as important as selecting appropriate materials. Avoid mealtimes and visiting hours.

Pamphlets and Brochures

Pamphlets and brochures are attractive, readily available, and often free. You can use them before, during, or after a presentation. Clients can hold them and use them to study and learn at their own pace so they can exercise more control over the learning experience. Voluntary health organizations are a rich source of printed materials, and many are provided in both English and Spanish. Examples include the American Cancer Society, the American Heart Association, and the

American Lung Association. Virtually every disease that affects a specific population is served by an organization that provides public education and written materials.

Some websites offer print-on-demand health information that is current and cost effective. For example, health information is available from The Joint Commission (TJC) through the Speak Up initiative (The Joint Commission, 2009). These brochures can be downloaded and used as needed. They are not copyrighted; however, The Joint Commission requires that TJC be credited as the source of the material. The topics are varied; examples include medication safety, preventing infection, pain management, and preventing medical mistakes.

It is important to give careful consideration to the timing of pamphlet distribution if you are using them in a class. If the pamphlets contain the actual information you wish to discuss, use them as advance organizers and a substitute for note taking. If you decide they are distracting, keep them out of sight until the presentation is completed.

Instructional Handouts and Patient Education Pathways

Instructional handouts refer to information specifically prepared for a client or group of clients served by a specific physician or healthcare institution or agency. They typically cover preparation for diagnostic procedures, following treatment regimens, and follow-up care after a treatment or a procedure. If you are preparing these handouts, you need to have a final draft approved by the physician or your employer. Follow the guidelines for writing instructional materials. Place this information on video or audio media for clients who have low health literacy (Roberts, 2008).

Patient education pathways are instructional tools that facilitate client education. They inform clients about what to expect in their course of treatment and their role in recovery and restoration of health, which are both major goals of the pathways. When they are shared with clients, pathways are personal educational tools that encourage participation in self-care routines and symptom management. Pathways assume that clients who are well informed and knowledgeable about their treatment are more likely to adhere to the treatment plan. The information provided in the pathways is comprehensive, consistent, and specific to the treatment a client is undergoing. It covers every aspect in the course of treatment; for example, diet, tests, treatments, medications, activities, education, and discharge planning. Patient education pathways are similar to the multidisciplinary critical pathway tools used to manage a client's hospital stay (Clarke, 2002).

Bulletin Boards

Bulletin boards supplement health education. Depending on clients' needs and health topics of interest, bulletin boards can display a variety of information. For example, they can highlight accident prevention, advertise national health awareness months, and announce health fairs. Specific health-related topics are often of interest, such as the nature of heart disease, cancer, and diabetes. Information can be related to the season of the year, such as preventing the common cold and flu during the fall months and healthful eating during holidays. Not only do bulletin boards supplement health education, but they also reinforce information you have taught. The display reminds clients of the important points of your presentation.

Bulletin boards are a type of *informal learning* that allows clients to learn at their own pace. Place them in conspicuous spots that are suitable for browsing. Keep in mind that pausing and glancing are the usual activities of browsers. Information that is deep or wordy will languish unread or may disappear if someone wishes to really delve into it. High-traffic areas are good places for bulletin boards, such as waiting rooms (hospital, clinic, and office), hallways, and cafeterias.

If the bulletin board is to be read by children or clients using wheelchairs, lower the height of the board from the normal erect adult's eye-level position.

Bulletin boards display pictures, photographs, tables, graphs, and cartoons, as well as text information. The content, text, and graphics should be simple, clear, and at a reading level appropriate for the target population. Determine the *central message* for the bulletin board and then organize the content to support that message. Organizers, such as headings, should be clearly marked and easy to differentiate from the body of the text.

The *font* used for headings should be larger than the font for text. The lines of the text should be short enough to scan with sufficient space to separate distinct messages. Paragraph and sentence length should be short and easy to read. Block-style fonts, such as Times New Roman, Gothic, and Verdana, are easier to read than script fonts or italics, which resemble handwriting. Use both upper- and lowercase lettering. Avoid using all capital letters because they are difficult to read (Thomas, 2007). They are also perceived as shouting.

Avoid cluttering the board with too much text or graphs and tables. Too much information, and information that is too complex, are difficult for clients to quickly grasp. Display just the essential information and avoid extraneous information that detracts from your message. The display and text should be current and updated as necessary.

Although bright, primary colors attract children, these colors are difficult for older adults to read. Age-related changes in the eyes make it difficult for older adults to discriminate shades of blue, green, and violet. The warm *colors* of red, orange, and yellow are easier for older adults to see (Linton, 2007). Make the background of the bulletin board a light color to avoid the glare that occurs with white backgrounds. Dark-colored text on a light-colored background is easier for older adults and others to read (Thomas, 2007).

If you have handouts or pamphlets to distribute that reinforce the message on the bulletin board, place them in a folder attached to a lower corner of the board. If the handouts or pamphlets are too bulky or heavy, consider placing a small table next to the bulletin board.

Posters

Many of the suggestions pertaining to bulletin boards also apply to the preparation of posters. *Posters* are another effective way to communicate health information. They can accompany a presentation or be located in conspicuous places for viewing. Posters are easy to make and also commercially available. They are especially useful for limited periods of time to communicate a specific message such as a health month, a workshop announcement, or safety precautions. If posters remain in place too long or are overused, they lose their ability to attract attention and can lead to boredom (Pittman, 2009). Posters are low cost, portable, and allow for self-paced learning.

Posters should use only *key words* to communicate a message, rather than complete sentences. Use bullets or list the essential information by numbers for brevity. If you use a picture, figure, or cartoon, it should be clear and large enough to be understood immediately. Illustrations should appeal to the age, gender, socioeconomic status, and cultural characteristics of clients. Sensitivity and delicacy are important, especially if you inject humor.

As with bulletin boards, use appropriate *colors* and *block-style fonts* rather than script fonts for ease of reading. If your clients are older, use large, bold fonts. If you are using a poster with a presentation, remember the 6-W formula. It means that the last row of the audience should be no farther from the poster than six times the width of the poster. For example, if the poster is 2 feet wide, the last row of viewers should be no farther than 12 feet from the poster. For a larger audience, transform the poster into a transparency, slide, or PowerPoint slide.

Flip Charts

A *flip chart* is versatile because it is *portable* and is used like a whiteboard or chalkboard. Creative uses of flip charts include composing instantaneous posters, gathering and preserving audience contributions, and having clients write out their thoughts. A flip chart combines the advantages of posters and whiteboards or chalkboards. You can plan ahead and prepare your charts, or you can have the blank pages available while teaching for spontaneous use.

If you prepare the flip chart ahead of time, take the time you need to prepare exactly what you want: written information, pictures, cartoons, or a combination thereof. A flip chart also is used as an *advance organizer* because it allows you to write your outline and have the clients follow along as you move through the presentation.

If you plan to use a flip chart spontaneously as you teach, have a good supply of colorful pens on hand. Spontaneous use is appropriate when you want to elicit responses from the audience or when you want your clients to work in small groups and write their contributions down to be shared later with a larger group. If you use this method, hang the finished charts around the room. When you do this, clients feel like valued contributors to the teaching and learning process. Your flip charts also can be saved for future use. The material you have collected can be transcribed and sent to all the participants. The major disadvantage to using a flip chart is you must have at least some artistic talent to be effective. Also your audience must be small enough so everyone can see the flip chart.

Whiteboards or Chalkboards

A whiteboard or chalkboard is available in most classroom settings. It is valuable for making a *spontaneous drawing, diagram*, or *illustration*. You can add to or take away from the drawing while using it to explain the meaning or purpose of the topic under discussion. A whiteboard or chalkboard is an excellent device for involving clients. To promote contributions, ask a question and then write down the responses from the clients. Most individuals find it reinforcing to see their words written on the board. The best questions to ask first are those to which everyone can respond, such as questions about personal experience. For example, you can ask, "How can you tell when you are stressed out? What do you do, or what have you seen others do, when they are stressed out?"

The whiteboard or chalkboard also helps with *organizing information*. You can link ideas in a circle or list problems on one side and solutions on the other. The board also allows you to compare and contrast various points of view or to organize contributions from the audience into whatever schema you choose. Whenever possible, transfer complicated ideas to a handout that clients can refer to during your presentation.

When using the whiteboard or chalkboard, determine if your cursive writing is more legible than your printing, and use the more readable style. Write a brief notation on the board, then step aside and face the audience. This allows you to maintain contact with your clients and receive their feedback on the clarity of your point. By stepping aside, you also allow clients to copy the message, which means they can integrate both visual and auditory stimuli. Stepping aside also keeps you from becoming so involved with your creation on the board that you start talking to the board instead of the clients.

Preparing Your Own Written Materials

Consider preparing your own written materials if nothing suitable is available. When preparing your own, it is important to write at the *sixth-grade reading level or lower* to benefit clients

(Winslow, 2001). Do this by shortening words with multiple syllables, eliminating extraneous words, and simplifying sentence structure. Use everyday, plain language consistent with the client's vocabulary; avoid using medical jargon that clouds the health message.

Plain Language (n.d.) is a U.S. government initiative emphasized by President Clinton in 1998 when he issued an executive memo requiring federal agencies to write in plain language. It requires written materials to be understandable the first time individuals read or hear it so they can (1) find what they need, (2) understand what they find, and (3) use what they find to meet their needs. Plain language is grammatically correct with accurate word usage and complete sentence structure. It is clear writing that tells clients exactly what they need to know without using unnecessary words. Plain language makes information more informative and easier for clients to understand.

Begin preparing your own teaching materials by assessing the clients carefully. Know who you are writing for and what their needs are. Consider involving selected members of your target audience as a focus group. Also involve selected healthcare providers who plan to use the material. There may be a difference between what the healthcare providers think is most important for clients to know and what the clients actually want to know.

After you identify the content to communicate, focus on the two to three most important points. Begin developing the most important point first, and then develop the others one at a time. Do not overload clients with too much information; decide what is essential and focus on that. If you must use technical terms such as the names of diagnostic procedures, be sure to define exactly what you mean. Keep the message and examples concrete because they are easier for clients to understand. Abstract messages may be difficult to grasp for those with low health literacy (Seligman et al., 2007; Zarcadoolas et al., 2006). It is important that your information is accurate and updated as necessary. As your focus groups (clients and providers) review your material, make changes based on their feedback.

The layout and presentation of your materials are important (Pittman, 2009). Consider the general appearance of the text and margins. The text should be limited so the material does not appear crowded, and the margins should be ample. The material should have a clear title that indicates its purpose. Use headings, subheadings, and bullets to present the information in a logical and organized format. Using different fonts, bold fonts, highlighting, bullets, and numbers make the text more readable. Add pictures, illustrations, and diagrams to illustrate important points. They often communicate health messages more effectively than text (Bryan, 2008). Be sure the material is appropriate for the age, gender, and culture of your target audience. Color always livens up a message if it is cost effective to add it. The goal in preparing your own written material is to simplify the message while communicating essential health information. **Box 12-1** lists guidelines for writing your own instructional materials.

Evaluating Printed Materials

Printed information must be *accurate* and from a *reliable source*. This is important for all printed materials, whether in the form of pamphlets, brochures, or instructional handouts. If the purpose of the printed material is to assist clients with treatment choices about a health problem, you can use the DISCERN (n.d.), an online tool to evaluate the quality of the printed healthcare information. It was a project funded from 1996 to 1997 by the British Library and the National Health Service (NHS) Executive Research and Development Programme and is available to health professionals. Nurses as educators can use the tool to evaluate written materials they develop or to evaluate printed materials already available. The tool rates, from 1 to 5, printed material in three areas: the reliability of the material, the specific details of the information about treatment choices, and an overall quality rating of the printed material.

Box 12-1 Guidelines for Writing Instructional Materials

Planning:

- Identify the purpose of the materials.
- Identify the most important points to communicate (two or three).
- Assess the characteristics and needs of the target audience.
- Involve selected members of your target audience as a focus group.
- Involve selected healthcare providers who will use the materials.

Organizing:

- Group like information together.
- Develop each point or group one at a time.
- Keep paragraphs brief.

Writing:

- Use short, simple sentences that express only one idea.
- Use plain language and familiar words with only one or two syllables.
- Be consistent in how you define and use words.
- Avoid medical jargon, technical terms, abbreviations, and acronyms.
- Write at the fourth- to sixth-grade reading level.
- Use conversational style with an active voice.
- Use concrete, not abstract, examples.
- Avoid extraneous words.
- Update the material as necessary to maintain currency and relevance.

Appearance and layout:

- Add pictures, illustrations, and colors that support the message.
- Use pictures and illustrations that are appropriate to the age, gender, and culture of the clients.
- Use attractive spacing and layout with generous white space.
- Use 12-point type for text.
- Use larger type, bold, or underlines to separate headings and subheadings.
- Use bold fonts; avoid script fonts and italics.
- Use highlighting, bullets, and numbers as appropriate.
- Use upper- and lowercase lettering; avoid all caps.

Always consider the source of the printed materials. Many health- and disease-related brochures that healthcare institutions or agencies use are prepared by voluntary healthcare organizations. Examples of reputable voluntary healthcare organizations are the March of Dimes and the American Heart Association. These are accurate and reliable sources of information.

Instructional handouts are usually prepared by a committee in the healthcare institution or by a physician who has approved the content. These are also accurate and reliable sources. In contrast, newspaper and magazine advertisements are less reliable, although they are not necessarily inaccurate. Each source must be evaluated on its own merits.

Multimedia

Video Media

Videos are excellent instructional tools. They show action images with sound. It is the closest substitute to the actual experience because it stimulates both hearing and sight. Videos evoke imagery and intense emotion because they invite clients to experience the scenes along with the actors. Visual images are more likely to be remembered than information clients read or hear (Doak et al., 1996).

Videos allow clients to observe action without being direct participants, which is consistent with Bandura's social cognitive theory (1986, 2001) of how people learn. The actor models the desirable behavior; for example, child-rearing practices or performing a procedure. Videos are also excellent for generating an affective response in the audience and for promoting discussion. Videos can be stopped to discuss a particular action or generate problem-solving options from the audience. They help clients anticipate experiences for which they must prepare, such as childbirth. Visual images are also effective with non-English-speaking clients.

When selecting video media, consider the client's age and preferred way of learning. Younger clients, Millennials, and Gen Z are adept at using social media, whereas older clients may prefer a traditional way of learning. For older clients, face-to-face with the nurse educator or watching videos in the privacy of one's home may be preferable. Health education topics are widely available on a variety of platforms. Video may be from a streaming source direct to the client's computer, watching YouTube videos, or watching via a personal digital assistance such as smartphones. Clients will need an Internet connection and a device to view video media.

Consider making your own video on your smartphone. It can be designed for a specific client's needs. It is relatively easy to make. You can then send the video to the client for their viewing. After watching it, they can converse with you through video conferencing for clarification and questions. Video chat and video conference are also available via the client's healthcare provider.

As with any learning experience, videos are most valuable if they are prefaced by advance organizers. An introduction includes a title, the length of the video, a synopsis of the message or story, and what you expect clients to gain from the viewing. It is helpful to tell clients specifically what they should notice and what they are expected to do with the experience afterward, such as discuss the plot or perform the procedures. If unfamiliar words are used, introduce them beforehand. Put the words on a transparency, handout, or a whiteboard or chalkboard before the video is shown.

Audio Media

Audio media delivers information through the means of sound. It includes the spoken word and music. Examples of audio media are recorders, radio, audio conferencing, MP3s, and podcasts. As with video media, consideration of the age, experience, and preference of the client user is important.

Podcasts are popular programs available in digital format for listening that can be downloaded from the Internet to the client's computer or mobile devise such as a smartphone. Podcasts are available via smart speakers such as Amazon Eco, Google smart speaker, and apps such as the Spotify and Apple Podcasts app. Audio podcasts are also available from streaming services such as Audible (Amazon) and Spotify.

Podcasts focus on specific themes such as health issues, topics of interest, and music. Audio media are especially useful when clients must learn an auditory skill, such as teaching the parents of an asthmatic child to recognize various breath sounds. By listening to different types of breathing patterns on YouTube, parents can learn which types of breathing require an emergency response and which types can be improved with routine treatment.

Audio media are useful for hearing directions when the client cannot look at the speaker. Consider a client who is lying prone while following directions for exercise or relaxation. Many people find it easier to concentrate when their eyes are closed or when they listen to soothing music or directions for creating healing images (Pittman, 2009). Clients can listen to their favorite therapeutic music on streaming services such as Spotify and Pandora.

In these days of early discharge, clients often leave the hospital before they or their families are confident of the procedures they must perform at home. Audio recording of health instructions for use after discharge reminds clients of the information they were taught. For example, by recording your voice on their smartphone during the client's final teaching session, you can talk the client through a procedure with a minimum of extra time and effort.

When you are in community health settings and clients live far away, such as in rural settings, consider audio conferencing between home visits. Podcasts and smartphones containing reminders, complicated instructions, and so forth could be available for the family.

Podcasts have many advantages. They are free or inexpensive, readily available, and can be tailor-made in the client's language. Also, they help clients develop listening skills. Audio media capture nuances of speech that are impossible to convey in written communication. However, audio media have drawbacks as well. Listeners find it difficult to listen for more than 15 minutes without other stimuli because they get bored.

Computer-Assisted Instruction

Many health maintenance organizations and healthcare institutions or agencies have special areas where clients can access interactive software to supplement health education. Computer-assisted instruction (CAI) is an excellent resource for self-paced learning. It does not become impatient; its pace can be controlled by the client, and it gives immediate, objective, and consistent feedback. The software allows clients to repeat all or part of a lesson and progress at their own rate. Clients acquire information in private, and no one else has to know what they think or how long they take to obtain the expected knowledge. CAI is useful for clients of any age, especially if they can control the pace at which they progress. For younger clients, CAI may evoke the fun and excitement of an arcade game. Self-paced learning takes initiative on the part of clients. The CAI may lead you to expect too much independent learning from clients. If CAI is provided in a healthcare setting, be available to answer questions from clients and assist them with the software as the need arises.

Many interactive websites are available on the Internet. For example, the website MedlinePlus is a service of the National Library of Medicine (NLM) and National Institutes of Health (NIH). The site offers easy-to-read instructional materials that are available in more than 40 languages and has interactive health tutorials on topics in the following categories: diseases and conditions, tests and diagnostic procedures, surgery and treatment procedures, and prevention and wellness (U.S. National Library of Medicine and National Institutes of Health, 2012). The Centers for Disease Control and Prevention (CDC) government website is also an excellent source of information. These sites can be accessed from a client's home.

Interactive bulletin boards serve as a continuing education resource for updating health team members (Flournoy, Turner, & Combs, 2000). Short, succinct lessons, messages, and updates can be created for health team members. It is self-paced learning that health team members use when they have the time and interest.

Digital Camera and Photographs

Digital cameras have largely replaced their older counterpart, the 35-mm camera. A digital camera takes video or still photographs by recording images on an electronic imaging sensor. Images are displayed immediately after they are recorded and can be stored or deleted as desired. Images can be printed on photo printers or taken to any commercial print service.

Digital photos can be displayed with an LCD projector, which is suitable for large groups. Everyone in your audience sees the same photo at the same time. Single photographs are best used on an individual basis or in a small group. When they are passed around, however, they may be distracting to the audience.

Slides

Film 35-mm slides may still be available for health education purposes in some healthcare institutions or agencies. The slides are placed in a carousel and require a slide projector to view them. They can also be inserted into a PowerPoint presentation. A slide presentation is excellent for visual learners and helps to clarify your comments. The order of slides can be replaced or rearranged in the carousel if you change the nature of your presentation. You need to prepare a script to accompany the slide presentation. Slides are easy to store and transport. Because 35-mm film is no longer common, it is wise to learn to use a digital camera.

Objects and Models

Objects should be used for demonstration when possible. For example, use a real syringe when you teach self-injections, and use a real dressing when you teach how to change a dressing. Models are used when the real object, such as a heart, is not available or not feasible to use. Three types of models are replicas, analogies, and symbols.

Replica

A replica is a model that resembles a real object. It is a scaled construction that magnifies the features of the original object. The increased size of the features makes demonstration easier. This type of model can be picked up and manipulated and helps convey the concept of dimensions. Replicas are useful for kinesthetic clients who learn better with hands-on opportunities. For example, clients can take a model of a kidney apart and put it back together again, thus getting a better idea of how the kidney works. By handling the replica, clients can control the pace of learning.

A replica can be used to help clients develop a skill. Learning to clean a central line or to examine breasts for lumps are challenging procedures that are best learned on something other than a human being. Replicas exist for practicing these skills, but they are expensive, fragile, and require storage space.

Replicas best serve only a few clients at a time. Compensate for this by using team teaching and placing different replicas at different stations. Such an arrangement divides the larger group into several smaller ones and allows each station to become an area of concentrated focus with fewer competing stimuli.

Analogy

An analogy is something that has features similar and a likeness to something else (*Webster's*, 2013). It compares known things to better understand or clarify something unfamiliar. It makes an abstract idea concrete. Analogies are suggestive but not definitive (Browne & Keeley, 2007. Analogies build on clients' existing knowledge to communicate complex medical concepts. They emphasize a shared quality that helps make something unfamiliar become more understandable.

When teaching clients, determine the need for analogy. A good analogy is familiar, short, clear, and visual. When you create an analogy, the unfamiliar concept is the target, and the familiar concept you use for comparison is the analog. The target and the analog are connected with the words *like* or *as*. For example, you could explain that the action of the heart is like a pump that moves water. Confirm that the client understands the analogy. You could say, "Tell me how you understand what I said"; then have the client state in their own words what you explained. If indicated, provide an in-depth explanation along with printed materials to supplement your teaching.

If the analogy lacks similarity in other aspects, point out its limitations. For example it is true that the brain is like a computer, but there are differences that the client should be aware of. Select analogies that are within the frame of reference, language and cultural experience of the client. They should be readily grasped and understandable by the client.

Analogies demand conceptual sophistication and an ability to understand how things are alike and different. Because not everyone perceives things the same way, practice using the analogy on others to find out if they understand the point and if it fits the message you intend to convey.

Symbol

A symbol stands for something else that it represents by association or resemblance. Often, a printed or written sign is used to represent an operation, element, quantity, quality, relation, or something invisible (*Webster's*, 2013). The treble clef sign and notes on lines are examples of musical symbols. Words are examples of symbols. They are combinations of circles and lines arranged in special patterns to convey a certain meaning. The meaning varies according to the language familiar to the speaker, writer, listener, and reader.

Words are symbolic models that you use to convey a concept or idea to clients. Words are such familiar symbols that you no longer perceive the circles and lines with which words are drawn unless you are dyslexic. If fact, unless you have a photographic mind, you could not even report the exact words on this page. You would probably report the ideas, general concepts, and meanings you attached to what you read.

You may draw diagrams, signs, or cartoons, all of which are attempts to convey meaning through the use of symbols. International traffic signs are examples of such symbols. The picture conveys the meaning. Circles have many meanings. If they are arranged on top of each other and colored red, yellow, and green, they would be perceived in the United States as parts of a traffic light. Smiley faces are recognized by most people in this culture as conveying happiness or approval.

The practice of representing something by symbols is so widespread in this culture that it is difficult to describe by example. The symbol + means plus, and the symbol = means equal to. Stick figures can be used by a teacher to symbolize people regardless of artistic talent. The figure can help you focus a client's attention on the desired point. Distinct symbols are used in health care to distinguish between male and female people.

Symbols are gaining widespread application in areas that cater to multilingual groups and international travel. Examples include airports, roadway traffic signs, lodging and food, and handicapped parking symbols. You should avoid using abbreviations that are common among healthcare personnel but are not common to clients. These abbreviations include NPO, PO, and PRN. Although these abbreviations convey meaning to certain groups, they might add confusion to other groups. **Figure 12-1** illustrates some common symbols.

Figure 12-1 Common Symbols
© AbleStock (left); © WilleeCole/Shutterstock (right)

Transparencies

Transparencies remain a popular choice for illustrating a presentation and are used as backup to other media, such as PowerPoint presentations. They can be seen with the room lights on. They are useful to highlight important points in a verbal presentation. The highlights can be in the form of brief, well-spaced outlines, pictures, simple drawings, or cartoons. You can prepare transparencies in advance or on the spot in response to interaction with the clients.

You can prepare permanent or nonpermanent transparencies in several ways. To create permanent transparencies, construct a drawing or write text on paper, copy the material in a copy machine, then run the copy together with a blank transparency through a thermal fax machine. The thermal fax and carbon on the copy interact to make the transparency in the presence of heat. The same process is used to create picture transparencies. To create nonpermanent transparencies, use nonpermanent, washable color marking pens. This works well for illustrating as you are presenting. The transparency is reusable because the ink will wash off. Transparencies are relatively inexpensive to purchase and can be stored flat in pocket envelopes that fit a standard note binder.

Transparencies are projected onto a screen via an overhead projector, and they are useful for any size audience. A projector is bulky and has a long arm with a mirror and lens that focus and redirect light forward onto a screen. When a transparency is placed on the projector, the image is directed onto the screen. The projector has a very bright halogen lamp, a fan to cool the machine, and a storage place for additional lamps.

An overhead projector needs to be adjusted before the presentation to ensure a good projected image on the screen. This means adjusting the size of the screen and the distance from the projector to the screen. We recommend that you stand to one side of the projector and look at the audience when giving a presentation. Place the projector so you can face the audience. The audience looks at the screen while you look at the transparency on the projector to see what the audience sees.

PowerPoint Slides

Microsoft PowerPoint is a presentation software program widely used by educators. It is useful for large audiences and requires an LCD projector to display the images onto a screen for viewing. The presentation can be accessed from the computer, a disc, or a flash drive. The room may need to be darkened for best viewing.

Box 12-2 Guidelines for Creating and Using PowerPoint Slides

- Choose a format that best illustrates your points with headings and subheadings.
- Choose a plain background to limit the distractions on the slides.
- Choose a soft background color that contrasts with the lettering.
- Use bullets or numbers to separate the information.
- Use upper- and lowercase lettering; avoid all capitalized lettering.
- List as few words as possible to communicate the message.
- Limit the amount of information on each slide; avoid overcrowding.
- Limit the number of slides so the audience focuses on your comments.
- Advance the slides to match your comments.
- Be sure the hardware and software are operating properly before your presentation.
- Give a copy of the slides to the audience to reinforce learning.

Identify what you want to illustrate through PowerPoint slides. You can input text, graphics, movies, or other objects on the slides and arrange and rearrange them as you wish. The software provides a template with a variety of formats and backgrounds to create the slides. You can navigate through the slides as you make your presentation. The slides can be printed, or you can display the presentation live on a computer. The software is easy to use but requires the proper equipment. See **Box 12-2** for help in preparing your presentation.

Storyboards

A *storyboard* is a visual presentation of text or graphic information. Storyboards tell a story or explain sequential information (Pittman, 2009). Microsoft PowerPoint software is commonly used for creating storyboards. The software provides many options for layout, text, and graphics.

Storyboards are easy to develop, edit, and distribute for client education purposes. They are low cost and provide consistent, current information to clients. The development of storyboards begins by selecting a health-related topic followed by identifying the essential information to include. A committee can help determine the topic, content, and accuracy. After they are developed, storyboards can be distributed via email, they can be printed, or they can be made into posters with the correct type of printer (Kisak & Conrad, 2004).

Cartoons

Cartoons can be transferred to a transparency or PowerPoint slide and projected for large groups; or cartoons may be circulated among members of a small group or shared with an individual. Humorous cartoons provide comic relief and make a point much more clearly than many words. Before you decide to use humor, test it out on people similar to your intended audience. Drawings that are intended to be humorous also can evoke unexpected reactions among clients who may perceive the material differently than you do. Cartoons are not necessarily cross-cultural, so you should show prospective cartoons to someone from the target culture and have them critique it for you. As with photographs, cartoons can be placed in clear plastic covers for protection.

Mobile Devices

The ownership and use of mobile devices have increasingly become how we communicate and access information both within the United States and around the world. They are rapidly replacing landline telephones with their powerful computing and battery capabilities and expanding wireless broadband networks. A goal of Healthy People 2020 is to "use health communication strategies and health information technology (IT) to improve population health outcomes and healthcare quality, and to achieve health equity" (HealthyPeople.gov, 2014, para. 1). Mobile devices are useful tools for educating clients, promoting the use of preventive services, managing chronic conditions, and improving overall health.

In addition to the web-based delivery of health education and e-health interactive tutorials, mobile devices can also serve as an interface between clients and healthcare providers by the real-time transmission of information about vital body functions such as blood sugar levels, and heart and respiratory rates. For example, iPhones were used to monitor adolescents with type 1 diabetes. One group kept a food diary, whereas another used the cell phone camera to record their dietary intake. The photographs were downloaded and analyzed, along with the food diaries. Although there was no significant difference between the two groups, it demonstrates a novel use of the cell phone to monitor clients (Donald, Franklin, & Greene, 2009). Text messaging was effective in improving self-efficacy and adherence in adolescents with type 1 diabetes (Franklin, Waller, Pagliari, & Greene, 2006), and mobile devices were effective in monitoring client vital signs (Mark, 2013). Many healthcare institutions and agencies provide telephone numbers for clients who have concerns. Health advice lines are also available. Telephones are used to follow up with clients to offer encouragement and help with any problems they have in adhering to a treatment regimen.

The Internet and World Wide Web

The Internet is a huge global network that connects computers for the purpose of transferring information from one computer to another. It connects millions of private, public, academic, business, and government computers. The Internet is the infrastructure that supports the web. The web is a network of hypertext documents called webpages that are accessed via the Internet. Webpages may contain text, images, videos, audio, and other multimedia. Users can easily navigate these pages with a touch screen or the click of a mouse. The web was created to display information, whereas the Internet was created to exchange information. The Internet and the web are not synonymous terms, although they are often used as if they were (Sopczyk, 2008; Wikipedia, 2014).

To access the web, clients must have a computer, or have access to one, with a telecommunication link and special software to connect to an Internet service provider (ISP). Clients navigate the web through a browser such as Microsoft Edge Google Chrome, Apple Safari, and Mozilla Firefox. When a person is on the Internet, search engines such as Google and Microsoft Bing allow users to search for specific information. Wikipedia is a free online encyclopedia, "created and edited by volunteers around the world and hosted by the Wikimedia Foundation" (https://www.wikipedia.org).

Technology and supporting software are developing rapidly and changing daily. By the time you read this, today's technology will have advanced, and the number of health-related websites will have greatly expanded. Nurses who work with this technology need to keep abreast of these changes to assist clients who need health education.

Because so many clients access the Internet, you should ask them if they are looking at health-related websites. If so, ask which ones they find useful and evaluate if they are accessing reliable sources of information. By listening to what clients have learned about health issues, you have the opportunity to evaluate that knowledge. You can refer clients to reliable websites if that is indicated. Clients may have questions about what they are learning, or they may be overwhelmed with the amount of information they are finding. Urge clients to use online health information to supplement that given by their healthcare provider, not act as a substitute. Many clients misunderstand or misinterpret health information and require clarifying explanations.

E-Health Websites

The web is the newest source for interactive health information, often referred to as e-health. Electronically available health information includes access to personal health records online, health education libraries, professional health journals, and self-assessment tools. When health information is so widely available and accessible, it has the potential to improve the quality of health if used by clients. It also has the potential to create problems for clients and providers if the health information is inaccurate and influences their decision making and healthcare practices.

The Internet is advantageous for clients because it is accessed in private in their own homes. Information is read at the clients' speed and convenience. Taking advantage of this technology is more effective for clients with adequate health-literacy skills. Those at low health-literacy levels may find accessing and understanding health information on websites more challenging.

Clients without a personal computer have free access through public libraries, community centers, or senior centers. Those persons enrolled in health maintenance organizations, such as Kaiser Permanente, have access to onsite interactive health education software. Electronic sources of health information are available from The Joint Commission through the Speak Up initiative (The Joint Commission, 2009) and Medline Plus, both described earlier in this chapter.

The web has become a source of information and an educational tool for clients with a variety of health issues (Hawn, 2009; Jacobi et al., 2007; Scharer, 2005; Schultz, Stava, Beck, & Vassilopoulou-Sellin, 2003). It puts information and power into the hands of consumers, especially those with chronic diseases. Half of clients with a chronic disease or disability go online. Of this number, 86% have searched for information about health topics (Fox, 2007). Millard and Fintak (2002) found that clients with chronic illnesses frequently accessed websites to get information about their illness and engaged in self-care and self-diagnosis. In a large study, they found that users were skeptical about health care in general. Some users were not satisfied or had experienced problems with access to the healthcare system. Others lacked insurance coverage or found it difficult to obtain healthcare services. Favored health websites were those designed specifically for health topics, medical journals, advocacy groups, and academic websites. Other ways that clients can access health-related information include YouTube, podcasts, and streaming video. A difficulty with websites is that clients do not know if the information is reliable.

Evaluating Website Information

Almost anything can be found on the web, so it is important to evaluate each site for accuracy and reliability. Although websites can be a source of excellent information, they also can be misleading and provide misinformation. It is your responsibility to thoroughly evaluate each website you recommended to clients. Monsivais and Reynolds (2003) and MedlinePlus offer guidelines for evaluating websites:

- What is the *source of the information*? Is it from an individual or an organization? Examples of reliable sources of information include local, state, and federal government sites, U.S. colleges and universities, professional organizations, and voluntary health organizations. Look at the About Us webpage for this information. Is there a way to contact the webmaster?

- What is the *quality of the information*? The writers of the information should be identified and may be found in the About Us webpage or in the mission statement. Who are they? Are they recognized experts in the field about which they are writing? Be skeptical; quackery thrives on the Internet. Look for claims that sound too good to be true, such as promises about new cures and secret ingredients.
- What *evidence is offered* to support the claims? Is it based on medical research conducted by properly credentialed researchers at known healthcare institutions, scientific laboratories, or universities? Is the evidence based on personal testimony and opinion? If so, are the persons and their credentials identified? Is there a way to contact them? Be skeptical of anonymous testimonials that claim cures and promote treatments.
- How *current* is the information? Note the date the information was posted and the last time the site was updated. Credible sites provide dates. Does the site provide references and maintain hyperlinks to other credible sites?
- Is the information *biased*? What is the purpose of the site, and who is sponsoring and funding it? Is it supported by public funds, donations, or commercial advertising? The distinction between health information and advertisements should be clear. Websites can appear to be credible, but a careful observer may discover otherwise. The purpose of many websites is to sell a product or recommend a particular treatment (Butler & Foster, 2003). Such a site would not be considered an objective source of information.

The National Library of Medicine (2020) offers a helpful web-based tutorial. The five-section tutorial teaches clients how to evaluate health information found on the Internet. It is found at https://medlineplus.gov/webeval/webeval.html.

When clients search for information on the web, many options appear, and choosing among them is confusing. Talk with clients about how to find credible websites. Also urge clients to talk with their healthcare providers about the accuracy of health information they are finding on the web.

Social Networking Websites

Boyd and Ellison define social network sites as "web-based services that allow individuals to (1) construct a public or semi-public profile within a bounded system, (2) articulate a list of other users with whom they share a connection, and (3) view and traverse their list of connections and those made by others within the system. The nature and nomenclature of these connections may vary from site to site" (2007, p. 2). Although social network websites are popular, it is not known how many adults use them to gather or share health information. Most users who access these sites share updates about themselves or their friends (Fox & Jones, 2009). Facebook, Instagram, X, Threads, TikTok, and Reddit are examples of social networking sites used by clients to share information.

Email, short for electronic mail, is used by both healthcare providers and clients, especially in rural areas. It increases the speed of communication and the ability to keep in contact with other clients and providers. Electronic communication also has disadvantages (Sopczyk, 2008). It lacks context, such as facial expression and tone of voice. Email is an efficient way to communicate; service has improved as the networks and speed have expanded. Instant messaging is also effective but more information can be communicated via email than with instant messaging. Response time to email and instant messaging are dependent on the promptness of the intended receiver. With email, there is a written record of the information shared or the advice given. It is important that this be accurate and appropriate and a copy of it be placed in the client's record. Although healthcare institutions and agencies take steps to ensure privacy in electronic communications and have guidelines for their use, you can never assume that the communications are private.

Hawn (2009) anticipates that social networking sites will become increasingly used by clients and healthcare providers. Hawn reports that through email, instant messaging, or video chat, some clients can now contact their physicians directly. It is a way for clients to stay in touch with their physicians. Email access to personal physicians and nurse practitioners is now available through some health maintenance organizations, such as Kaiser Permanente and Palo Alto (California) Medical Group. Clients can also make appointments, refill prescriptions, and see their personal test results online. Some physicians are establishing their own Facebook-like profiles and communicating with clients via secure email message networks. Some are also writing blogs about common health topics (Hawn, 2009).

Electronic discussion boards have been useful for clients who are experiencing similar health issues and share common concerns. Clients post their experiences and thoughts on the site and gain the support of other clients who are experiencing similar problems. Clients exchange helpful messages with each other. It is an effective, relatively inexpensive way to provide social support to clients. Discussion boards are also a promising health resource (Scharer, 2005; Schultz et al., 2003). HealthBoards.com is an example of a social support site (http://www.healthboards.com/). Clients have access to more than 150 message boards that cover a wide range of health topics. This resource may be especially helpful for clients with disabilities or chronic illnesses.

Selecting Instructional Materials

When selecting instructional materials, review the learning objectives, teaching content, and teaching strategies, and ask how you can best supplement these. Consider the characteristics of your clients and which media would best help them learn. In **Box 12-3**, we have summarized some questions to ask in this process.

Table 12-1 summarizes the advantages, disadvantages, and helpful hints for using the various types of instructional materials. We hope this is helpful to you in making a selection.

Box 12-3 Choosing a Medium

Questions to ask yourself when choosing a medium:
1. What medium is most appropriate given the learning objectives, teaching content, and teaching strategies?
2. Is sound necessary, or can a silent medium be used?
3. Is motion important, or can still pictures convey the ideas?
4. Is color important, or is black and white more advantageous?
5. Is individual study encouraged?
6. Is the focus on learning as a group?
7. How often is the material likely to need updating?
8. Do you have the technical competence to use this medium?
9. Can you handle common problems with this medium?
10. Do you know where to get help with it?
11. What is realistic for you to accomplish given your budget and time constraints?
12. What resources are necessary in the learning environment to use this equipment, such as a screen, podium, and electrical outlets?

Table 12-1 Features of Instructional Materials

Type	Advantages	Disadvantages	Helpful Hints
Video media	■ Good substitute for actual experience ■ Easily obtainable ■ Easy to remake and update ■ Can be stopped and rerun ■ Familiar to many	■ Size of monitor limits audience distance ■ Technical skill needed ■ Expensive initial investment ■ Connectivity	■ Need compatible equipment ■ Can take longer than expected to produce a video ■ Store properly
Audio media	■ Can be used with individuals or groups ■ Good for developing listening skills ■ Accessible ■ Inexpensive ■ Can be tailor-made, erased, or remade	■ Can be dull if used by itself or for too long a period ■ Need proper equipment ■ Connectivity	■ Store properly ■ Should be of high audio quality to maintain interest
Computer-assisted instruction	■ Client controls the pace ■ Correct responses reinforced immediately ■ Incorrect responses retaught immediately ■ Good for sequential thought processes ■ Allows client to repeat the lesson if necessary	■ Depends on client initiative ■ Time consuming for client ■ Time consuming for nurse to monitor ■ Limited value if nurse is not available for questions ■ Clients must be visual learners and computer literate ■ Can be boring	■ Select the most user-friendly software available ■ Spend time with client to ensure comfort with the program
Digital camera and photographs	■ Images can be displayed and printed immediately ■ Images easily stored and deleted ■ Can be used with taped narration or music	■ Expensive initial investment ■ Single photographs distracting if passed around during presentation ■ Show no movement	■ Synchronize with a presentation
Objects and models	■ Depict the real thing as closely as possible ■ Can be handled and studied at client's pace ■ Replicas are static ■ Analogies are dynamic ■ Appeal to kinesthetic learners	■ Can be bulky and heavy ■ Inconvenient to transport ■ Require storage space ■ Time consuming ■ Expensive and fragile ■ Analogies require conceptual sophistication	■ Require advance planning if borrowed ■ Work well with several stations around a teaching area ■ Require a teacher at each station

Type	Advantages	Disadvantages	Helpful Hints
Transparencies	■ Versatile, inexpensive, and reusable ■ Teacher can face learners ■ Eliminate verbal repetition ■ Can be used with the lights on ■ Can be used with overlays ■ Good backup for PowerPoint	■ Overhead projector is bulky and needs to be adjusted to the screen ■ Use bulbs that often burn out ■ Transparencies are time consuming to prepare	■ Protect transparencies from hand oils and fingerprints ■ Use multicolor, washable pens
PowerPoint slides or storyboards	■ Easy to format, create, use, and store on disc or flash drive ■ Show still images, motion, and sound ■ Stimulating to audience ■ Allow audience to follow the presentation	■ Require expensive equipment and screen ■ Slides are time consuming to prepare ■ Must have operational LCD projector and screen	■ Be sure equipment is available and working properly ■ Important to sequence slides and storyboard
Instructional handouts and education pathways	■ Developed for specific clients or healthcare institutions ■ Easily changed and updated ■ Clients can review at their pace	■ Takes time to prepare and update ■ Duplicating takes time	■ Require storage space ■ Keep materials organized and handy for use
Pamphlets and brochures	■ Portable and attractive ■ Can be used before, during, and after a presentation ■ Can be studied at client's pace ■ Readily available ■ Often free	■ May overwhelm clients if too many ■ May contain outdated or irrelevant information ■ May be culturally inappropriate	■ Distribute at the most propitious time ■ Check for currency of information
Bulletin boards	■ Clients can process at own pace ■ Attract browsers	■ Can get cluttered and outdated ■ Unsuitable for long or complex information	■ Change often ■ Keep attractive, lively ■ Contain a minimal number of messages
Posters	■ Portable and attractive ■ Attract browsers ■ Can be used before, during, and after a presentation ■ Can be studied at client's pace ■ Readily available ■ Often free	■ Time consuming to make ■ Provide limited viewing ■ Need a prop ■ Bulky to carry and store ■ Useful only to readers	■ Change often ■ Keep attractive, lively ■ Contain a minimal number of messages

(continues)

Table 12-1 Features of Instructional Materials   (*continued*)

Type	Advantages	Disadvantages	Helpful Hints
Flip charts	▪ Versatile, portable ▪ Use like a whiteboard or chalkboard ▪ May be prepared before or created spontaneously during presentation	▪ Require artistic talent and good handwriting ▪ Clients may have a limited view	▪ Have a good supply of black and colored pens ▪ Use masking tape or adhesive to affix flip charts to wall
Whiteboards or chalkboards	▪ Widely available ▪ Useful for spontaneous illustration at the time of the client's concern ▪ Offer reinforcement to respondents ▪ Erasable ▪ Allow teacher to add to and take away from illustration ▪ Good backup aid	▪ Two dimensional ▪ Messy ▪ Require pen or chalk and an eraser ▪ Require good lighting ▪ Can be time consuming to use ▪ Require legible writing skills	▪ May need to supply pens or chalk and eraser ▪ Chalk is messy, especially on dark clothing ▪ Write high on board to avoid writing below clients' line of vision ▪ Divide in half for lengthy lists

Clients with Disabilities

Clients with hearing and visual impairments present special challenges when it comes to the selection of instructional materials and media. Insofar as possible, materials and media should be adapted to the particular needs of each client. It helps to involve the client's family, significant other, or caretaker if that is appropriate and the client is agreeable. They may have suggestions that will facilitate your health teaching.

Depending on the client's degree of impairment, you need to identify the best way to communicate with clients who have hearing and visual impairments. We offer some practical suggestions here.

Many clients who are hearing impaired are able to benefit from print media and video recordings. If a client is receptive to print media, choose materials that are appropriate in terms of readability and information, such as pamphlets and brochures. If the client knows how to write and has the strength to do it, providing paper and pencil may be an effective way to communicate. If the client is computer literate and a laptop computer is available, this may be helpful. Many health-related videos are commercially available and also available online. You can also custom-make videos to suit the special needs of your client.

Visual impairments can be mild, moderate, or severe, or the client may be blind. You need to know each client's specific capabilities to make an appropriate selection of instructional materials and media. Many clients who are visually impaired benefit from auditory media and video magnifiers where the screen is enlarged. If the client is not a reader or has poor literacy, Pittman (2009) recommends using audio media. Examples of current audio media include MP3s, podcasts, audio

---

Box 12-4 Evaluating Effectiveness of Instructional Materials

In the client education plan, were the instructional materials:

- Appropriate to the learning objectives?
- Appropriate to the teaching content?
- Complementary to the teaching strategies?

For the learners, were the instructional materials:

- Appealing to visual, auditory, and/or kinesthetic learners?
- Appropriate to the client's level of comprehension?
- Age, gender, and culturally appropriate and sensitive?
- Engaging to the client?

Was the selection of instructional materials:

- Visually pleasing?
- Suitable to the time constraints of the learning activity?
- Visible in terms of contrast, size, and location?
- Easy to use?
- Accurate and up to date?
- Cost effective and within budget constraints?

---

books, audio conferencing, audio streaming services, and email with audio. The technology continues to evolve and its usage is challenging to the older population.

Clients with limited visual impairment may benefit from print media if the font size is sufficiently large. The background and font colors can be altered to increase readability. Magnifying lamps and handheld lighted magnifiers are also available to assist these clients.

Evaluating the Effectiveness of Instructional Materials

Evaluate the effectiveness of all instructional materials. Evaluation tools should be specific to the type of materials you are using to supplement health education. **Box 12-4** provides some criteria for evaluating the effectiveness of instructional materials.

Copyright Issues in Using Instructional Materials

Copyright laws in the United States protect intellectual property and original works of authorship when they are fixed in a tangible form. This protection exists for both published and unpublished works (U.S. Copyright Office, 2009). Knowing about copyright restrictions is important if you are using certain instructional materials, such as text and images. Instructional materials may be copyrighted or they may be in the public domain. Depending on their source, it is important to know the difference and respond accordingly. If you have any questions about copyright issues, it is best to consult with your employer's legal counsel.

Instructional materials taken from professional journals, magazines, and other published sources always carry a copyright. To make multiple copies, you must seek written permission from the publisher or the owner of the materials. When making the request, allow plenty of time and ask how the copyright owner wants the materials cited. It is important to comply with the copyright owner's citation format (Kisak & Conrad, 2004). Copyright law permits an individual to make one copy of a copyrighted document for their own personal use without requesting permission.

Instructional materials in the public domain are not protected by copyright and therefore do not require permission. Examples of materials in the public domain include those first published in a U.S. government document. It also includes commonly used materials in which the ownership is unknown or questionable. Some images are also in the public domain and are available for use. Even though no permission is required, credit should always be given to the source of the information.

If you are downloading information from websites, be sure to check the copyright information provided on that website. Clear guidelines are provided that identify what is and what is not copyrighted and any restrictions on the use of the information (Kisak & Conrad, 2004). For example, on The Joint Commission website, there are no copyright or reprinting permissions required for the Speak Up materials. However, the website stipulates that The Joint Commission must be credited as the source of the materials.

Summary

In this chapter, we introduced health literacy and assessing and engaging with clients when considering the readability and appropriateness of written materials. We discussed instructional materials under three broad headings: printed materials, multimedia, and Internet and World Wide Web. Instructional materials are designed to help you achieve the learning objectives and supplement your teaching strategies. The materials you select should be appropriate to you as the teacher and to the clients as learners. Each type of instructional material has advantages and disadvantages that must be considered when making a selection.

Clients with disabilities include those with auditory and visual impairments who need special consideration. Instructional materials and websites need to be evaluated in terms of being reliable and accurate sources of information. Criteria were provided to help in the evaluation process. It is important to remember that some instructional materials are protected by copyright. These implications were discussed.

Exercises
Exercise I: Assessing Health Literacy

Purpose: Assess the impact of health literacy on client care.
Directions:

1. Select a client you have cared for and who was confronted with a major health decision. Identify that decision.
2. List the literacy and decision-making skills the client needed to make a good, informed decision.
3. Share your thoughts with the class.

Exercise II: Writing Health Information

Purpose: Prepare health information for distribution to clients.

Directions: Work in pairs and prepare a handout that includes the purpose, description, rationale, benefits, and instructions for clients for one of the following procedures. Evaluate your written instructions using the Free Text Readability Consensus Calculator.

1. Mammogram
2. Immunizations
3. Colonoscopy
4. Chest X-ray
5. Blood test

Exercise III: Writing Health Information

Purpose: Increase awareness of client perceptions of medical jargon.

Directions:

1. On paper, draw four columns. List the following words in the left-hand column: ambulate, edema, peristalsis, hypertrophy, jaundice, urinate, biopsy, hypertension, vital signs, and NPO.
2. In the middle column, write what a client might think the words mean. If you cannot think of a possible client meaning for the word, ask friends who do not have medical backgrounds or clients who could use some entertainment.
3. In the third column, write the medical meaning.
4. In the last column, write an alternative word or phrase that conveys the desired meaning.
5. What words would you add to the list that clients might not know the meaning of?

Exercise IV: Rewriting Health Information

Purpose: Evaluate health information.

Directions:

1. Bring a health-related written advertisement for a product or medication to class.
2. Identify the central message of the advertisement. What is explicit? Implicit?
3. What assumptions does the advertisement make about the client's health literacy?
4. At what reading level is the advertisement?
5. Share your observations with others in your class.

Exercise V: Evaluating Misinformation

Purpose: Assisting clients with below-basic health literacy skills to evaluate both the source and accuracy of information.

Directions:

1. Select a sample of misinformation related to COVID-19 or any similar topic. Your client has below-basic health literacy skill. Guide the client to identify both the source and accuracy of that information. How is the client interpreting the information? How would you go about addressing the misinformation? Would verbal clarification be effective? Would written information be effective? Draft a written sample to provide accurate information.

Exercise VI: Misinformation and Disinformation

Purpose: Challenging misinformation and disinformation
Directions: Meet with a small community group and select a health topic of interest pertinent to that community, such as vaccine hesitancy, physical distancing, or mask wearing.

1. Identify information sources that members use (doctor, websites, newspapers, public bulletins, neighbors, family member, TV, radio, iPhone, local health department, schools, church, etc.).
2. Explain the preference for that source.
3. Discuss ways to determine if information source(s) are trustworthy and accurate. Provide evidence to support the credibility of a preferred information source.
4. Give an example of misinformation that members have experienced or are aware of. What are the underlying assumptions of that misinformation?
5. Give an example of disinformation that you've experienced or are aware of. What are the underlying assumptions of that disinformation?
6. Why do people spread misinformation and disinformation?
7. Identify trusted, accurate sources of information.
8. Identify what you can do to correct misinformation and spread accurate information.
9. Summarize your findings in a written report.

Exercise VII: Evidence-Based Nursing Practice

Purpose: Apply evidence-based nursing research to client education.
Directions:

1. Search the literature for nursing research applicable to instructional materials related to health education.
2. Describe how the findings could be applied to your practice in educating clients.

References

Bandura, A. (1986). *Social foundations of thought and action: A social cognitive theory*. Englewood Cliffs, NJ: Prentice Hall.
Bandura, A. (2001). Social cognitive theory: An agentic perspective. *Annual Review of Psychology, 52*, 1–26.
Benoit, S. L., & Mauldin, F. F. (2021). The "anti-vax" movement: A quantitative report on vaccine beliefs and knowledge across social media. *BMC Public Health*, 2021(21), 2106.
Boyd, D. M., & Ellison, N. B. (2007). Social network sites: Definition, history, and scholarship. *Journal of Computer-Mediated Communication, 13*(1), article 11. Retrieved from http://jcmc.indiana.edu/vol13/issue1/boyd.ellison.html
Browne, M.N. & Keeley, S. M. (2009). *Asking the right questions: A guide to critical thinking* (9th ed.). Pearson Prentice Hall.
Bryan, C. (2008). Provider and policy response to reverse the consequences of low health literacy. *Journal of Healthcare Management, 53*(4), 230–241.
Butler, L., & Foster, N. E. (2003). Back pain online: A cross-sectional survey of the quality of web-based information on low back pain. *Spine, 28*(4), 395–401.
Clancy, C. M. (2008). *Navigating the health care system. What's your health literacy score?* Retrieved from http://www.ahrq.gov/CONSUMER/cc/cc052008.htm
Clarke, L. K. (2002). Pathways for head and neck surgery: A patient-education tool. *Clinical Journal of Oncology Nursing, 6*(2), 78–82.
DISCERN. (n.d.). Welcome to DISCERN. Retrieved from http://www.discern.org.uk/index.php
Doak, C. C., Doak, L. G., & Root, J. H. (1996). *Teaching patients with low literacy skills* (2nd ed.). Philadelphia, PA: Lippincott.

Donald, H., Franklin, V., & Greene, S. (2009). The use of mobile phones in dietary assessment in young people with type 1 diabetes. *Journal of Human Nutrition and Dietetics, 22*(3), 256–257.

Falvo, D. R. (2011). *Effective patient education: A guide to increased adherence* (4th ed.). Sudbury, MA: Jones & Bartlett Learning.

Flournoy, E., Turner, G., & Combs, D. (2000). Critical care nurses read the writing on the wall: Use interactive bulletin boards to teach your nurses. *Nursing Management, 31*(2), 46–47.

Fox, S. (2007). *E-patients with a disability or chronic disease.* Retrieved from http://www.pewinternet.org/Reports/2007/Epatients-With-a-Disability-or-Chronic-Disease.aspx

Fox, S., & Jones, S. (2009). *The social life of health information.* Retrieved from http://www.pewinternet.org/~/media//Files/Reports/2009/PIP_Health_2009.pdf

Franklin, V. L., Waller, A., Pagliari, C., & Greene, S. A. (2006). A randomized controlled trial of sweet talk, a text-messaging system to support young people with diabetes. *Diabetic Medicine, 23*(12), 1332–1338.

Hasselkus, A. (2009, January 20). Health literacy. *The ASHA Leader,* 28–29.

Hawn, C. (2009). Report from the field. Take two aspirin and tweet me in the morning: How Twitter, Facebook, and other social media are reshaping health care. *Health Affairs, 28*(2), 361–368.

HealthyPeople.gov. (2014). *Health communication and health information technology.* Retrieved from http://healthypeople.gov/2020/topicsobjectives2020/overview.aspx?topicId=18

Jacobi, C., Morris, L., Beckers, C., Bronisch-Holtze, J., Winter, J., Winzelberg, A. J., & Taylor, C. B. (2007). Maintenance of Internet-based prevention: A randomized controlled trial. *International Journal of Eating Disorders, 40*(2), 114–119.

Kisak, A. Z., & Conrad, K. J. (2004). Using technology to develop and distribute patient education storyboards across a health system. *Oncology Nursing Forum, 31*(1), 131–135.

Levy, M., & Royne, M. B. (2009). The impact of consumers' health literacy on public health. *The Journal of Consumer Affairs, 43*(2), 367–372.

Lewis, J. R. (2020). What is driving the decline in people's willingness to take the COVID-19 vaccine in the United States? *JAMA Health Forum, 1*(11), e201393.

Linton, A. D. (2007). Age-related changes in the special senses. In A. D. Linton & H. W. Lach (Eds.), *Matteson and McConnell's gerontological nursing concepts and practice* (3rd ed., pp. 600–627). St. Louis, MO: Saunders Elsevier.

Mark, A. J. (2013). Universal access to essential vital signs monitoring. *Anesthesia & Analgesia, 117*(4), 883–890.

McCormack, L., Thomas, V., Lewis, M. A., & Rudd, R. (2017). Improving low health literacy and patient engagement: A social ecological approach. *Patient Education and Counseling, 100*(1), 8–13.

McLaughlin, G. H. (1969). SMOG grading: A new readability formula. *Journal of Reading, 12*(8), 639–646.

Millard, R. W., & Fintak, P. A. (2012). Use of the Internet by patients with chronic illness. *Disease Management and Health Outcomes, 10*(3), 187–194.

Monsivais, D., & Reynolds, A. (2003). Developing and evaluating patient education materials. *The Journal of Continuing Education in Nursing, 34*(4), 172–176.

Mooney, A., & Prins, E. (2013). *Addressing the health literacy needs of adult education students.* Goodling Institute for Research in Family Literacy, Penn State College of Education.

Murthy, V. (2001). Confronting health misinformation: U.S. Surgeon General's advisory on building a healthy information environment. Office of the U.S. Surgeon General. Retrieved on April 17, 2023, from https://pubmed.ncbi.nlm.nih.gov/34283416..

National Center for Education Statistics. (2003). *National assessment of adult literacy (NAAL).* Retrieved from http://nces.ed.gov/naal/health_results.asp

Pittman, T. J. (2009). Teaching tools. In A. J. Lowenstein, L. Foord-May, & J. C. Romano (Eds.), *Teaching strategies for health education and health promotion: Working with patients, families, and communities.* Sudbury, MA: Jones & Bartlett Learning.

Plain Language. (n.d.). Improving health literacy. Retrieved from http://www.plainlanguage.gov/populartopics/health_literacy/index.cfm

Pohl, M. L. (1981). *The teaching function of the nurse practitioner.* Dubuque, IA: Wm. C. Brown.

Roberts, D. (2008). Nursing antidotes for poor health literacy. *MEDSURG Nursing, 17*(2), 75.

Scharer, K. (2005). An Internet discussion board for parents of mentally ill young children. *Journal of Child and Adolescent Psychiatric Nursing, 18*(1), 17–25.

Schultz, P. N., Stava, C., Beck, M. L., & Vassilopoulou-Sellin, R. (2003). Internet message board use by patients with cancer and their families. *Clinical Journal of Oncology Nursing, 7*(6), 663–667.

Seligman, H. K., Wallace, A. S., DeWalt, D. A., Schillinger, D., Arnold, C. L., Shilliday, B. B., Delgadillo, A., Bengal, N., & Davis, T. C. (2007). Facilitating behavior change with low-literacy patient education materials (Suppl. 1). *American Journal of Health Behavior, 31,* S69–S78.

Sopczyk, D. (2008). Technology in education. In S. B. Bastable (Ed.), *Nurse as educator: Principles of teaching and learning for nursing practice* (pp. 515–552). Sudbury, MA: Jones & Bartlett Learning.

The Joint Commission. (2009). *Speak up initiative. Brochures and infographics.* Retrieved from http://www.jointcommission.org/topics/speakup_brochures.aspx

Thomas, C. M. (2007). Bulletin boards a teaching strategy for older audiences. *Journal of Gerontological Nursing, 33*(3), 45–52.

U.S. Copyright Office. (2009). *Copyright in general.* Retrieved from http://copyright.gov/help/faq/faq-general.html#what

U.S. Government Publishing Office. (2010). *Patient protection and Affordable Care Act.* Retrieved from http://www.gpo.gov/fdsys/pkg/BILLS-111hr3590enr/pdf/BILLS-111hr3590enr.pdf

U.S. National Library of Medicine and National Institutes of Health. (2012). *Interactive health tutorials.* Retrieved from http://www.nlm.nih.gov/medlineplus/tutorial.html

Webster's All-in-One Dictionary and Thesaurus (2nd ed.). (2013). Springfield, MA: Federal Street Press.

Wikipedia. (2014). *History of the Internet.* Retrieved from http://en.wikipedia.org/wiki/History_of_the_Internet

Wilson, F. L., Mood, D., & Nordstrom, C. K. (2010). The influence of easy-to-read pamphlets about self-care management of radiation side effects on patients' knowledge. *Oncology Nursing Forum, 37*(6), 774–781.

Winslow, E. H. (2001). Patient education materials: Can patients read them, or are they ending up in the trash? *American Journal of Nursing, 101*(10), 33–38.

Wood, M. R., Kettinger, C. A., & Lessick, M. (2007). Knowledge is power: How nurses can promote health literacy. *Nursing for Women's Health, 11*(2), 180–188.

Zarcadoolas, C., Pleasant, A. F., & Greer, D. S. (2006). *Advancing health literacy: A framework for understanding and action.* San Francisco, CA: Jossey-Bass.

PART V

Client Education Outcomes

CHAPTER 13

Formative Evaluation

OBJECTIVES

Upon completion of this chapter, you will be able to do the following:

- Describe the history of assessment.
- Identify at least three purposes for evaluation.
- Distinguish between formative and summative evaluation.
- Identify the three components of formative evaluation in the Miller–Stoeckel Client Education Model.
- Describe the evaluation of a client education plan in terms of concept comprehension and motivation.
- Describe evaluation of the learning environment in terms of the delivery format and technology.
- Describe the evaluation of the nurse–client relationship in terms of engagement and communication.

CHAPTER OUTLINE

Introduction

The final step of the teaching and learning process and the client education plan is evaluation. *Evaluation* means to determine the value, significance, worth, or condition of something by careful appraisal and study (Merriam-Webster, 2013). Applied to health education, evaluation is the process of judging the effectiveness of your teaching efforts from beginning to end. Everything you have studied up to this point has a bearing on evaluation. The Miller–Stoeckel Client Education

Model is the conceptual framework for this text, and in this chapter we address the final component of the model: client education outcomes. The model shows two distinct aspects of client education outcomes: *formative evaluation* and *summative evaluation*. This chapter describes different forms and purposes of evaluation and how they fit into the Miller–Stoeckel Client Education Model. The main focus of this chapter is to discuss formative evaluation.

Evaluation

Evaluation is important for nurses as educators, clients as learners, health team members, and educational program managers because it informs them about their progress in learning and the effectiveness of the teaching and learning process. Evaluation is feedback that tells clients and educators if their time and effort together have been well spent (Slavin, 2015).

Evaluation is about judging and providing a basis for making those judgments (Morrison et al., 2007). It tells us the degree to which the learning goals and objectives have been met or not met, and if they were appropriate (Falvo, 2011). Evaluation tells us whether or not the content was suitable and if the teaching strategies and instructional materials were effective. Evaluation in health education provides evidence about the following:

- Client learning
- Effectiveness of the teaching and learning process
- Teacher effectiveness
- Cost–benefit of health education programs

Redman (2007) identifies additional purposes of evaluation, noting that it can motivate clients and reinforce their correct behavior, as well as reinforce educators for effective teaching. Evaluation is also useful in working with health team members. It helps to determine if health team members are knowledgeable, safe, and competent to deliver nursing care and perform nursing procedures.

Evaluation provides credibility and accountability to individual client education efforts and to health education programs taught to groups. It is vital to the institution's education department to document the importance and effectiveness of teaching and learning. This includes documenting client learning, the time teaching takes, and the positive, cost-effective results of the time investment. In addition to the preceding political and financial factors, nurses as educators need to be aware of the legal responsibilities of documentation. Documentation also provides for continuity of teaching efforts because it serves as a communication tool among health team members (Rankin et al., 2005).

The process of evaluation has evolved over time and is divided into two broad categories: *formative* and *summative*. Scriven (1967) made the initial distinction between the two types of evaluation. He stated that formative evaluation is intended to promote improvement within an ongoing activity, person, or program, and summative evaluation is used to assess whether the end goals of the activity, person, or program had been met. Scriven placed more emphasis on summative evaluation to determine the appraisal of the final product. Saettler (1990) further defined the two types of evaluation by saying that formative evaluation is used to refine goals and evolve strategies. Summative evaluation is used to determine the impact of educational practice. He pointed out that formative evaluation can give more detailed information, but it takes longer and is labor intensive.

> **Box 13-1** **Client Education Outcomes: Formative Evaluation**
>
> **Evaluation of the client education plan:**
> - Concept comprehension
> - Motivation
>
> **Evaluation of the learning environment:**
> - Delivery format
> - Technology
>
> **Evaluation of the nurse–client interaction:**
> - Engagement
> - Communication

Box 13-1 presents the formative evaluation portion of client education outcomes for the Miller–Stoeckel Client Education Model. It is the framework for this chapter and addresses three areas: *evaluation of the client education plan*, *evaluation of the learning environment*, and *evaluation of the nurse–client interaction*.

Formative Evaluation: Evaluation of the Client Education Plan

Formative evaluation can be thought of as an assessment *for* learning, as opposed to summative evaluation, which is assessment *of* learning. It begins with evaluation of the client education plan based on the learning outcomes and objectives. Learning outcomes and objectives inform clients and educators of the criteria for success and are part of a feedback loop designed to provide information about the learning experience. Evaluation strategies help determine the effectiveness of learning objectives on learning experiences (**Figure 13-1**).

Concept Comprehension

Formative evaluation of the client education plan includes determining concept comprehension based on the learning objectives. Tools and techniques exist for both clients and educators to assess how well they are meeting the learning objectives. They are not used to grade or determine the end results of learning. Mastery is not expected when concepts are first introduced. The purpose of formative evaluation strategies is to assess concept comprehension along the way and provide information needed to adjust teaching and learning while still occurring. Evaluation of the client education plan helps identify gaps in knowledge, fosters self-study, and informs the client of misunderstandings. Examples of formative evaluation tools include quizzes; direct observation; simulations; concept maps; and Classroom Assessment Techniques (CATs), such as the 1-minute paper, think-pair-share, and case-based learning. The construction of a portfolio also serves as formative evaluation. A portfolio is defined as a collection of evidence gathered to show a person's learning journey over time and progress toward a learning goal (Butler, 2006). Formative assessment tools inform clients of their progress and help them identify strengths and weaknesses.

Figure 13-1 Learning Objectives Feedback Loop

Formative evaluation of educators is used to provide information and feedback about their teaching for the purpose of learning, developing, and improving. Examples of formative evaluation tools for educators include peer observation, use of a checklist or narrative feedback form, one-on-one teaching consultations, and questionnaires. Formative evaluation of the educator is designed to assist in making refinements and adjustments midway through teaching to better meet the learning objectives and needs of clients (Falvo, 2011). It is also helpful in analyzing the usefulness of instructional materials. The *Suitability Assessment of Materials (SAM)* tool measures how well materials fit your clients; it compares different materials and selects those most suitable for your clients. It helps you tailor existing materials to a particular population, sets standards, and guides development and testing of culturally and linguistically appropriate materials.

As you are teaching, it is important to know if you are responding appropriately and effectively to clients. This means monitoring your ability to observe behavior and ask pertinent questions. Observing client behavior in face-to-face encounters includes awareness of verbal and nonverbal cues as you are teaching (O'Brien, 2007). Demonstration and return demonstration is an effective way to observe the client's progress in mastering psychomotor skills. It is an opportunity for you to reinforce what the client is doing right and correct mistakes. Direct questioning is another way to assess client progress in learning. By asking questions, you pick up any gaps or misunderstandings and can clarify the information. Using open-ended questions that require clients to think through an answer is preferred over questions that result in a simple yes or no answer. The client and educator discuss and negotiate ways to improve the educational experience. This highlights the embedded concept of negotiation in the Miller–Stoeckel Client Education Model.

Motivation

While going through the learning process, a client decides whether or not to pay attention. In formative evaluation it is important to determine if the client is paying attention. If the learning objective is judged as important and doable, then the client is motivated to engage in it. If the task is presented as having little relevance to the client or is perceived to have a low probability of success, client motivation may be negatively affected. A negative effect is generated and motivation to complete the learning task is low. Response to teaching is also influenced by individual experiences, behaviors, and attitudes about health behaviors. These influences should be a part of an ongoing formative evaluation of motivation.

The Pender Health Promotion Model provides a framework for describing health-promoting lifestyles. It seeks to interpret healthy behavior of individuals and groups through understanding biophysical processes that motivate them to engage in behaviors directed toward health enhancement (Pender, 2011). The model posits that cognition, action, and environment influence individuals' health-promoting behaviors. It assists the nurse educator with formative evaluation of client motivation in adhering to the education plan.

Nurse–client relationship

- Present health status?
- Previous health-related actions?
- Perceived benefits to act?
- Perceived barriers to act?
- Confidence to act?
- Excitement/apathy to act?
- Environmental influences on action?

Nurse as educator   **Client as learner**

Figure 13-2 Evaluation of Client Motivation to Act

Data from Pender, N. J. (1996). *Health promotion in nursing practice*. Norwalk, CT: Appleton-Century-Crofts.

Promoting healthy behavior through education is not isolated to understanding a person's characteristics; it is also interactive with the environment. The environment is not limited to the physical space occupied; it includes the cultural and social influences within the community. Due to this environmental influence, behaviors that may deter the success of health education must be addressed through formative evaluation. The nurse as educator uses the concepts of the model to develop, modify, and deliver health promotion education to individuals, families, and groups.

The Health Promotion Model provides a lens through which the nurse as educator can evaluate clients' capacity for self-care with the goal to promote, retain, and restore health. The process of evaluating motivation and the willingness to act is ongoing and implies that nurses as educators will adjust the client education plan to accommodate changes in the patient's health status, beliefs, and environmental circumstances. **Figure 13-2** shows the adaption of the Pender Health Promotion Model to the nurse–client relationship concept of the Miller–Stoeckel Client Education Model.

Kirkpatrick (1994) states that formative evaluation should include how well the client liked a particular learning process. It is important that clients and family are satisfied with the health education process. Satisfaction surveys give feedback to assist and improve the educational experience (Falvo, 2011; Rankin et al., 2005). Dansky and Miles (1997) suggest that satisfied clients are more likely to maintain relationships with providers. Other important outcomes are that satisfied clients are more likely to keep appointments, comply with treatment, and refer other patients to their providers (Chung et al., 1999).

If formative evaluation reveals that the client education plan is not relevant to the client, it means effort is needed to revamp the design and presentation of the learning process. The design of the client education plan should promote the learning process rather than just making it entertaining. If the client education plan is built on sound purpose and design, it should motivate the client to learn and support improved performance. Evaluation of motivation and concept comprehension gives you information for improving and evaluating the learning process.

Formative Evaluation: Evaluation of the Learning Environment

Learning environments include the delivery format of the client education plan and the technology that supports the plan. Formative evaluation assesses the delivery format, which includes evaluation of the traditional classroom, distance learning, or a blended format. Traditional classroom learning involves educators in face-to-face situations, whereas in distance education the vast majority of teaching takes places with the educator and client apart. Distance learning uses teaching methods that deliver education through the computer, the Internet, software programs, electronic conferencing, or other approaches. Blended learning combines both classroom and online education so the client may both attend class and independently complete online learning components. The delivery format should be evaluated to determine its appropriateness and effectiveness in delivering content.

Technology resources are all the tools and resources used to support education. Technologies should meet the needs of the client. When they are combined with the appropriate delivery format, they should create an effective and rich learning environment. Formative evaluation includes assessing comfort and the ease of use of delivery formats and technologies.

Delivery Format

Formative evaluation of the delivery format involves assessing the type of delivery format—whether it is face to face, distance learning, or blended—and if it meets the needs of the client and educator. When teaching at a distance, you must address different challenges than when teaching in a traditional classroom. Individual preferences for different formats should be acknowledged, and efforts should be made to promote a positive learning environment.

The classroom evaluation includes both physical and psychological aspects. Questions to ask clients include the following: How does the delivery format support your ability to learn? Do you feel that the physical environment is safe and comfortable? Describe the classroom culture. Is there a culture of mutual respect and understanding? What is the comfort level of interacting with the instructor and other clients? Distance learning formats are evaluated with questions such as the following: What is your comfort level with the method of distance instruction? What is the appropriateness of the online content and assignments? Do the activities support learning? Are there adequate support services for distance learners?

Technology

Formative assessment of technology includes examining the resources used during client education. Learning technologies provide different channels of communication, such as text, audio, visual, and motion, and runs the gamut from slide shows and videos to PowerPoint presentations and hyperlinks. Technologies selected for learning should be effective, efficient, and appealing in meeting the needs of clients. An important part of formative evaluation is that the technology should focus on the needs of the client instead of being used because of an "expectation for technology integration." Questions to ask clients include the following: Is the technology helping you learn? Is the technology user-friendly? What is the best approach to helping you learn? Questions to ask educators include the following: Are you comfortable using the technology? Is the technology engaging clients and supporting the learning objectives?

Formative Evaluation: Evaluation of the Nurse–Client Interaction

Positive relationships are the heart of successful teaching and learning, whether they are defined in terms of respect and rapport, therapeutic interactions, or personal relationship building (Danielson, 2007; Saphier et al., 2008). The Miller–Stoeckel Client Education Model includes the nurse–client relationship as an interaction between nurses and clients to promote, retain, and restore health. It is a professional and planned relationship between client and nurse that focuses on the client's needs, feelings, problems, and ideas. Formative evaluation examines the interaction as it progresses from inception of the client education plan to the point of summative evaluation. The level of engagement and communication between the client and nurse are evaluated to determine if changes are needed to make the interaction more supportive of learning.

Engagement

The nurse–client interaction is directed by the nurse and involves engaging clients in their care, providing information and explanations, and answering questions. Engagement is defined as "an agreement to meet or be present at a specified time and place" (Merriam-Webster, 2013). This implies that clients and educators take initiative and make the effort to participate. For learning to occur, the client and educator must engage in the learning process. Client engagement can be evaluated by determining if the client is present and showing interest in learning activities. Questions for engagement evaluation include the following: Are clients paying attention? Do clients participate in the teaching sessions? Do clients exhibit interest and curiosity about what is being taught? Taking attendance in a classroom setting or showing up to one-on-one teaching sessions helps reveal who is engaged and who is not. Engaged clients will attend and participate in activities, including asking questions. Online engagement can be determined by the number of times the client views or participates in the learning activities, such as online discussions.

Educator engagement can be evaluated in similar ways. Questions to evaluate educator engagement include the following: Is the educator paying attention? Does the educator ask and respond to questions in class or online? Does the educator show enthusiasm and interest in what they are teaching? A formative evaluation can assist both clients and educators to address ways to increase or maintain engagement as part of the nurse–client interaction.

Communication

Communication is the exchange of meanings between individuals through a common system of symbols (Merriam-Webster, 2013). Communication is an essential concept in the Miller–Stoeckel Client Education Model. Clients and educators communicate by speaking and writing and through body language or nonverbal means. Communication is a two-way process that involves getting your message across and understanding what others have to say. It involves active listening, speaking and writing, and observing. The communication process loop reviews how communication takes place; the sender gives the message to the receiver, and the receiver gives feedback to the sender (**Figure 13-3**).

Figure 13-3 Communication Loop

Table 13-1 Helpful and Unhelpful Feedback

Unhelpful Feedback	Reason	Helpful Feedback	Reason
Your nonverbal behavior was not good as you interacted with the client.	Judgmental	I observed you looking at the computer screen, not at the client, as she was answering your questions.	Identifies a specific behavior
You were not empathetic toward the client.	Nonspecific	To show empathy, acknowledge the problems that the client has in dealing with her husband's illness.	Identifies a different solution to a specific problem
You were very abrupt in your response to the client.	Nonspecific	I noticed that when the client was talking about her family, you interrupted her.	Identifies a specific behavior
It would be better if you did it this way.	Does not support critical thinking	Have you thought about trying it in a different way?	Helps generate alternatives
You did not see how upset the client was.	Judgmental	Did you notice that at one point the client was looking down and appeared upset, but you continued to question her?	Describes specific, detailed behavior to encourage reflection
You did a really good job.	Nonspecific	You started the interaction with open-ended questions and allowed the client time to tell her story by remaining silent and attentive.	Describes positive feedback that is specific and descriptive

Data from Wood, D. (2007). *Understanding medical education formative assessment* (p. 15). Edinburgh, Scotland: Association for the Study of Medical Education.

Clients communicate feedback about learning, and educators communicate clear direction and encouragement for continuous improvement. Both clients and educators are expected to speak with respect, listen for understanding, and speak so that others can understand. Both clients and educators should evaluate communication skills by asking the following questions: What are the barriers that keep us from understanding each other's ideas and thoughts? How am I coming across in the way I interact? Am I stating my message clearly? An important type of communication for nurses as educators is giving effective feedback. Nurses should ask themselves if they are giving effective feedback. Feedback should be supportive, behavior specific, and nonjudgmental. **Table 13-1** provides examples of helpful and unhelpful feedback.

During the process of formative evaluation, nurses need to be adaptable. If communication is ineffective, consider what would be a better approach, and change what you are doing as you are doing it.

Case Example: Mrs. Rosa Lopez

Formative evaluation of the interaction with Mrs. Rosa Lopez begins with reviewing the learning objectives and critiquing the teaching and learning process as it is ongoing. For example, by the end of the lesson, the cognitive objective is to have Mrs. Lopez correctly verbally explain to the nurse from memory how excessive salt intake affects blood pressure. An example of midcourse correction might be to notice that Mrs. Lopez preferred the video instruction to viewing charts and pamphlets. Consequently, we would focus on the video and reinforce its message.

In evaluating the affective objective—the client will choose to limit sodium intake by preparing a low sodium dietary plan for one week—we would ask, "How do you plan to incorporate these changes into your meal planning and usual diet?" Note the strength of Mrs. Lopez's desire and willingness to limit excessive sodium intake. Depending on her response, we would follow up with suggestions for how she could accomplish this. We would also ask how these dietary changes would help control her high blood pressure. We would reinforce Mrs. Lopez's correct responses and reteach if her responses demonstrate a lack of understanding. It also might be helpful for Mrs. Lopez to talk to clients who have a similar diagnosis to gain practical meal planning suggestions.

The psychomotor objective is the client will demonstrate how to accurately obtain her own blood pressure reading using a digital monitor without guidance from the nurse. We would have Mrs. Lopez read the equipment directions as we demonstrate how to take the blood pressure using her own digital equipment. Mrs. Lopez would then perform a return demonstration and record the findings following the procedure checklist. She would be given a checklist of the steps to follow at home in obtaining her blood pressure, after which she would be given an opportunity to evaluate her own performance. During this time Mrs. Lopez would be allowed an opportunity to ask questions and be given feedback to guide her learning.

In the formative evaluation process, we would encourage Mrs. Lopez, listen to her concerns, correct misunderstandings, and assure accurate skill performance. When necessary, misinformation would be corrected by reviewing and reteaching any missed or misunderstood content.

Summary

This chapter begins the discussion of the final phase of the teaching and learning process: evaluating client education outcomes. Evaluation of client education has two components: formative and summative. This chapter discussed formative evaluation. Formative evaluation is ongoing during the process of teaching and learning. Clients, educators, health team members, and program managers conduct formative evaluations to improve the learning experience. The Miller–Stoeckel Client Education Model identifies specific aspects of formative evaluation to consider, and they apply to all categories of evaluation.

As the educator, you continuously monitor the effectiveness of the client education plan with attention to concept comprehension and motivation of clients. You also evaluate the learning environment as it relates to the delivery format and technology used for learning. The nurse–client interaction is evaluated by determining the level of engagement and communication. These components of formative evaluation begin at inception of the teaching intervention and conclude at the point of summative evaluation. **Figure 13-4** highlights the key difference between formative and summative evaluation.

The desired outcome of all health education is client learning. Formative evaluation asks, How are we doing in the process of learning? Answering that question and facilitating client learning by making necessary changes during the process of teaching and learning are your responsibilities as educator.

	Formative evaluation (Ongoing, *for* learning)	Summative evaluation (After instruction, *of* learning)
Evaluation of education plan:	Concept comprehension, motivation	Measures learning
Evaluation of environment:	Delivery format, technology	Measures effectiveness of programs
Evaluation of nurse–client interaction:	Engagement, communication	Measures accountability
Tools for evaluation:	CATs, simulation, surveys, self-assessments, portfolio	Testing, surveys, rubrics, exams, checklists
Purpose:	Feedback for improvement	Final assessments

Intervention inception ⟶ Midway ⟶ End

Figure 13-4 Formative and Summative Evaluation Continuum

Data from McTighe, J., & Wiggins, G (1999). *The understanding by design handbook*. Alexandria, VA: Association for Supervision and Curriculum Development.

Exercises

Exercise I: Evaluation of the Client Education Plan

Purpose: Apply formative evaluation to the client education plan.

Directions: Discuss the following situations and describe, as the educator, how you would handle each one.

1. You are teaching a hospitalized client who is ready for discharge about the importance of taking an antibiotic as prescribed. The learning objectives are for the client to explain the purpose of the antibiotic and how to take the medication. You want to conduct a formative evaluation to determine concept comprehension as you teach. Give an example of a tool or other evaluation method that will inform you as to whether the client education plan is working (such as CAT, quiz, role-play). Explain why you have chosen this method. What types of feedback would indicate that you need to make changes to your approach?

2. You are teaching a series of classes to a group of older clients about the benefits and types of exercise to improve stamina. You notice at the second class that some clients are not participating and seem to withdraw from the group. Give examples of questions you will ask to determine motivation to act as part of formative evaluation of the client education plan. What are possible barriers to participation in the client education plan?

Exercise II: Evaluation of the Learning Environment

Purpose: Apply formative evaluation to the learning environment.

Directions: With a partner, discuss the following situations and describe how, as the educator, you would handle each one:

1. You are teaching a group of parents at the clinic about how to care for ill toddlers. Many of the parents bring their children and tend to them during the class. As the class progresses, you wonder if the other parents are comfortable with the learning environment. What kinds of questions would you ask to determine if the environment is conducive to learning as part of a formative assessment? How would having this information help you make improvements in the class?
2. You are leading a bereavement discussion group in the hospital and have arranged for several videos to be shown on the experience of loss. You notice that some clients are leaving in the middle of the videos and not returning until the lights are turned on. How will you conduct a formative evaluation to determine how technology is affecting learning in this class? Why is it important to evaluate the learning environment in this class?

Exercise III: Evaluation of the Nurse–Client Interaction

Purpose: Apply formative evaluation to the nurse–client interaction.

Directions: Divide into small groups. Discuss the following situations and describe how, as the educator, you would handle each one:

1. To evaluate the educator–client interaction, have each person share a personal experience about learning new information or a skill. Then identify helpful and unhelpful feedback that you received during the experience. Describe what makes the communication helpful and not helpful.
2. Think of a class in which you did not participate and felt uncomfortable giving feedback. Describe what made you disengage and how things could have been changed to make you want to interact with other students and the instructor.

Exercise IV: Evidence-Based Nursing Practice

Purpose: Apply evidence-based nursing research to client education.

Directions:

1. Search the literature for nursing research applicable to formative evaluation related to health education.
2. Describe how the findings could be applied to your practice in educating clients.

References

Butler, P. (2006). *Review of the literature on portfolios and e-portfolios.* Retrieved from http://www.eportfolio practice.qut .edu.au/docs/Butler%20-%20Review%20of%20lit%20on%20ePortfolio%20research%20-%20 NZOct%202006.pdf

Chung, K. C., Hamill, J. B., Kim, H. M., Walters, M. R., & Wilkins, E. G. (1999). Predictors of patient satisfaction in an outpatient plastic surgery clinic. *Annals of Plastic Surgery, 42*(1), 56–60.

Danielson, C. (2007). *Enhancing professional practice: A framework for teaching* (2nd ed.). Alexandria, VA: Association for Supervision and Curriculum Development (ASCD).

Dansky, K. H., & Miles, J. (1997). Patient satisfaction with ambulatory healthcare services: Waiting time and filling time. *Hospital and Health Services Administration, 42*, 165–176.

Falvo, D. R. (2011). *Effective patient education: A guide to increased compliance* (4th ed.). Sudbury, MA: Jones & Bartlett Learning.

Kirkpatrick, D. L. (1994). *Evaluating training programs.* San Francisco, CA: Berrett-Koehler.

Merriam-Webster. (2013). *Webster's All-In-One Dictionary and Thesaurus* (2nd ed.). Springfield, MA: Federal Street Press.

Morrison, G. R., Ross, S. M., Kemp, J. E., & Kalman, H. K. (2007). *Designing effective instruction* (5th ed.). Hoboken, NJ: John Wiley and Sons.

O'Brien, P. G. (2007). Patient and family teaching. In S. L. Lewis, M. M. Heitkemper, S. R. Dirksen, P. G. O'Brien, & L. Bucher (Eds.), *Medical-surgical nursing* (7th ed., pp. 53–65). St. Louis, MO: Mosby.

Pender, N. (2011). *The health promotion manual.* Retrieved from https://deepblue.lib.umich.edu/bitstream /handle/2027.42/85350/HEALTH_PROMOTION_MANUAL_Rev_5-2011.pdf

Rankin, S. H., Stallings, K. D., & London, F. (2005). *Patient education in health and illness* (5th ed.). Philadelphia, PA: Lippincott Williams & Wilkins.

Redman, B. K. (2007). *The practice of patient education: A case study approach* (10th ed.). St. Louis, MO: Mosby Year Book.

Saettler, P. (1990). *The evolution of American educational technology.* Englewood, CO: Libraries Unlimited.

Saphier, J., Haley-Speca, M. A., & Gower, R. (2008). *The skillful teacher: Building your teaching skills* (6th ed.). Acton, MA: Research for Better Teaching.

Scriven, M. (1967). The methodology of evaluation. In R. W. Tyler, R. M. Gagne, & M. Sciven (Eds.), *Perspectives of curriculum evaluation* (pp. 39–83). Chicago, IL: Rand McNally.

Slavin, R. E. (2015). *Educational psychology theory and practice* (10th ed.). Boston, MA: Pearson.

Wood, D. (2007). *Understanding medical education: Formative assessment.* Edinburgh, Scotland: Association for the Study of Medical Education.

Summative Evaluation

OBJECTIVES

Upon completion of this chapter, you will be able to do the following:

- Identify the three components of summative evaluation in the Miller–Stoeckel Client Education Model.
- Distinguish between measurement and evaluation.
- Describe the evaluation of client learning using direct and indirect measurement methods.
- Describe four sources of error in measurement.
- Select measurement methods best suited for cognitive, affective, and psychomotor objectives.
- Describe the evaluation of educational effectiveness as it relates to course and program evaluation.
- Describe the evaluation of the integration of learning into clients' daily living as it relates to adherence and the impact on the community.
- Describe the ecological perspective on client adherence.

CHAPTER OUTLINE

Introduction

In this chapter, we discuss summative evaluation and its purpose in accomplishing the goal and purpose of the Miller–Stoeckel Client Education Model. Each chapter in the book focused on specific aspects of health education and now it is time to evaluate the effectiveness of our health education efforts. How effective have we been in promoting, retaining, and restoring client health and the health of the community?

Summative evaluation occurs at the conclusion of teaching and learning and how to use the results to promote client learning and adherence, and to improve courses and programs. Summative evaluation focuses on three areas: *evaluation of client learning*, *evaluation of educational effectiveness*, and *evaluation of integration of learning into daily living* (**Box 14-1**). This chapter explores each of these areas. The ultimate test of our educational efforts is improvement in clients' health and the health of the community.

Summative Evaluation: Evaluation of Client Learning

After any teaching effort, it is important for nurses as educators to pause, look back, and reflect on what has been accomplished and what they can learn from their efforts. Did clients achieve the knowledge, attitudes, and skills specified in the learning objectives? What evidence do we have of client learning? Were the objectives, content, teaching strategies, and instructional materials suitable and effective for the clients? Would different instructional materials be more effective— for example, would having models and equipment to manipulate be more effective than watching videos? Summative evaluation involves making comparisons between what is effective and what is not. To begin our discussion of summative evaluation, we must first focus on measurement and the difficulties of measuring learning.

Measurement

Evaluation is about judging and determining the value, significance, worth, or condition of something. It is how we support that evaluation, and it establishes the criteria by which to judge something. *Measurement* means gauging the dimensions, quantity, or capacity of something by

---

Box 14-1 Client Education Outcomes: Summative Evaluation

Evaluation of client learning:
- Measurement
- Direct measurement methods
- Indirect measurement methods

Evaluation of educational effectiveness:
- Course evaluation
- Program evaluation

Evaluation of integration of learning into daily living:
- Client adherence
- Impact on the community

Figure 14-1 Direct and Indirect Measurement Continuum

comparing it with some kind of standard (*Webster's*, 2013). Measurement ranges from the concrete, such as clients learning to take their own pulse, to the abstract, such as learning better ways to handle stress. Both phenomena are important; however, the former is much easier to measure than the latter. Methods of measurement are ordered along a continuum from direct to indirect at opposite ends (**Figure 14-1**).

Measurement involves both observation and recording behavior, regardless of whether the measurement is direct or indirect. *Direct measurement* is the most accurate when it takes place in the actual situation and, ideally, when it occurs over time. It is direct observation of the behavior being measured. For example, nurses make observations at the hospital bedside, in the home, or at the work site. Direct observations are also obtained from equipment and monitors that measure things such as vital signs, oxygen levels, blood glucose, and so forth.

Indirect measurement is not as accurate as direct measurement. It occurs when the educator creates substitute situations or takes incomplete samples of behavior. For example, if you role-play with clients, you create substitute situations that imitate, or substitute for, the real one. When you give clients paper-and-pencil tests, you attempt to measure cognitive processes indirectly. No one knows what thinking is or what it looks like. Therefore, you must infer from what clients write whether or not they have thought about, retained, and gained the knowledge and understanding you hoped they would grasp.

Measurement methods are also categorized as being objective or subjective (Lorig et al., 2001). Examples of *objective measures* include observable factors such as vital signs, weight, blood glucose, cholesterol levels, wound healing, hospital readmissions, and class attendance. *Subjective measures* are data from human observers (clients, providers, educators) and are therefore considered biased measures. These measures are less reliable because there are multiple explanations for client behavior. There may be extenuating circumstances that affect whether the client can successfully meet the objectives, and these circumstances may be unknown to the observer. For example, a nurse reports that a client who is overweight has little interest in weight reduction, when in fact the client does not understand how to diet. The nurse assumes the client is not motivated to learn about weight reduction because the client discarded reading material they were given, when in fact the client has low health literacy skills. The client can also be a subjective observer. For example, the client who chain smokes reports that they stopped smoking, when in fact they cut down to one to two cigarettes per day.

Sources of Error in Measurement

Error is always possible in measurement, and the more indirect the measurement, the more likely errors will occur. Redman (2007) notes the following common sources of error: indirect measurement, the complexity of behavior, observer bias, and sampling error. A brief description of each source of error follows.

Indirect Measurement

Indirect measurement provides a false picture of how a client would react unless the nurse observes that person in the actual situation. The saying "he talks a good game" indicates that many people know the difference between talking about a situation and actually handling it. Because your time with clients is limited, your only choice may be to measure the learning objectives by indirect means, such as oral quizzes and paper-and-pencil tests. Keep in mind that these methods are indirect and you infer the degree of client learning from them.

Complex Behavior

Behavior, by nature, is complex. The causes of behavior, especially thought patterns, feelings, and attitudes, are difficult to identify for both the observer and the client who exhibits the behavior. As an educator, you may not be able to discover what, if any, impact the learning had on clients. A client may act agreeable just to please you, or they may choose not to tell you all the variables involved in a failure to learn. Indeed, clients themselves may not be fully aware of all the factors that help or hinder their learning.

Observer Bias

Humans are limited in the amount of stimuli they can notice. Observers draw conclusions based on their own perceptions, culture, and past experiences. This can lead to erroneous inferences and conclusions about client learning. One advantage of working with colleagues is that it can help balance the perceptions of individual clients. How others see a particular client influences your perceptions. When you team teach, you and your colleagues give balanced views of the clients. If a colleague tells you a client, a family, or a team member is difficult to deal with, you are likely to approach that individual in a different manner. This can lead to bias, but it can also lead to a collaborative effort to help the client learn. Approach each individual with openness.

Sampling Error

Sampling is obtaining a small picture of the client's behavior that is representative of all the learning you provided. From this sample, you infer that the client has or has not mastered the learning objectives. Sampling error occurs when the sample you choose to measure is not representative of client learning. Clients may have learned A, B, and C; but if you measure D, E, and F, you get a false picture of the client's learning and achievements.

The period of time during which you choose to measure the behavior can also be misleading. For example, you form a different perception of your client's willingness and ability to do range-of-motion exercises if you test them early in the morning rather than waiting until later in the day. It is not possible to observe all the required behaviors. Therefore, your task is to select behavioral samples that are as representative as possible and relevant to the variables that are most critical. In general, you can compensate for measurement errors by using a variety of measurement methods.

Direct Measurement Methods

Measurement methods must be consistent with the learning objectives. You cannot test everything you have taught or that clients have learned, so you must select a representative sample to test

(Slavin, 2015). *Direct measurement* of behavior is achieved through observation of behavior, video recordings, rating scales, checklists, evaluation rubrics, and anecdotal notes.

Observation of Behavior

Direct observation occurs when the nurse observes clients demonstrating mastery of psychomotor skills. For example, you observe a client properly using crutches with no axillary pressure and no loss of balance. Another example is observing how skillfully a client removes a dressing, cleans the wound, and applies a fresh dressing without contamination. Both examples are direct observations of client behavior.

Direct observation also involves nurses using the senses. For example, the nurse listens to breath sounds through a stethoscope after a guided session of turning and deep breathing. Or the nurse counts the client's pulse and respiration rate to observe the impact of a relaxation exercise. Direct observations of client responses are documented by using a checklist designed for specific procedures, which is discussed later in this chapter.

Video Recordings

Direct observation of behavior is also achieved through video recordings. Video recordings offer the advantage of accuracy. The video camera observes and records what happened, rather than depending on the nurse's interpretation of what happened. The recording is useful in that the nurse and client get accurate feedback by watching it. This is especially useful when teaching health team members new psychomotor skills. The recording can be studied repeatedly and at length for feedback to improve performance.

Video recordings are helpful when clients role-play new affective behaviors, such as improving interpersonal communications. Families who are puzzled by their communication difficulties can sometimes gain insight into their patterns when viewed from a different perspective. Video recording helps decrease defensiveness and increases objectiveness as they watch themselves.

Video recordings are effective for teaching health team members how to interact with clients who are depressed, anxious, or hostile. They are also effective for nurses who are new in the role of educator and for experienced nurses who want to improve their teaching performance. It is much easier to accept feedback from observing a video recording of one's performance rather than an instructor's critique.

Rating Scales

Rating scales on surveys and questionnaires use a Likert-type scale to rate client responses. For example, one rating scale asks if clients strongly agree, agree, disagree, or strongly disagree with a number of specific items. Another rating scale asks how clients would evaluate items on a scale that ranges from 1 to 5, in which 1 means no confidence and 5 means total confidence. There are a variety of responses for this scale, depending on what you want to know. The meaning of the numbers can also vary but should be clearly identified in the legend. For example, 1 could mean "did not help me" at the low end, and 5 could mean "helped me a great deal" at the high end of the scale.

Rating scales are given to clients to fill out at the conclusion of a teaching session, course, or program to evaluate their satisfaction with the teaching experience. They provide insight into the clients' perceptions of learning effectiveness. They also provide helpful feedback to improve the teacher's performance. Rating scales are used for statistical purposes. Collating the results

Exhibit 14-1 Sample Form to Evaluate Learning Objectives

List each learning objective here	0	1	2	3	4	5
1.						
2.						
3.						
4.						

Descriptors for the key can vary.
For example, the stem can read "To what degree did this course help you achieve the learning objective?" and the key could be a 3-point rating scale: not at all, somewhat, and a lot.

Key:
0 = not applicable
1 = did not help me achieve this objective
2 = helped me less than I expected
3 = helped me about what I expected
4 = helped me more than I expected

and determining the mean and standard deviation for each item on the rating scale provides instructive information. These data collected over time provide useful feedback to evaluate clients' perceptions of teaching and learning effectiveness. **Exhibits 14-1** and **14-2** are sample rating scales used to evaluate learning objectives and teacher evaluations.

Checklists

Checklists are more precise than rating scales because they identify each of the desired behaviors and provide space for recording the presence or absence of each behavior. When you create a checklist, identify the critical elements of the desired behaviors, and exclude nonessential ones. For example, when you measure a parent's bonding behavior, include observations such as whether they look at, touch, and talk to the infant rather than whether they have the most updated equipment. Another example is teaching a client to give a self-injection. It is not critical how the client arranges the placement of equipment on a tray. It is critical, however, that the sterility of the equipment is maintained. **Exhibit 14-3** is a sample checklist of critical requirements for giving an injection. The learning domain is psychomotor, and the learning objective is as follows: the client will perform an injection accurately according to the steps of the procedure.

Assistance from colleagues is valuable in developing a checklist. They can try out the checklist to refine the items and wording. Because clients do not pass until they can do every step correctly, it is important to establish the number of times clients must exhibit the correct behaviors to ensure they have mastered the task.

Evaluation Rubrics

An *evaluation rubric* combines features of the rating scale and checklist that are useful for evaluating team members' performance when a team member is your client (**Exhibit 14-4**). The example

Exhibit 14-2 **Teacher Evaluation Form**

Teacher Evaluation Form

Key:
0 = not applicable
1 = definitely below average
2 = slightly below average
3 = average
4 = slightly above average
5 = definitely above average

Speaker:_____

Evaluator: _____

Objectives — Were the objectives:
    Clearly presented to the clients?
    Evident throughout the presentation?

Content — Was the content:
    Clearly explained?
    Accurate?
    At the right vocabulary level?
    Appropriate to the audience's background?

Strategies — Were the strategies:
    Appropriate for the content?
    Appropriate for the audience?

Teaching aids — Were the materials:
    Appropriate to the context?
    Appropriate to the objectives?
    At the client's level of comprehension?
    Pleasing to the eye?
    Visible (contrast, size, and location)?
    Used in a practiced manner?

Performance — Did the teacher:
    Dress appropriately to the clients and topic?
    Maintain eye contact with the audience?
    Speak in a clear, audible voice?
    Use a pace appropriate to the audience?
    Stay attuned to the audience?
    Give recognition for contributions?
    Allow time for questions?
    Seek feedback periodically?
    Show preparation by smooth performance?

0 1 2 3 4 5

Comments:

Data from Babcock, D., & Miller, M. (1994). *Client education: Theory & practice.* St. Louis: Mosby.

uses Benner's (1984) five levels of proficiency (novice, advanced beginner, competent, proficient, and expert) to evaluate nurses in their role as educators. The evaluator notes the level of proficiency at which the team member is performing each criterion. The evaluator then writes an anecdotal note in the space provided. An alternative rating scale that could be used instead of Benner's

Exhibit 14-3 Checklist for Giving an Injection

Name of Client: _____ Behavior	Dates					Comments
1. Selects appropriate equipment.						
2. Identifies action, use, side effects, and dosage range of medication.						
3. Maintains sterility: a. of equipment. b. in administration.						
4. Prepares accurate dosage: a. verifies dosage prescribed. b. draws up correct dose. 5. Selects acceptable injection site.						
6. Injects at appropriate angle: a. 30- to 60-degree angle for SQ b. 90-degree angle for IM 7. Aspirates plunger before injecting.						
8. Injects medication.						
9. Disposes of needle safely.						

levels is beginning, developing, proficient, and independent. Whichever rating scale is used, a committee of nurses in the healthcare institution should define the rating levels. There should be broad agreement of the definition of the scope of skills and responsibilities for each level. The criteria in the example are samples of what could be included in the rubric.

Anecdotal Notes

An *anecdotal note* is a brief vignette of a client's behavior at a particular moment in time. This type of note is used in psychiatric facilities because it helps observers detect changes in clients' behaviors over time and the circumstances under which changes occurred. For example, an adolescent client hospitalized for severe behavior problems was cooperative with their therapist away from the hospital, but was obstinate and defiant with caregivers on the psychiatric unit. The nurse must determine the following:

- What is the client's behavior with their family and friends?
- What is the gender of the therapist and other caregivers? Does the gender of the caregiver make a difference?
- How are the therapist's interactions with the client different from that of the staff?

It is crucial for various caregivers on the unit to use the observations as important data for evaluation. They should not automatically jump to a conclusion like, the client always acts fine for me. The hidden implication is, what are the rest of you doing wrong?

Anecdotal notes must be recorded consistently over time for the caregivers to pick up client behavior patterns and changes. They should be pertinent to the learning objectives with related

Exhibit 14-4 Evaluation Rubric

Criterion	Novice	Advanced beginner	Competent	Proficient	Expert	Notes
Communicates learning objectives				Yes		Clearly stated at outset
Presents accurate information		Yes				Much improved over previous session
Uses appropriate teaching strategies		Yes				Tried another strategy when the first was ineffective
Uses appropriate handouts			Yes			Distributed two handouts written in client's native language
Answers questions	No					Needs to take the time to answer questions
Seeks feedback periodically	No					Needs to pause and seek feedback
Maintains eye contact		Yes				Fairly consistent eye contact

Definitions of these terms should be created by a committee of professional nurses in the healthcare institution/agency using the tool: Novice, Advanced beginner, Competent, Proficient, and Expert.

comments. They should also clearly and specifically describe client behavior and be free of bias or derogatory terms.

The following example illustrates an inappropriate comment: the client is obnoxious and uncooperative. It would be better to restate such an observation as follows:

- The client refuses to get out of bed until . . .
- When client is reminded about the importance of exercise to their recovery, they avoid eye contact and do not respond.

The latter example may create a climate of investigation rather than disapproval. If nurses are curious rather than judgmental, they will more likely discover clues that help create a learning environment that is conducive to success. If they maintain an attitude of curiosity, they are more likely to discover if there are disparities between the client's and nurses' goals.

Indirect Measurement Methods

Indirect measurement methods must be consistent with the learning objectives. Develop questions that provide evidence of how well clients achieved the learning objectives. Indirect measurement of behavior includes direct questioning and written measurement.

Direct Questioning

Direct questioning is an effective way to determine a client's level of understanding of what you taught. It is useful in both formative and summative evaluation; however, it is more often used in formative evaluation when teaching is ongoing. Its use in summative evaluation is limited to oral quizzes, which have little application in health education. Direct questioning is also used to obtain oral feedback from clients at the conclusion of a teaching session or program to learn what was most and least helpful.

Written Measurement

So far, we have considered measurement involving direct transactions with clients in which you have observed the learning directly or asked clients for their perceptions of the learning that took place. A more indirect way to gather evidence of learning is *written measurement*; however, there are prerequisites to using this method for evaluation. For example, to use written measurement, clients must be able to read and have the ability to see. A client who is well educated but taking medications that cause double vision cannot participate in written measurement, nor can clients whose reading glasses are unavailable. Clients who are bilingual but read only in another language, or clients who are so weak they cannot write, are inappropriate subjects for written evaluations.

One of the main advantages of written measurement is its efficiency in terms of time and energy. One person (not necessarily the nurse educator) can distribute a written measurement tool to many people at once. The data can be analyzed at the evaluator's convenience and can be easily stored along with the conclusions. In this computer age, written measurements for evaluation are part of software educational programs.

Test Construction

To construct an effective test, you need to keep many variables in mind. A good test covers all of the relevant material and relates directly to the learning objectives. Because you cannot ask everything on a test, the test should include a representative sample of what was taught (Gronlund & Brookhart, 2009). Testing is sampling what clients have learned.

Any test should be relevant to the clients in terms of their life experience and health literacy level. If the clients' reading skills are limited, use very simple words and supplement them with pictures. If they are unable to understand written directions, give the directions orally. Reviewing a couple of sample items with clients helps them to understand your expectations. Many clients are more confident if you show them what you want them to do. Be aware that clients may read directions only as a last resort.

A good test uses different types of items, such as true or false, multiple choice, matching, fill in the blank, and short-answer essay to test learning in a variety of ways. True-or-false and fill-in-the-blank questions are good for testing knowledge of facts. Matching questions are good for testing recall of related concepts. Multiple-choice questions are good for distinguishing myths from reality and for measuring some levels of problem solving, inference, and making generalizations.

Box 14-2 Guidelines for Writing Test Questions

- Group questions according to type: true or false, matching, multiple choice, fill in the blank, and short-answer essay.
- State general directions at the beginning of the test; for example, "This test is designed to measure what you know about how to take care of yourself. It will help us plan further teaching." (For clients with low literacy say, "Please take this test. The results will tell us what else we need to teach you.")
- State specific directions before each group of questions.
- Indicate where to record the answer and provide a place for the clients' answers.
- Use vocabulary that fits the reading level of the clients.
- Make the directions as clear and as short as possible.
- Underline or bold the directions and special words.
- Make all multiple-choice options similar in length.
- Put the multiple-choice question and answer options on the same page.
- Make all multiple-choice options grammatically parallel.

Short-answer essay questions reveal the clients' thinking process. They also provide clues to the clients' use of the information you taught. See **Box 14-2** for guidelines to help you write test questions.

When preparing test questions, avoid using the exact words you used while teaching so that you measure understanding rather than memory. The use of giveaway words should also be avoided, although they can be used as distracters in the questions. The words *never, always,* and *all* usually indicate that the answer is false. The words *generally, mostly,* and *usually* commonly indicate that the answer is true. If words such as these are used, the test may measure the test-taking skills of clients rather than their attainment of the learning objectives. Be clear about what you want to measure.

True-or-false questions are good for testing common misperceptions about health and illness. These questions test recognition of information rather than recall. The advantage is that they are easy to write. The disadvantage is that clients have a 50% chance of selecting the correct answer regardless of their knowledge. If you use true-or-false questions, write out *T or true* and *F or false* in front of the question, and instruct clients to circle the correct answer. When clients have to write either T or F, sometimes it is difficult to decipher their handwriting.

Each *multiple-choice question* has three parts: the stem, the correct answer, and the distracters. The stem is the lead-in sentence or question to which the client must then fit the correct answer. Distracters are other possible but incorrect answers. Myths and plausible answers are good distracters. A good test question is grammatically consistent with all the possible answers. All answer options should be about the same length. Inconsistencies in length can give clues to the correct answer. Clients guess the right answer by looking for the best grammatical fit in matching or multiple-choice questions. If all of the options begin with the same word or phrase, that word or phrase should be stated only once at the end of the stem (**Box 14-3**). Try to avoid negatively stated items. If you use negative items, be sure to underline the negative. An example of this is the test question 2 in Box 14-3. A table of random numbers helps you list answers and distracters inconsistently; it is easy to slip into a predictable pattern for listing correct answers. Another way to randomize the sequence of choices in multiple-choice questions is to arrange answers alphabetically.

Box 14-3 Examples of Multiple-Choice Questions

---

1. Which of the following statements is true about parenthood? It is a/an:
   a. Impossible role for most couples
   b. Demanding but growth-enhancing experience
   c. Essential element of a healthy marriage
   d. Necessary element of a well-rounded, fulfilled life
2. Effective crutch walking includes all the following except:
   a. Avoiding slippery surfaces so that you remain stable
   b. Keeping the crutches snug in your armpits by leaning on them
   c. Practicing until you have developed a smooth rhythm
   d. Placing your most important items in a fanny pack

Matching questions have two columns. The first column gives a list of words that must be matched to the words or phrases in the second column. It is preferable to use phrases in the second column to discourage guessing, and it also makes the test a better measure of the client's knowledge. There should be more words or phrases listed in the second column than in the first column. The words or phrases in the second column will be a combination of correct answers and distracters. The goal is to test the client's knowledge, not their guessing ability.

Fill-in-the-blank questions should contain blanks that are all the same size. If the blanks vary in size, clients will try to guess what word you had in mind when you constructed the test. If you choose to provide a list of correct words, it should contain distracters.

Short-answer essay questions are good because clients can answer them in their own words. When you read the answers, you learn about the clients' perceptions about the health issue and gain insight into their thinking. For health education purposes, the answer to the question should take only a few sentences.

When preparing a test, group questions according to type because clients must switch mental processes to answer each type. For example, all true-or-false questions should be grouped together, and all multiple-choice questions should be together. If the test is likely to produce some anxiety, it may help to start it with some easy items. This helps to measure clients' learning rather than how they think when they are stressed.

Making test directions clear is a challenging task. A good way to clarify the directions is to have them critiqued by someone who knows the subject. Sometimes clients need help and hints. This is especially true when a written tool is used to test children. Include a grading scale if clients are to grade themselves; a key can be provided on the back of the page or upside down at the bottom of the page.

Pretests and Posttests

A pretest is useful for assessing the clients' current knowledge about a subject and their learning needs. The results of the pretest allow nurses to construct the knowledge base for teaching and avoid repeating what clients already know. Pretests are also good for piquing the curiosity of clients. One possible disadvantage of pretests is that they are often perceived as threatening. This threat may be outweighed by the fact that pretests are helpful as self-diagnostic feedback.

At the conclusion of the teaching session, administer a posttest. The posttest should be the same as the pretest to determine the gains made as a result of the teaching session. The results of both pre- and posttests are compared to measure client learning. Some test services design equivalent pretests and posttests. This means that although the tests are not exactly alike, they test the same knowledge or skills. The process for developing equivalent tests is lengthy, expensive, and must be done with populations of significant size. This involves sophisticated statistical analysis that is beyond the scope of this text.

Choosing Appropriate Measurement Methods

Cognitive, affective, and psychomotor learning objectives require different measurement methods. To determine which are best, ask which are most appropriate for the learning objective you are measuring. For example, which are most appropriate to measure *cognitive* learning? The most appropriate methods to use here are oral questions and written measurement. These methods are indirect because you cannot measure cognition (thinking) directly.

How do you measure changes in clients' *attitudes* or feelings? You may be able to question them directly if they trust you. Their willingness to share is affected by the quality of the nurse–client relationship. Direct observation is also an excellent method because you can infer much from clients' behavior. Clients are not always fully aware of or willing to admit their attitudes and feelings. However, a client's behavior may give clues if you are an astute observer. Video recordings done with a client's permission and anecdotal notes are two good ways to gather the needed data. Written measurement in the form of an attitude scale or opinion survey may also be useful. The use of open-ended questions is yet another way to measure attitudes and feelings. Many factors influence a person's willingness to admit attitudinal change or lack of change.

How do you decide whether or not clients can perform a *psychomotor* skill at a satisfactory level? Direct observation is the main method for evaluating the attainment of psychomotor skills. If performance is being evaluated, a video recording is excellent. Checklists and rating scales are also useful because they enable you to remain objective with a previously constructed and carefully formulated list. Checklists also reduce the likelihood that crucial elements of the desired performance will be neglected.

Evaluation of Health Team Members

Evaluating health team members is similar to evaluating clients, but the outcome for health team members is more consequential. Clients can choose to learn, partially learn, or ignore learning your health message to promote, retain, and restore health. Evaluation is different for health team members because they are required to learn what you are teaching and will be evaluated accordingly. It is important that the behavior and practice of health team members is aligned with the best practices of the profession and the employing healthcare facility.

The purpose of evaluating health team members is to ensure that each member is fully prepared, competent, safe, and knowledgeable to deliver health care to clients. The evaluation should be consistent with each state's statutes that govern nursing practice and the policies of the employing healthcare facility. The outcome of the evaluation ensures that clinical skills and knowledge are current. Team members must be skillful and have the latest understanding of nursing, healthcare actions, and rationales.

It is important to have conducted a thorough assessment of the health team member's knowledge and skills prior to evaluation. Although teaching can be done individually or in a group, evaluation of learning is based on each individual's performance. Health team members should be fully aware of what they are expected to know, the level at which they are expected to know it, and the knowledge and skills they must demonstrate prior to evaluation. Evaluation follows your teaching; you are evaluating what you taught and what you are expecting team members to learn.

Health team members' knowledge and skills are evaluated using many of the same measurement methods described in this chapter for clients. Direct measurement methods are used to evaluate skills and include direct observation of behavior while performing a skill on a client, a simulation manikin, or simulation models. Evaluation may include video recording of performance. Skill evaluation uses rating scales, checklists of critical steps, evaluation rubrics, and anecdotal notes. Indirect measurement methods are used to evaluate knowledge and include direct questioning and written methods such as quizzes and tests.

The level of knowledge and skill that health team members must demonstrate is higher and more consequential than expected of clients. Do team members need to perform all steps of a skill correctly and answer all questions on a knowledge test correctly? Or do they need to correctly answer most of them? Do they need to achieve a given percentage correctly, such as 90%? Are some skill steps or knowledge items more critical than others, so those items must be answered at 100% accuracy? These are questions that must be addressed in evaluating health team members.

Summative Evaluation: Evaluation of Educational Effectiveness

Evaluating educational effectiveness has two aspects: course evaluation and program evaluation. These are discussed in the following section.

Course Evaluation

The focus of course evaluation is limited to the specific teaching you did with a client or a group of clients. It is concerned with the learning objectives, subject matter content that was taught, teaching strategies used, and instructional materials used to supplement your teaching. You will also want to know how the clients viewed your effectiveness as a teacher. Some of this information is gathered using course evaluations, and some information is what you noted in your own evaluation of the course.

Evaluating learning objectives is done in one of several ways. Exhibit 14-1 illustrates a typical rating scale for evaluating learning objectives. The form is customized by listing each learning objective to be evaluated. Each learning objective is then rated on a 3- or 5-point scale. When you use a form like this, include open-ended questions and leave ample space for clients to provide written responses. A similar form could be created to have clients evaluate the teaching strategies and instructional materials.

Another evaluation method is comprised of open-ended questions. Such questions require clients to provide more thoughtful responses than on a rating scale or checklist. For example, to gain additional evaluative information from the clients, ask questions like these:

- What content was most helpful for you? (Variations: What was the most important thing you learned? Name the two most important things you learned.)
- What content was the least helpful for you? (Variations: What was the least important thing you learned? Name the two least important things that were taught.)
- What content was not covered that you think should have been? (Variation: What content would you like to see covered in this course in the future?)
- What would be helpful for us to know that would make the course better?

To evaluate your own performance as a teacher, see Exhibit 14-2. It covers how effectively you addressed learning objectives, the subject matter content, your teaching strategies, the teaching and instructional aids, and your performance. At the bottom of the evaluation form is an opportunity for clients to write their own impressions and comments. It should be administered at the same time as the form to evaluate learning objectives. We have used this form on numerous occasions and found it very helpful for nurses as educators. Administer both evaluation forms at the last class while everyone is still present. The forms should be administered by the department secretary or someone other than the nurse who taught the course. The nurse should leave the room when the forms are distributed. The responses are confidential, and clients should not be asked to provide their names on the forms. After clients have completed the forms, the responses can be tabulated and then shared with the nurse who taught the course and the head of the health education department.

Program Evaluation

Health teaching is often delivered through structured programs. A program is any group of related, complementary activities intended to achieve specific outcomes. The process of program evaluation includes the systematic gathering, analysis, and reporting of data about a program to assist in decision making. *Program evaluation* is usually broad in scope, covering an entire department or a specific program; however, it can also refer to a single course (Worral, 2014).

The purpose, scope, and context of evaluating a program must be clearly defined. In contemplating program evaluation, consider the questions you want answered (Lorig et al., 2001). Do you want to know about a program's overall effectiveness or the clients' perceptions of the degree to which the learning objectives were taught? Do you want to know the clients' level of satisfaction with the program or whether the cost of the program was worth the outcomes? Is the purpose of the evaluation to justify the expenditures of time and money by the health education department, or is it to identify the program's strengths and weaknesses?

Also consider the intended audience for the evaluation and how the evaluation report will be used. The report may be intended for the healthcare institution or agency management accreditation bodies, or it may be for internal use by the health education staff. The intended use of the program evaluation may be to improve services or justify additional funding.

The data you gather must be consistent with the questions the program evaluation is designed to answer (Lorig et al., 2001). For example, if a health education course was designed for staff to reduce hospital-acquired infections, you would collect data about the infection rate before and after the teaching intervention to determine its impact. If a program was designed to reduce hypertension in clients, you would collect blood pressure readings and medication usage before and after the teaching session to determine its impact.

Table 14-1 introduces you to a variety of program evaluation models. These models have been selected as the most useful approaches to program evaluation. It is not an exhaustive list of models; rather, we have selected ones that we think are most applicable. The table identifies the name of the model and its purpose and provides a summary of the unique application components to program evaluation.

To conduct a program evaluation, identify the purpose for the evaluation by identifying the goals and answering the questions we identified earlier in this section. Since resources for program evaluation are always limited, decision criteria are needed to help you determine who will use the results and what information will be most useful to them. Carefully consider how much time and how many resources are available for the evaluation. Then look at the choice of models in Table 14-1 and select the one that best helps you achieve that goal.

Table 14-1 Program Evaluation Models

Models for Program Evaluation	Application
Roberta Straessle Abruzzese (RSA) Education Model (1996)	■ Process evaluation ■ Content evaluation ■ Outcome evaluation ■ Impact ■ Total program evaluation
Alspach's Evaluation Model (1995)	■ Satisfaction ■ Learning ■ Application ■ Impact
Consumer-Oriented Evaluation Model (Scriven, 1967)	■ Formative: Improve development ■ Summative: Assess value, costs, merits, worth
Stake's Countenance Model (1967)	■ Antecedents ■ Transactions ■ Outcomes ■ Unexpected outcomes
Developmental Model for the Evaluation of Health Education Programs (Nutbeam et al., 1990)	■ Does it work? ■ Can it be repeated and refined? ■ Can it be widely implemented?
Improvement-Oriented Evaluation Model (CIPP) (Stufflebeam, 1971)	■ Context: The environment ■ Input: System capabilities ■ Process: Implementation ■ Products: Worth and merit
International Association for Continuing Education and Training's 10-Level Model (1991)	■ Assessment of learning outcomes ■ Program evaluation
Kirkpatrick's Four-Level Model (1994)	■ Reaction ■ Learning ■ Behavior ■ Results
Logic Model (Frye & Hemmer, 2012)	■ Inputs ■ Activities ■ Outputs ■ Outcomes
Haggard's Three Dimensions in Evaluating Teaching Effectiveness (1989)	■ Assimilation during teaching ■ Information retention after teaching ■ Use of information in day-to-day life
Object-Based Model (Tyler, 1967)	■ Satisfaction or dissatisfaction ■ Effectiveness of planning and actions ■ Fit between student performance and objectives ■ Methodology dependent on the evaluator's definition of measurement

Models for Program Evaluation	Application
Program Evaluation for Public Health (Centers for Disease Control and Prevention, 1999)	■ Engage stakeholders ■ Describe program ■ Focus the evaluation design ■ Gather credible evidence ■ Justify conclusion ■ Ensure use and share lessons learned
Rankin and Stallings's Five Levels of Evaluation of Patient Learning (Rankin et al., 2005)	■ Assessment of learning needs and influencing factors ■ Diagnosis of learning needs ■ Goal setting ■ Implementation of patient teaching ■ Evaluation of learning
Zhang and Cheng's Planning Development Process and Product Model (PDPP) (2012)	■ Planning ■ Development ■ Process ■ Product evaluation

Cost-effectiveness of health education programs is a growing concern and documenting it is increasingly important. Research has shown that cost-containment studies in health education can result in significant savings, better health with fewer complications, fewer hospitalizations, and reduced visits to the emergency room, clinics, and physician offices (Euro Med Info, n.d.). Nursing has contributed to this body of knowledge. For example, patients who received an additional telephone follow-up educational intervention after radical prostatectomy surgery had a better understanding of how to manage their care at home and used fewer healthcare resources (Inman et al., 2011). A health promotion education program for older adults was effective in improving their health promotion knowledge and behaviors (Huang et al., 2002).

Others have reported positive results on health education programs for diabetes patients (Abdo, 2010; Loveman et al., 2003; Norris et al., 2001; Odnoletkova et al., 2016). The effectiveness of health education programs has also been documented for computer-tailored education on physical activity and dietary behaviors (Kroeze et al., 2006); patient self-management programs for patients with chronic diseases (Warsi et al., 2004); a patient education hypertension intervention (Trogdon et al., 2012); and patient education for the prevention of falls in the hospital (Haines et al., 2013).

Summative Evaluation: Evaluation of Integration of Learning into Daily Living

This area of summative evaluation addresses client adherence. Adherence is the goal of the Miller–Stoeckel Client Education Model and is essential to promoting, retaining, and restoring health. All components of the Model lead to this point. The nurse educator needs to know whether clients have retained what they learned and are using their knowledge for more healthful living. It is also important to know if regimen changes are needed. The questions you should ask are: Have individuals, families, groups/communities, and health team members benefitted? Are individuals and families incorporating new learning into their daily lives, if not, why? Are community education programs effective in promoting health behaviors? In this section, we address client adherence, client nonadherence, promoting client adherence, and introduce an ecological perspective on medical adherence.

Client Adherence

Adherence as defined by the World Health Organization (Pruett, 2020) is the degree to which a person's behavior corresponds with the agreed recommendations from a healthcare provider. This definition suggests a collaborative relationship between nurses and clients, whereas the word compliance suggests a more authoritarian approach. A collaborative relationship respects clients as independent and autonomous individuals who are active participants in maintaining health.

Achieving and sustaining high levels of adherence to effective medical regimes improves health outcomes. Adherent clients abide by agreed-upon behaviors such as taking medications, obtaining immunizations, following treatment plans, keeping appointments, and following health promotion behaviors. Long-term adherence is theorized to occur when individuals successfully initiate behavior that meets their medical needs by (1) forming favorable treatment beliefs, (2) receiving favorable feedback that their beliefs are correct, and (3) repeating or practicing their routine long enough to develop a habit. The importance of habit formation is considered important to long-term treatment adherence. The steps are illustrated in **Figure 14-2**.

Treatment-specific *beliefs* have been shown to be especially predictive of treatment-specific *behaviors*. Research suggests that medical adherence is determined by complex factors. Models of adherence offer advantages by proposing relationships between factors that guide adherence promotion strategies. The Health Belief Model was addressed in Chapter 1 and views behavior as

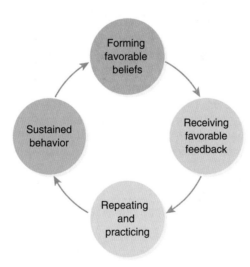

Figure 14-2 The Steps of Habit Formation

Data from Murali, K.M., & Lonergan, M. (2020). Breaking the adherence barriers: Strategies to improve treatment adherence in dialysis patients. *Seminars in Dialysis, 33*(6), 475-485. Wang, H., & Jiao, R. The relationship between career social support and career management competency: The mediating role of career decision-making self-efficacy. *Current Psychology.* Sep2023, Vol. 42 Issue 26, p23018-23027. 10p. DOI: 10.1007/s12144-022-03418-y.

a dynamic interaction between the possible barriers and benefits to engaging in a behavior. Patient adoption of recommended treatment depends on four factors: perceived susceptibility, perceived threat, perceived benefits, and perceived barriers (see **Figure 14-3**) (Murali & Lonergan, 2020).

When clients are confronted with the need to change behavior or adhere to a treatment regimen, they have decisions to make. Behavioral and lifestyle changes usually do not happen instantly; rather, change is a process that occurs over time. Prochaska et al. (2008) developed a Transtheoretical Model also known as the Stages of Change Model to explain the process of change. The model proposes that behavioral change progresses through the stages of precontemplation, contemplation, preparation, action, and maintenance. At any one-time, clients are in different stages of changing their behavior. During the journey through the various stages, individuals commonly relapse to their old behaviors or a lower level and several cycles of change may be required before the client stabilizes on the new behavior (Murali & Lonergan, 2020). The Health Belief Model and the Transtheoretical Model will be used as a theoretical base for the discussion of adherence in this chapter (see **Table 14-2**).

Figure 14-3 Reasons for Patient Adoption of Treatment and Medication
Data from Murali, 2020a, Health Belief Model.

Table 14-2 Transtheoretical Model

Stage	Characteristics	Nurse as Educator Role
Precontemplation	The client is unaware of the problem, but others are aware of it.	Supports and nurtures
Contemplation	The client is aware of the problem and thinks about changing within the next 6 months. The client contemplates the pros and cons.	Encourages client to examine the problem and gain insight
Preparation	The client intends to change soon, within the next month. The client has a plan of action but has not yet made a decision.	Serves as a coach as the client makes plans to change; suggests programs, such as weight loss, smoking cessation, etc.
Action	The client takes the time and makes an effort to modify the behavior. This stage lasts up to 6 months.	Serves as a consultant, providing advice and guidance
Maintenance	The client maintains the change and prevents relapse. This stage lasts longer than 6 months.	Serves as a consultant, providing advice and guidance
Termination	The client is fully committed to behavioral change and is 100% confident in his or her ability to maintain the change.	Reinforces success

Client Nonadherence

Nonadherence is defined as the behavior in which clients intentionally or unintentionally fail to follow a medically prescribed regime (NICE, 2010). Studies have shown that nonadherence varies by disease state and population (Unni & Bae, 2022). Most nonadherence is intentional and is when the client decides not to follow the treatment recommendation based on their personal knowledge, experience, and beliefs. There are various reasons why clients intentionally fail to follow medical plans. Clients often fear the side effects of medications and may be concerned about becoming dependent. These concerns may emanate from previous experience or from witnessing family or friends. Clients may also be concerned about the cost, particularly if they are taking multiple medications. Cost-related nonadherence is especially high in chronic diseases such as diabetes and hypertension (Unni & Bae, 2022). Clients often misunderstand why they are prescribed medications and may distrust the motives of the practitioner. If they are not experiencing symptoms, they may discontinue prescriptions when they do not feel different or see immediate change. Clients experiencing depression are much less likely to follow prescribed treatment. Nonadherence may also be driven by cultural or political beliefs. Adherence rates are lower among people of color and people of lower socioeconomic status (Scialli et al., 2021).

Unintentional nonadherence occurs when clients want to follow the agreed treatment but are prevented from doing so by barriers that are beyond their control. There are multiple barriers to unintentional nonadherence. Some of these are poor recall, memory loss, not understanding instructions, cultural differences, and inability to pay. It should be noted that poor medical adherence is a global issue especially for chronic disease. The estimated nonadherence rate for long-term therapy is 50%. From 20% to 30% of prescriptions are never filled, and only 50% of prescribed medications are taken as recommended (Unni & Bae, 2022). It is estimated that nonadherence costs the U.S. healthcare system $100–$300 billion annually (Wiley, 2018). Nonadherence can result in worsening of the client's health problem, it impacts the family, increases healthcare costs, and even results in preventable death (Rolnick et al., 2013; Wells, 2011). Nonadherence should also be seen as an opportunity for caregivers to consider different approaches to treatment (see **Table 14-3**).

Promoting Client Adherence

Achieving and sustaining high levels of adherence to medication and treatment regimens is essential to improving health outcomes. Empowering clients to adhere to medical regimes is a complex process influenced by client, family, the healthcare system, and community level factors. At the

Table 14-3 Reasons for Client Intentional and Unintentional Nonadherence

Intentional Nonadherence	Unintentional Nonadherence
■ Fear side-effects	■ Poor memory and recall
■ Dependency	■ Not understanding instructions
■ Cost	■ Cultural differences
■ Distrust	■ Inability to pay
■ Depression	■ Too many medications

Box 14-4 **The Morisky Medication-Treatment Adherence Scale**

---

1. Do you ever forget to take your (*name of health condition*) medicine/treatments?
2. Do you ever have problems remembering to take your (*name of health condition*) medication/treatments?
3. When you feel better, do you sometimes stop taking your (*name of health condition*) medicine/treatments?
4. Sometimes if you feel worse when you take your (*name of health condition*) medicine/treatment, do you stop taking it?

Data from De Las Cuevas, C., & Peñate, W. (2015). Psychometric properties of the eight-item Morisky Medication Adherence Scale (MMAS-8) in a psychiatric outpatient setting. *International Journal of Clinical and Health Psychology: IJCHP, 15*(2), 121–129. https://www.sciencedirect.com/science/article/pii/S1697260014000623?via%3Dihub

---

core of promoting adherence is the development of a partnership between the client and nurse (Pruette & Amaral, 2021). That relationship begins with building trust. A beginning strategy to build trust is to determine a client's past history of adherence with medications and treatments. The Morisky Medication-Taking Adherence Scale (De Las Cuevas & Penate, 2015) is a brief assessment that can give important clues to client past adherence. This can promote an honest discussion of barriers that the client has experienced before and gives the nurse a realistic place to start in planning adherence strategies. The four question scale in **Box 14-4** was adapted from the Morisky Scale and can assist nurses in assessing past adherence to medication and treatments.

Involving the client in decisions about taking medicines and treatments can promote trust and stimulate discussion to address barriers. Nonadherence in the past should not be seen as the client's problem. Nurses should use nonadherence as an opportunity to address problems such as cost, side-effects, and other identified issues. Rather than labeling a client as uncooperative or difficult, nonadherence should be seen as a message to the nurse that different treatment options and approaches are needed (Scialli et al., 2021).

Nurses should familiarize themselves with their clients. Assessment of additional personal factors should be completed. These six open-ended questions will assist the nurse in planning strategies for medication/treatment adherence (Pruette & Amaral, 2021):

1. Describe other diseases/medications you have.
2. Describe the highest level of formal schooling you completed.
3. Describe your ability to read and write and understand.
4. Describe any mental health problems you have experienced.
5. Describe your level of family support.
6. Describe your level of trust or mistrust of healthcare providers.

Listening to the client's concerns and working with them to design a mutually agreed-upon plan is the key to excellent health care. It is important to ask clients what they think. Clear, concise, respectful, and actionable communication is necessary. There is a delicate balance between the nurse providing sufficient communication and overcommunication. When we over-educate, we make the medical regime more complex, so we need to break it down to a basic level (Wiley, 2018).

The following is a comprehensive approach to developing a plan of care that promotes client collaboration (Adapted from Lowes, 1998):

1. Agree on the problem.
2. Negotiate reasonable goals.

3. Give general options for discussion that incudes pros and cons.
4. Decide on a reasonable regimen.
5. Agree how to measure results.

Once the plan is in place it is important to assess whether the plan is satisfactory to the client. Even though they have given initial input to the plan, specific beliefs have been shown to be especially predictive of adherence behaviors. **Box 14-5** outlines nine yes or no questions adapted from the Health Belief Model as a format for addressing possible adherence barriers after implementation of a medical plan (Murali & Lonergan, 2020).

Client-centered care relies on identification of specific deficiencies in factors that drive adherence. These factors can be operationalized and serve as the focus of modified intervention efforts and nurse–client reevaluation. Strategies to improve adherence depend on the situation, but could include approaches such as reducing the number or daily doses or organizing medications in a different way such as using pill boxes. The nurse should create a blame-free environment and praise goal achievement. The Transtheoretical Model also serves as a reminder that clients may relapse to old behaviors and beliefs and that behavior change occurs over time (Murali & Lonergan, 2020).

Direct and indirect methods are used to assess medication adherence (see **Table 14-4**). Direct methods such as observing medication use is ideal but not always possible. Blood analysis and other physiological measures are also considered direct, but these are not always practical. Indirect methods include client questionnaires, journals, pharmacy refills, pill counts, and noted physiological changes which are more common (Ho et al., 2009).

Box 14-5 Questionnaire to Assess Adherence Based on the Health Belief Model

- Do I believe my healthcare provider knows what I want regarding to my treatment/medication?
- Do I know the risks of not taking the treatment/medication?
- Do I know the benefits of taking the treatment/medication?
- Do I know the side-effects of the treatment/medication?
- Do I know how to take the treatment/medication?
- Do I have enough money to take the treatment/medication?
- Do I know how to record that I have taken my treatments/medications?
- Will taking the treatment/medication affect my normal daily routine?
- Will I take my treatments/medications?

Data from Murali, K.M., & Lonergan, M. (2020). Breaking the adherence barriers: Strategies to improve treatment adherence in dialysis patients. Seminars in Dialysis, 33(6), 475-485. http://doi-org.dml.regis.edu/10.1111/sdi.12925

Table 14-4 Direct and Indirect Methods to Access Medication Adherence

Direct Adherence Measures	Indirect Adherence Measures
Observe medication/treatment use	Client questionnaires, journals
Blood analysis and labs	Number of pharmacy refills
Pill counts	Physiological changes

Impact on the Community

The traditional approach to adherence has been to focus on individuals by promoting adherence at that level. While that is still an important, we want to present a larger picture here, regarding the ecological perspective on medical adherence. It examines the multiple interrelated and interacting aspects of communities that also impact individual adherence.

Ecological Perspective on Medical Adherence

Adherence to a prescribed medication or treatment regimen is influenced not only by characteristics of the individual client, but also by complex interactions among multiple factors within the client's environment. The social ecological model is a visual depiction of a systems approach to show dynamic relationships among individuals, groups, and their environments. The social ecological model, first advanced in the 1947 Constitution of the World Health Organization, has been widely adopted and applied to a number of health issues (Sallis et al., 2008; Israel et al., 2003; Wallerstein et al., 2003). Health is a complex interplay among factors at each level, because they are interdependent, interacting, and interrelated in influencing health behavior. Health-promoting interventions taken at several levels are more effective than those targeting only one level (Kumar et al., 2012).

The Socio-Ecological Model of Adherence presented in **Figure 14-4** is adapted from the CDC social ecological model and uses a four-level framework that addresses adherence factors (CDC, 2012). Those factors are the *Individual Focused*, *Family Social Relationship Focused*, *Community Cultural Focused*, and *Systems Societal Focused*.

Individual Focused

The individual level comprises characteristics such as age, knowledge, self-efficacy, and attitudes. This level incorporates the developmental history of the individual and their knowledge and

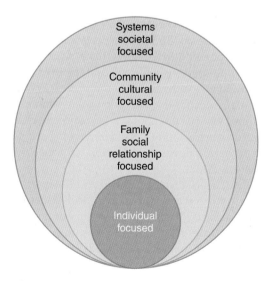

Figure 14-4 Socio-Ecological Model of Adherence

Data from the CDC social ecological model (CDC, 2012).

skills. Intentional and nonintentional reasons for non-adherence affect this level and were covered previously. The level can be influenced by individual-level strategies such as educational and skill-building programs.

Family Social Relationship Focused

This level includes the client's social circle that includes family, friends, peers, and neighbors. The level encompasses factors related to interpersonal or face-to-face relationships with healthcare professionals, as well as social support by peers. It includes our social groups, and social media platforms (Facebook, X, Instagram, YouTube). It is the network and friends with whom we value and associate. This level can be influenced by enhancing the client provider relationship and social networks and not forcing technology on patients who are unlikely to use it.

Community Cultural Focused

The community level includes environments where clients live, work, and get health care, such as hospitals, schools, places of employment and worship, neighborhoods, sports teams, and volunteer groups. Characteristics of these organizations impact the lives and health of clients. Some diseases present differently among races and cultures and perceptions of those illnesses vary among different groups. The Community Cultural Level is influenced by changes to rules, regulations, and policies within community organizations.

Systems Societal Focused

The societal level is the larger public domain which includes local and state governments. These governing bodies are in charge of prevention efforts. They also conduct research. The Systems Societal Focused level is important because it affects a larger portion of the population than the other levels. Issues such as politics, insurance, and drug access are paramount. This level is influenced by changing laws, policies, and social norms.

Before nurse educators use the Socio-Ecological Model of Adherence to promote client adherence, it is important to consider research findings that have an impact on planning. An important finding from a meta-analysis reported that the intervention used most often to improve medication adherence was education. Despite making significant improvements in education, the study revealed treatment and medication adherence did not improve (Conn et al., 2009). Berben et al. (2012) also found that, despite evidence that educational interventions could support long-term behavioral change, health professionals did not have the required skills, such as motivational interviewing, to initiate needed changes. Motivational interviewing is defined as "a client-centered, directive method for enhancing the intrinsic motivation to change by exploring and resolving ambivalence" (Miller & Moyers, 2002).

Studies also showed that clients frequently failed to fill new prescriptions for medication for hypertension, asthma, rheumatoid arthritis, epilepsy, and diabetes (Scialli et al., 2021). The studies concluded that new drugs may be risky because a newer drug may have more side-effects and lack a safety record. These drugs may be heavily pushed by pharmaceutical companies. In addition, a study at the Cleveland Clinic (Ryan et al., 2017) revealed that clients may not accurately report their medication use. This was demonstrated by inconsistent concentrations of the medication in their blood. A meta-analysis showed that clients who comply with prescribed medication and treatment regimens may also have adopted healthy behaviors that result in better health outcomes. These clients referred to as "healthy adherers" often showed improvement due to lifestyle changes rather than to increased medication or treatment adherence (Ho et al., 2009).

The Socio-Ecological Model of Adherence was used to develop an assessment tool that could assist the nurse in viewing client adherence from a broad perspective. The Socio-Ecological Model of Adherence Tool emphasizes the importance of working across levels to address factors that influence individuals and populations. In the past, it was common for the nurse to address only the individual level with emphasis on more education. **Table 14-5** addresses the levels of adherence, risks to adherence, and general adherence strategies, and uses the tool to address a specific problem: vaccine hesitancy. The World Health Organization declared vaccination hesitancy as one of the global threats to public health (Braverman, 2021). Use of the tool demonstrates how the nurse can bring together factors that impact nonadherence among individuals, groups, communities, and society to find solutions.

The Socio-Ecological Model of Adherence Tool encourages a more "upstream downstream" approach that looks broadly at individuals through societal factors influencing adherence. It addresses the importance of interventions directed at changing interpersonal, organizational, community, and public policy. The most effective approach is to target multilevel interventions that promote long-term behavior change to promote, retain, and restore health.

Table 14-5 Socio-Ecological Model of Adherence Tool

Levels	Risks to Adherence	Adherence Strategies	Anti-vaccine Strategies
Individual	■ Intentional/ Nonintentional nonadherence- political beliefs, culture, cost, side-effect ■ Lack of trust in healthcare providers	■ Listen to clients ■ Review questions before during and after adherence planning ■ Use motivational interviewing and clear communication ■ Avoid a paternalistic approach ■ Acknowledge risks	■ "Individualism" Fear of medical procedures/ management of phobia ■ Refusal to accept what they do not understand. ■ Have patience, give time to make decisions. ■ Honest respectful dialogue with two-way communication
Family Social Relationship Focused	■ Poor communication with healthcare providers; language barriers ■ Lack of trust with providers ■ Misinformation about health practices ■ Family and friends' resistance to treatment	■ Improve self-management support through local health programs ■ Improve family and social network interventions through better communication ■ Be patient when giving information ■ Information from peers is better accepted	■ Anti-vax use of "medicine like terminology"/lack of ability to distinguish reliable sources/ refer to reputable sources ■ Information from peers better accepted/positive families interact with anti-vax families

(continues)

Table 14-5 Socio-Ecological Model of Adherence Tool   *(continued)*

Levels	Risks to Adherence	Adherence Strategies	Anti-vaccine Strategies
Community Cultural Focused	▪ Unclear about caregiver options who are in their cultural group ▪ Unaware of community programs to help with adherence ▪ Vaccine hesitancy	▪ Promote continuity of care ▪ Provide adequate skill mix of the healthcare team ▪ Training of practitioners in motivational interviewing ▪ Give honest accurate information online ▪ Encourage questions	▪ Conspiracy theories often spread through Internet/ help to distinguish misinformation ▪ Promote vaccination through employment and use of celebrities and religious leaders ▪ Positive online campaigns to explain research and vaccine development
Systems Societal Focused	▪ Lack of insurance ▪ Lack of reimbursement of medications ▪ Lack of trust in governmental programs and policies	▪ Improve insurance coverage and prescription drug coverage ▪ Support legislation to lower cost to drugs ▪ Support federal and state programs that promote accurate scientific information	▪ Forcing vaccination may increase conspiracy theories and anti-government attitude ▪ Support scientific approaches through legislation.

CDC, 2021.

Case Example: Mrs. Rosa Lopez

We now illustrate how to measure each of the learning objectives for Mrs. Lopez. The cognitive objective—the client will correctly verbally explain to the nurse from memory how excessive salt intake affects blood pressure—can be measured in several ways. We would ask Mrs. Lopez to verbalize the relationship or give her a brief paper-and-pencil test. The test questions could be true or false, multiple choice, short-answer essay, or fill in the blank (**Box 14-6**).

The affective objective—the client will choose to limit sodium intake by preparing a low-sodium dietary plan for 1 week—would be evaluated in several ways. A short-term measure would be to have Mrs. Lopez fill out an attitude scale, as seen in **Box 14-7**. Another approach would be to have her construct a meal plan from a list of foods to determine her choices. The long-term measure would be whether or not she makes the dietary changes resulting in lower blood pressure. To determine this, she records her blood pressure on a chart. Dietary changes should result in lowered blood pressure readings. The ability to take her own blood pressure is a psychomotor skill, so the chart measures her success in the affective domain.

The psychomotor objective—the client will demonstrate how to accurately obtain her own blood pressure reading using digital monitor without guidance from the nurse—can be evaluated by observing Mrs. Lopez's performance. The steps of the procedure are shown in the checklist in **Box 14-8**.

Box 14-6 Sample Test Questions for Mrs. Rosa Lopez

Sample True-or-False Questions
Directions: Circle T if the statement is true. Circle F if any part of the statement is false.
T F 1. It is OK to add a small amount of salt to my food at the dinner table.
T F 2. Processed and canned foods are low in sodium.
T F 3. Excess sodium intake can cause body fluid retention.
T F 4. Excess fluid retention can result in the elevation of blood pressure.

Sample Multiple-Choice Question
Directions: Put an X in front of the one best answer.
1. A sodium-restricted diet is important in the treatment of hypertension because it:
  _____ a. Minimizes excess fluid retention.
  _____ b. Results in fluid accumulation.
  _____ c. Expands the blood capillaries.
  _____ d. Increases urinary output.

Sample Short-Answer Essay and Fill-in-the-Blank Questions
Directions: Fill in the blanks to make the statement correct. The missing words are listed at the bottom.

1. Although _____ sodium in your _____ is important to make a regular part of your _____ routine, it may not _____ the need for medication. Dietary changes will help you to control _____ accumulation and may help you _____ your blood _____.
Possible missing words:
    daily
    pressure
    diet
    limiting
    style of life
    eliminate
    rate
    fluid
    reduce
2. In 25 words or less, describe the relationship among sodium, fluid retention, and hypertension.

Mrs. Lopez would be considered successful when we observe her complete each step of the procedure correctly. We would have her perform the procedure once initially to check her familiarity with the procedure. She would be tested once. If she does not perform correctly, then we would repeat the procedure until she is accurate and is comfortable with the procedure.

Mrs. Lopez would use the chart shown in **Box 14-9** to record her daily blood pressure readings. Each time she comes in for a weekly checkup, her readings would be reviewed and her blood pressure would be checked to assess her progress. We would expect to find similar readings to our own. If they are similar, we would consider her performance successful. Because some digital blood pressure equipment also calculates the pulse rate, we have included a row on the chart to record the pulse.

Adherence for Mrs. Lopez

If Mrs. Lopez adheres to the client education plan, she would incorporate the dietary changes into her meal planning and daily diet. She would also be taking her blood pressure and recording it daily. At her clinic visits, we would take her blood pressure and compare our readings with hers.

Box 14-7 **Alternative Sample Attitude Scale for Mrs. Rosa Lopez**

Directions: Place an X in the column that most closely describes your feelings toward each of the statements. Be as honest as you can; this information is for you.

Statement	Agree	Neutral	Disagree
I am too busy to worry about meal planning.			
Altering my diet requires making too many changes.			
I can tell when my blood pressure is up.			
I am worried about stroke or heart disease.			
Everyone must die of something sometime.			
Proper diet can have a positive effect on my life.			
My children are cooperating with my dietary changes.			
I like salty snacks when I watch television.			

Box 14-8 **Sample Checklist for Taking Blood Pressure**

_____ Reads digital blood pressure equipment directions.
_____ Arranges the digital blood pressure equipment on a table by a chair.
_____ Locates the brachial artery.
_____ Places arm in the cuff.
_____ Inflates the cuff according to equipment directions.
_____ Releases air in the cuff according to equipment directions.
_____ Records the systolic and diastolic pressure, the pulse, and the date.

Box 14-9 **Sample Chart for Recording Blood Pressure**

Systolic reading										
Diastolic reading										
Pulse										
Date										

If Mrs. Lopez tells us she is not adhering, our first response would be to reinforce her honesty and talk about the perceived barriers. After listening to her story, we would help her identify options to surmount the problems. As we identify these options, we might preface them with a question such as, Have you thought about . . ., or, How would . . . work for you?

For illustrative purposes, we have created a problem that interferes with Mrs. Lopez's adherence. She says she is too busy with her employment, her children, and volunteering to implement all of the dietary changes. She removed the salt shaker from the table, adds no salt in cooking, avoids canned or processed foods that are high in sodium, and uses low-sodium seasonings such as herbs and spices in her cooking, but she enjoys munching on salty snacks in the evening as she watches television. We would focus on her enjoyment of salty snacks. Some options include finding snacks that are satisfying but devoid of the sodium content. We would do this by giving her a handout that lists low-sodium snacks or showing her how to search the Internet for such listings. For example, we would suggest unsalted nuts, crackers, rice cakes, granola bars, and fresh and dried fruits. We might also suggest keeping her mind and hands busy with a craft as she watches television, such as knitting or embroidery, or by taking a walk every evening.

Summary

Summative evaluation is the final step in the teaching and learning process. Summative evaluation focused on three areas: evaluation of client learning, evaluation of educational effectiveness, and evaluation of integration of learning into daily living. It is important to use the results of evaluation to improve health education and your effectiveness as an educator.

Summative evaluation of client learning addressed measurement itself and introduced a variety of direct and indirect measurement methods to use. Selecting specific measurement methods is based on the domain (cognitive, affective, and psychomotor) of the learning objectives. A variety of methods is available to choose from. The evaluation of health team members is more consequential than evaluating clients, and those differences were discussed.

Summative evaluation of educational effectiveness covered course and program evaluations and their importance in adapting materials to the needs of clients. Summative evaluation of integration of learning into daily living focused on client adherence, client nonadherence, promoting client adherence, and introduced the *Socio-Ecological Model of Adherence*. The *Socio-Ecological Model of Adherence Tool* complements the model and expands our thinking about adherence to include the community, culture, and society. The ultimate goal of the Miller–Stoeckel Client Education Model is to promote, retain, and restore the health of individuals and the community.

Exercises
Exercise I: Evaluate a Test by Finding the Flaws

Purposes:

- Make an inference about the purpose of this test.
- Apply guidelines for proper test construction.

Directions:

1. Find all the flaws in this test, and state your rationale for each.
2. Rewrite the test to improve the form, clarify questions, and maintain the purpose of the test.
3. Share your perceptions of the test's purpose with your peers.
4. State the rationale for your conclusion.

Critical Care Unit in the Hospital of St. Anywhere

Directions: Circle the statements you think are true:

1. The damage in a heart attack is caused by:
   a. Too much fat in the blood.
   b. Too much blood in the heart chambers.
   c. Too little blood to the heart muscles.
   d. There is no heart damage; the only damage is a clot in a blood vessel.
2. The pain involved in a heart attack is from:
   a. Heart irritability.
   b. Too little oxygen to the heart muscle.
   c. Too little blood to the heart chambers.
   d. Damaged heart muscle.
3. The damage to the heart muscle from a heart attack is:
   a. Similar to a deep cut.
   b. Similar to a muscle sprain.
   c. Similar to a bruise.
4. The healing of the heart following an attack is:
   a. Never really complete because there is always a scar that is subsequently weaker than the natural heart muscle.
   b. Totally complete, leaving no trace or damage.
   c. Shown by a scar.

Directions: Mark T for true or F for false:

_____ 5. After a heart attack, a client will not return to their previous level of physical activity.

_____ 6. After a heart attack, one's sex life always has to be reduced (in future years).

_____ 7. It was my last meal that led to my heart attack.

_____ 8. Even an occasional cocktail is bad for your heart.

_____ 9. High blood cholesterol signals a proneness to heart attack.

10. About medication:

   _____ a. You should not become dependent on them as a crutch.

   _____ b. It may help to carry nitroglycerin tablets in your pocket.

   _____ c. After you leave the hospital, medications you are given in the hospital are not to be changed in the future by your doctor.

Exercise II: Program Evaluation

Purpose: Investigate program evaluation in a healthcare institution or agency.

Directions:

1. Working in pairs, interview the head of the education department in a local healthcare institution or agency.
2. Prepare interview questions that are consistent with the content discussed in this chapter. Some sample questions you can ask are as follows:
   a. How do they conduct program evaluation?
   b. Do they have a program evaluation model that they frequently use?
   c. What common indicators do they track?

    d. Describe the health education program being evaluated. What is the purpose of this particular evaluation? What do they hope to learn by the report? Who will read the evaluation report? What types of decisions will be based on the report?

3. Report your findings in class.

Exercise III: Client Adherence

Purpose: Gain insight into client adherence issues.
Directions:

1. Working with your instructor, identify a client for whom you have provided nursing care and health education.
2. Obtain permission to do a follow-up interview with the client either by telephone or by visiting the client at home.
3. Prepare interview questions that are directly related to the health education you provided.
4. Interview the client.
5. Report in class your findings about the client's adherence to the health education recommendations you provided. Was the client adhering to the recommendations? If not, why? If not, did the reasons surprise you? Were the reasons different from those described in this chapter?

Exercise IV: Evidence-Based Nursing Practice

Purpose: Apply evidence-based nursing research to client education.
Directions:

1. Search the literature for nursing research applicable to health education related to summative evaluation.
2. Describe how the findings could be applied in educating clients in your practice.

References

Abdo, N. M. (2010). Effectiveness of health education program for type 2 diabetes mellitus patients attending Zagazig University Diabetes Clinic, Egypt. *Egypt Public Health Association, 85*(3–4), 113–130.

Abruzzese, R. S. (1996). *Nursing staff development: Strategies for success* (2nd ed.). St. Louis, MO: Mosby.

Aliotta, S. L., Vlasnik, J. J., & Delor, B. (2004). Enhancing adherence to long-term medical therapy: A new approach to assessing and treating patients. *Advanced Therapy, 21*(4), 214–231.

Alspach, J. G. (1995). *The educational process in nursing staff development.* St. Louis, MO: Mosby.

Bandura, A. (1986). *Social foundations of thought and action: A social cognitive theory.* Englewood Cliffs, NJ: Prentice Hall.

Benner, P. (1984). *From novice to expert.* Menlo Park, CA: Addison-Wesley.

Berben, L., Dobbels, F., Engberg, S., Hill, M. N., & De Geest, S. (2012). An ecological perspective on medication adherence. *Western Journal of Nursing Research, 34*(5), 635–653. https://doi.org/10.1177/0193945911434518

Braverman, A. (2021). Ecological model of health behavior as a methodology for reducing anti-vaccination trends. *Wiener klinische Wochenschrift, 133*(13-14), 721–723. https://doi.org/10.1007/s00508-021-01817-

Centers for Disease Control and Prevention. (1999). Framework for program evaluation in public health. *Morbidity and Mortality Weekly Report, 48*(No. RR-11).

Centers for Disease Control and Prevention. (2007). The social-ecological model: A framework for prevention. Atlanta (GA): Centers for Disease Control and Prevention. Retrieved May 11, 2023, from http://www.cdc.gov/ncipc/dvp/social-ecological-model_DVP.htm.

Centers for Disease Control and Prevention. (2021). The Social-Ecological Model: A framework for prevention. *Violence Prevention, Centers for Disease Control and Prevention.* Retrieved on June 21, 2021, from www.cdc.gov/violenceprevention/about/social-ecologicalmodel.html.

Centers for Disease Control and Prevention. (2022). *COVID-19 vaccine equity for racial and ethnic minority groups*. March 29, 2022.

Chisholm-Burns, M. A., & Spivey, C. A. (2008). Pharmacoadherence: A new term for a significant problem. *American Journal Health-Systems Pharmacists, 65*, 661–667.

Conn, V. S., Hafdahl, A. R., Cooper, P. S., Ruppar, T. M., Mehr, D. R., & Russell, C. L. (2009). Interventions to improve medication adherence among older adults: Meta-analysis of adherence outcomes among randomized controlled trials. *Gerontologist, 49*, 447–462.

De Las Cuevas, C., & Peñate, W. (2015). Psychometric properties of the eight-item Morisky Medication Adherence Scale (MMAS-8) in a psychiatric outpatient setting. *International Journal of Clinical and Health Psychology, 15*(2), 121–129. https://doi-org.dml.regis.edu/10.1016/j.ijchp.2014.11.003

Dezii, C. M. (2000). Medication noncompliance: What is the problem? *Managed Care, 9*(Suppl. 9), 9–12.

DiGiacomo, M. (2008). Patient adherence: Sharing the responsibility. *PT Magazine, 16*(7), 28–30.

DiMatteo, M. R. (2004). Variations in patients' adherence to medical recommendations: A quantitative review of 50 years of research. *Medical Care, 42*(3), 200–209.

Euro Med Info. (n.d.). *The growing need for patient teaching*. Retrieved from http://www.euromedinfo.eu/the-growing-need-for-patient-teaching.html/

Falvo, D. R. (2011). *Effective patient education: A guide to increased compliance* (4th ed.). Sudbury, MA: Jones & Bartlett Learning.

Frye, A. W., & Hemmer, P. A. (2012). Program evaluation models and related theories: AMEE guide no. 67. *Medical Teacher, 34*, e288–e299.

Golden, S. D., McLeroy, K. R., Green, L. W., Earp, J. A., & Lieberman, L. D. (2015). Upending the social ecological model to guide health promotion efforts toward policy and environmental change. *Health Education & Behavior: The Official Publication of the Society for Public Health Education, 42*(1 Suppl), 8S–14S. https://doi.org/10.1177/1090198115575098

Gronlund, N. E., & Brookhart, S. M. (2009). *Gronlund's writing instructional objectives* (8th ed.). Upper Saddle River, NJ: Pearson Education.

Haggard, A. (1989). Evaluating patient education. In A. Haggard (Ed.), *Handbook of patient education* (pp. 159–186). Rockville, MD: Aspen.

Haines, T. P., Hill, A. M., Brauer, S. G., Hoffmann, T., Etherton-Beer, C., & McPhail, S. M. (2013). Cost effectiveness of patient education for the prevention of falls in hospital: Economic evaluation from a randomized controlled trial. *BMC Medicine, 11*, 135. doi:10.1186/1741-7015-11-135

Ho, P. M., Bryson, C. L., & Rumsfeld, J. S. (2009). Medication adherence: Its importance in cardiovascular outcomes. *Circulation, 119*(23), 3028–3035. https://doi.org/10.1161/CIRCULATIONAHA.108.768986

Huang, L., Chen, S., Yu, Y., Chen, P., & Lin, Y. (2002). The effectiveness of health promotion education programs for community elderly. *Journal of Nursing Research, 10*(4). doi:10.1097/01.JNR.0000347607.68424.f9

Inman, D. M., Maxson, P. M., Johnson, K. M., Myers, R. P., & Holland, D. E. (2011). The impact of follow-up educational telephone calls on patients after radical prostatectomy: Finding value in low-margin activities. *Urologic Nursing, 31*(2), 83–91.

International Association for Continuing Education and Training. (1991). *A practical handbook for assessing learning outcomes in continuing education and training*. Washington, DC: Author.

Kirkpatrick, D. L. (1994). *Evaluating training programs*. San Francisco, CA: Berrett-Koehler.

Kroeze, W., Werkman, A., & Brug, J. (2006). A systematic review of randomized trials on the effectiveness of computer-tailored education on physical activity and dietary behaviors. *Annals of Behavioral Medicine, 31*(3), 205–223.

Kumar, S., & Preetha, G. (2012). Health promotion: An effective tool for global health. *Indian Journal of Community Medicine: Official Publication of Indian Association of Preventive & Social Medicine, 37*(1), 5–12. https://doi.org/10.4103/0970-0218.94009

Lorig, K., & Associates (2001). *Patient education: A practical approach* (3rd ed.). Thousand Oaks, CA: Sage.

Loveman, E., Cave, C., Green, C., Royle, P., Dunn, N., & Waugh, N. (2003). The clinical and cost-effectiveness of patient education models for diabetes: A systematic review and economic evaluation. *Health Technology Assessment, 7*(22), 1–190.

Lutfey, K. E., & Wishner, W. J. (1999). Beyond "compliance" is "adherence." *Diabetes Care, 22*(4), 635–639.

Magai, C., Consedine, N., Neugut, A. I., & Hershman, D. L. (2007). Common psychosocial factors underlying breast cancer screening and breast cancer treatment adherence: A conceptual review and synthesis. *Journal of Women's Health, 16*(1), 11–23.

Miaskowski, C., Shockney, L., & Chlebowski, R. T. (2008). Adherence to oral endocrine therapy for breast cancer: A nursing perspective. *Clinical Journal of Oncology Nursing, 12*(2), 213–221.

Miller, J. H., & Moyers, T. (2002). Motivational interviewing in substance abuse: Applications for occupational medicine. *Occupational Medicine, 17*, 51–65, iv.

Mosher, H. J., Lund, B. C., Kripalani, S., & Kaboli, P. J. (2012). Association of health literacy with medication knowledge, adherence, and adverse drug events among elderly veterans. *Journal of Health Communication, 17*, 241–251.

Murali, K. M., & Lonergan, M. (2020). Breaking the adherence barriers: Strategies to improve treatment adherence in dialysis patients. *Seminars in Dialysis, 33*(6), 475–485. http://doi-org.dml.regis.edu/10.1111/sdi.12925.

NICE. (2010). Medicines adherence. Involving patients in decisions about prescribed medicines and supporting adherence. *National Guideline Clearinghouse*, 1–21.

Norris, S. L., Engelgau, M. M., & Narayan, V. (2001). Effectiveness of self-management training in type 2 diabetes. A systematic review of randomized controlled trials. *Diabetes Care, 24*(3), 561–587.

Nutbeam, D., Smith, C., & Catford, J. (1990). Evaluation in health education. A review of progress, possibilities and problems. *Journal of Epidemiology and Community Health, 44*, 83–89.

Odnoletkova, I., Ramaekers, D., Nobels, F., Goderis, G., Aetgeerts, B., & Annemans, L. (2016). Delivering diabetes education through nurse-led telecoaching. Cost-effective analysis. *PLoS ONE, 11*(10), e0163997. doi:10.1371/journal.pone.0163997

Osterberg, L., & Blaschke, T. (2005). Adherence to medication. *New England Journal of Medicine, 353*, 487–497.

Prochaska, J. O., & Norcross, J. C. (2001). Stages of change. *Psychotherapy, 38*(4), 443–448.

Prochaska, J. O., Redding, C. A., & Evers, K. E. (2008). The transtheoretical model and stages of change. In K. Glanz, B. K. Rimer, & K. Viswanath (Eds.), *Health behavior and health education: Theory, research, and practice* (4th ed., pp. 97–122). San Francisco, CA: Jossey-Bass.

Pruette, C. S., & Amaral, S. (2021). Empowering patients to adhere to their treatment regiments: A multifaceted approach. *Pediatric Transplantation, 25*(1), 1–10. https://doi.org/10.1111/petr.13849

Rankin, S. H., Stallings, K. D., & London, F. (2005). *Patient education in health and illness* (5th ed.). Philadelphia, PA: Lippincott Williams & Wilkins.

Redman, B. K. (2007). *The practice of patient education: A case study approach* (10th ed.). St. Louis, MO: Mosby Year Book.

Robinson, J. H., Callister, L. C., Berry, J. A., & Dearing, K. A. (2008). Patient-centered care and adherence: Definitions and applications to improve outcomes. *Journal of the American Academy of Nurse Practitioners, 20*, 600–607.

Rolnick, S. J., Pawloski, P. A., Hedblom, B. D., Asche, S. E., & Bruzek, R. J. (2013). Patient characteristics associated with medication adherence. *Clinical Medicine & Research, 11*(2), 54–65.

Ryan, T. P., Morrison, R. D., Sutherland, J. J., Milne, S. B., Ryan, K. A., Daniels, J. S., Misra-Hebert, A., Hicks, J. K., Vogan, E., Teng, K., & Daly, T. M. (2017). Medication adherence, medical record accuracy, and medication exposure in real-world patients using comprehensive medication monitoring. *PloS one, 12*(9), e0185471. https://doi.org/10.1371/journal.pone.0185471

Sallis, J. F., Owen N., & Fisher E. B. (2008). Ecological models of health behavior. *Health Behavior and Health Education, 4*, 465–485.

Scialli, A. R., Saavedra, K., & Fugh-Berman, A. (2021). The benefits and risks of adherence to medical therapy. *JoSPI, 3*(1). doi:10.35122/001c.21386

Scriven, M. (1967). The methodology of evaluation. In R. Tyler (Ed.), *Perspectives of curriculum evaluation*. Chicago, IL: Rand McNally.

Slavin, R. E. (2015). *Educational psychology: Theory and practice* (10th ed.). Boston, MA: Pearson Education.

Stake, R. E. (1967). The countenance of educational evaluation. *Teachers College Record, 68*(7), 523–540.

Stufflebeam, D. L. (1971). *Education evaluation and decision making*. Itasca, IL: F. E. Peacock.

Substance Abuse and Mental Health Services Administration (SAMHSA). (2021). A guide to SAMHSA's strategic prevention framework. *Substance Abuse and Mental Health Services Administration*. Retrieved on April 23, 2023, from www.samhsa.gov/sites/default/files/20190620-samhsa-strategic-prevention-framework-guide.pdf

Trogdon, J. G., Larsen, B., Larsen, D., Salas, W., & Snell, M. (2012). Cost-effectiveness evaluation of collaborative patient education hypertension intervention in Utah. *Journal of Clinical Hypertension, 14*(11), 760–766. doi:10:1111/jch.12013.

Trust for America's Health. (2008). *Prevention for a healthier America*. Retrieved from http://healthyamericans.org/reports/prevention08/

Trust for America's Health. (2013). *F as in fat: How obesity threatens America's future*. Retrieved from http://healthyamericans.org/report/108/

Tyler, R. (1967). *Perspectives of curriculum evaluation*. Chicago, IL: Rand McNally.

Unni, E., & Bae, S. (2022). Exploring a new theoretical model to explain the behavior of medication adherence. *Pharmacy (Basel, Switzerland), 10*(2), 43. https://doi.org/10.3390/pharmacy10020043

Vermeire, E., Hearnshaw, H., Van Royen, P., & Denekens, J. (2001). Patient adherence to treatment: Three decades of research. A comprehensive review. *Journal of Clinical Pharmacy and Therapeutics, 26*, 331–342.

Wang, H., & Jiao, R. (2023). The relationship between career social support and career management competency: The mediating role of career decision-making self-efficacy. *Current Psychology, 42*(26), 23018-23027. https://doi .org/10.1007/s12144-022-03418-y

Warsi, A., Wang, P. S., LaValley, M. P., Avron, J., & Solomon, D. H. (2004). Self-management education programs in chronic disease. *Archives of Internal Medicine, 164*(15), 1641–1649.

Webster's All-in-One Dictionary and Thesaurus (2nd ed.). (2013). Springfield, MA: Federal Street Press.

Wells, J. R. (2011). Hemodialysis knowledge and medical adherence in African Americans diagnosed with end stage renal disease: Results of an educational intervention. *Nephrology Nursing Journal, 38*(2), 155–162.

Wiley, F. (2018, October). Adherence improvements: An individualized approach is key to helping patients. *Drug Topics, 162*(10), 20+. https://link-gale-com.dml.regis.edu/apps/doc/A567633901/ITBC?u=regis&sid=ebsco&xid=132487b1

World Health Organization. (2014). *Adherence to long-term therapies: Evidence for action.* Retrieved from http://apps.who .int/medicinedocs/en/d/Js4883e/6.html#Js4883e.6.1.1

Worral, P. S. (2014). Evaluation in healthcare education. In S. B. Bastable (Ed.), *Nurse as educator: Principles of teaching and learning for nursing practice* (4th ed., pp. 601–636). Burlington, MA: Jones & Bartlett Learning.

Zhang, W., & Cheng, Y. L. (2012). Assurance in e-learning: PDPP evaluation model and its application. *International Review of Research in Open and Distance Learning, 13*(3), 66–82.

CHAPTER 15

Application of the Miller–Stoeckel Client Education Model

CHAPTER OUTLINE

Introduction

We offer this summary of the Miller–Stoeckel Client Education Model as a ready resource for nurse educators. The model is a holistic approach to health education and has multiple applications in a wide variety of situations and settings. It is our desire that the model be useful to busy nurse educators.

We also hope that aspiring doctoral students in nursing will conduct research on selected aspects of the model to further demonstrate its value. We expect that aspects of the model will change through the years as nurse educators apply it to their practice. As technology develops, it will change the delivery of health care and, consequently, health education. The model is flexible and can readily be adapted to incorporate changing health education practices.

Overview of the Miller–Stoeckel Client Education Model

Purpose

The purpose of the model is to assist nurses and other healthcare professionals in becoming effective health educators. It is a conceptual model that guides users in gaining a comprehensive understanding of the essential, interrelated concepts of health education.

History

The model was initially envisioned by colleagues Pamella Rae Stoeckel, Mary A. Miller, and Dorothy E. Babcock in 2005/2006. Dorothy E. Babcock passed away in 2007.

Pamella Rae Stoeckel and Mary A. Miller further developed and refined the model, naming it the Client Education Model. It was first published by Jones and Bartlett Publishers in the first edition of the textbook *Client Education: Theory and Practice* (2011).

The second edition of the textbook, *Client Education: Theory and Practice* (2016), renamed the model by including the authors' names. It became the Miller–Stoeckel Client Education Model.

The third edition of the textbook, *Client Education: Theory and Practice* (2019), includes significant additions to the model: the embedded concepts of cultural caring, communication, negotiation, and collaboration.

Brief Description

The Miller–Stoeckel Client Education Model (Model) (**Figure 15-1**) identifies the essential players in health education: the Nurse as Educator and the Client as Learner. Between them exists the all-important Nurse–Client Relationship. The goal of the entire health education enterprise is the Client Education Outcomes. Within and among these major concepts are the embedded concepts of cultural caring, communication, negotiation, and collaboration.

Conceptual and Theoretical Support

The Model has support in the conceptual and theoretical literature. As a conceptual model, the Model identifies the concepts and conceptual links that exist in providing health education. Conceptual models give direction for action and suggest solutions to practical problems (Fawcett, 2005).

The theoretical basis for the Model is drawn from theories of nursing and education: Hildegard Peplau's interpersonal relations theory (1952); Ida Jean Orlando's nursing process discipline theory (1972); Nola Pender's health promotion model (2011); Josepha Campinha-Bacote's model of cultural competence in the delivery of healthcare services (1998); Christine Tanner's model of clinical judgment in nursing (2006); Bernadette Melnyk and Ellen Fineout-Overholt's process of evidence-based practices (2011); and Malcolm Knowles's adult learning theory—andragogy (1990). These concepts and theories provide the support for the Model and are applied throughout the text.

Figure 15-1 Miller–Stoeckel Client Education Model

Definition of Major and Embedded Concepts in the Model

Major Concepts

- **Nurse as Educator**: Nurses are professionals who plan, organize, teach, and direct health education to promote, retain, and restore health in a variety of settings. They include nurses in healthcare institutions, public health, and health education programs.
- **Client as Learner**: Clients are consumers of health education and include individuals, families, groups/communities, and health team members.
- **Nurse–Client Relationship**: The Nurse–Client Relationship creates the environment for the interaction that focuses on the achievement of health education goals. It includes the nursing process, the teaching/learning process, clinical judgment, and evidence-based nursing practice.

- **Client Education Outcomes**: Client Education Outcomes are the result of health education efforts. This concept has two foci: formative evaluation and summative evaluation. *Formative evaluation* includes evaluation of the client education plan, the learning environment, and the nurse–client interaction. *Summative evaluation* includes evaluation of client learning, educational effectiveness, and integration of learning into daily living.

Embedded Concepts

- **Cultural Caring**: Behaviors and attitudes exhibited by the nurse who respects and values diversity.
- **Communication**: The exchange of information in spoken, written, and nonverbal forms that is the foundation for clients to understand and act on health information.
- **Negotiation**: The give-and-take within the relationship that acknowledges the client as a partner with the nurse in achieving mutually acceptable goals.
- **Collaboration**: Sharing, planning, setting goals, solving problems, and working cooperatively together to achieve the goals of health education.

Propositions of the Model

- The Nurse as Educator and the Client as Learner come together in the Nurse–Client Relationship to achieve Client Education Outcomes to promote, retain, and restore health.
- The environment created by the Nurse–Client Relationship is influenced by the embedded concepts of Cultural Caring, Communication, Negotiation, and Collaboration.

Assumptions of the Model

- Health status can be improved for most clients through health education.
- Health status is affected by a variety of factors, including lifestyle, heredity, environment, culture, and availability of health care.
- Clients can learn positive behaviors.
- Clients are responsible for choices under their control that affect their health.
- Nurses are primary providers of health education in a variety of settings.

Application of the Model

We provide the following format for applying the Model in these two health education situations.

Example: One-on-One Client Education

Directions: Identify an appropriate client for whom health education is indicated.

1. Which assessment factors are most important in this particular teaching/learning situation?
   Psychological factors (perception, motivation, emotional status)
   Biological factors (health status, developmental stage, physical challenges)
   Social factors (culture/support system, socioeconomic status, generational differences)
   Intellectual factors (educational level, willingness to learn, background knowledge)
   Environmental factors (type of setting, physical and emotional atmosphere)

2. Develop the client education plan
   Perform a gap analysis
   Determine the learning outcomes and objectives (cognitive, affective, and psychomotor
      domains)
3. Selection of content
   Identify/select age-appropriate content
   Identify/select content appropriate to health status (promote, retain, restore)
   Select evidence-based research if available
4. Teaching strategies
   Determine/select which category of teaching strategies is most appropriate:
      Teacher-directed strategies
      Teacher-facilitated strategies
      Learner-directed strategies
5. Instructional materials
   Determine/select which type of instructional materials is most appropriate:
      Printed materials
      Multimedia
      Internet and the World Wide Web
6. Evaluation methods
   Identify the formative and summative evaluation methods most appropriate to the situation:
      Formative (client education plan, learning environment, nurse–client interaction)
      Summative (client learning, educational effectiveness, integration of learning into
         daily living)

Example: Group/Community Client Education

Directions: Identify the group for whom health education is indicated. Identify the general characteristics of the group—for example, the age range of the group, the reasons for health education,
and the similarity of health issues. Based on this summary, follow the same format for preparing
a client education plan.

1. Which assessment factors are most important for this particular group?
   Psychological factors (perception, motivation, emotional status)
   Biological factors (health status, developmental stage, physical challenges)
   Social factors (culture/support system, socioeconomic status, generational differences)
   Intellectual factors (educational level, willingness to learn, background knowledge)
   Environmental factors (type of setting, physical and emotional atmosphere)
2. Develop a client education plan suitable for the characteristics of this group:
      Perform a gap analysis
      Determine the learning outcomes and objectives (cognitive, affective, and psycho-
         motor domains)
3. Selection of content
   Identify/select group-appropriate content
   Identify/select content appropriate to health status (promote, retain, restore)
   Select evidence-based research if available
4. Teaching strategies
   Determine/select which category of teaching strategies is most appropriate for this group:
      Teacher-directed strategies

Teacher-facilitated strategies

Learner-directed strategies

5. Instructional materials

Determine/select which type of instructional materials is most appropriate for this group:

Printed materials

Multimedia

Internet and the World Wide Web

6. Evaluation methods

Identify the formative and summative evaluation methods most appropriate for this group and this situation:

Formative (client education plan, learning environment, nurse–client interaction)

Summative (client learning, educational effectiveness, integration of learning into daily living)

Summary

We conclude this chapter and textbook by offering the Model to the nursing profession and to all who teach clients. The Model is currently used in the education of nursing students, but we believe the Model has untapped potential to guide practicing nurses in clinical and community practice.

Our purpose is to enhance client education in the healthcare environment and highlight the importance and essence of the nurse–client relationship that is at the heart of the Model. We believe this holistic approach to health education has multiple applications in a wide variety of situations and settings. We encourage the use of the Model with a multitude of clients of different cultures to positively impact global health.

References

Campinha-Bacote, J. (1998). *The process of cultural competence in the delivery of healthcare services: A culturally competent model of care* (3rd ed.). Cincinnati, OH: Transcultural C.A.R.E. Associates.

Fawcett, J. (2005). The structure of contemporary nursing knowledge. In *Contemporary nursing knowledge: Analysis and evaluation of nursing models and theories* (2nd ed., pp. 1–48), Philadelphia, PA: F.A. Davis.

Knowles, M. S. (1990). *The adult learner: A neglected species* (4th ed.). Houston, TX: Gulf.

Melnyk, B. M., & Fineout-Overholt, E. (2011). *Evidence-based practice in nursing and healthcare: A guide to best practice*. Philadelphia, PA: Lippincott Williams & Wilkins.

Orlando, I. J. (1972). *The discipline and teaching of nursing process: An evaluative study.* New York, NY: G. P. Putman's Sons.

Pender, N. (2011). *The health promotion manual.* Retrieved from http://research2vrpractice.org/wp-content/uploads/2013/02/HEALTH_PROMOTION_MANUAL_Rev_5-2011.pdf

Peplau, H. E. (1952). *Interpersonal relations in nursing.* New York, NY: G. P. Putnam's Sons.

Tanner, C. (2006). Thinking like a nurse: A research-based model of clinical judgment in nursing. *Journal of Nursing Education, 45*(6), 204–211.

Index

Note: Page numbers followed by *b*, *f*, and *t* indicate materials in boxes, figures, and tables respectively.

V

W